TUTORIALS IN
DIFFERENTIAL
DIAGNOSIS

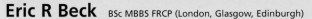

Eric R Beck BSc MBBS FRCP (London, Glasgow, Edinburgh)
Emeritus Consultant Physician
Whittington Hospital, London;
Professional Development Spine (PDS) Academic Lead
Royal Free and University College School of Medicine, London

Robert L Souhami MD FRCP FMedSci
Emeritus Professor of Medicine
University College London;
Director of Clinical Research Development and Training
Cancer Research UK, London

Michael G Hanna BSc(Hons) MBChB(Hons) MD FRCP (UK)
Consultant Neurologist
National Hospital for Neurology and Neurosurgery, Queen Square, and Middlesex Hospital,
University College London Hospitals NHS Trust, London;
Reader in Clinical Neurology, University College London

Diana R Holdright MD FRCP FESC MBBS BSC DA
Consultant Cardiologist
The Heart Hospital, University College London Hospitals, London

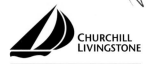

CHURCHILL
LIVINGSTONE

EDINBURGH LONDON NEW YORK OXFORD PHILADELPHIA ST LOUIS SYDNEY TORONTO
2003

CHURCHILL LIVINGSTONE
An imprint of Elsevier Science Limited

First edition 1974
Second edition 1982
Third edition 1992
Fourth edition 2003

ISBN 0443 061572
International edition 0443 061580

British Library Cataloguing in Publication Data
A catalogue record for this book is available from the British
Library

Library of Congress Cataloging in Publication Data
A catalog record for this book is available from the Library of
Congress

Notice
Medical knowledge is constantly changing. Standard safety
precautions must be followed, but as new research and clinical
experience broaden our knowledge, changes in treatment and
drug therapy may become necessary or appropriate. Readers
are advised to check the most current product information
provided by the manufacturer of each drug to be administered
to verify the recommended dose, the method and duration of
administration, and contraindications. It is the responsibility of
the practitioner, relying on experience and knowledge of the
patient, to determine dosages and the best treatment for each
individual patient. Neither the Publisher nor the authors
assumes any liability for any injury and/or damage to persons
or property arising from this publication.
The Publisher

Preface

In the course of our experience of undergraduate and postgraduate teaching, we have noticed that although many students have a wide theoretical knowledge they often lack the ability to apply this to individual clinical problems. Symptoms and signs are the raw material of medicine. Even though screening programmes may lead to diagnoses in asymptomatic people, patients usually present to doctors with symptoms. From their first day on the wards as students, and throughout their professional lives, doctors make a diagnosis by combining the patient's symptoms and signs with judicious investigations.

While patients present with symptoms, most textbooks are written in the form of descriptions of diseases. This book attempts to give a symptom- rather than a disease-orientated approach. Each chapter discusses a common symptom or sign. It attempts to relate this to normal and abnormal function so as to give a basis for understanding. The clinical features which are important in the differential diagnosis are emphasised and there is a discussion of those investigations which will help to establish the diagnosis. Subjects have been selected which are either important in the day-to-day practice of general medicine, or which are poorly understood by students and postgraduates. At the end of each chapter there is an illustrative case history with questions followed by a detailed discussion of the case. These problems serve as a challenge to the reader's diagnostic ability and as a test of comprehension of the chapter. They will be of value to those taking the MRCP (UK) examinations, which contain this type of case problem.

Diagnostic methods continue to increase in sophistication and power, while at the same time becoming progressively less invasive. The newer imaging techniques in particular have revolutionised the approach to many diagnostic problems. They are given due weight and their incorporation into diagnostic protocols is clearly demonstrated.

The book is intended for students, for postgraduates studying for higher examinations, and for all those who wish to refresh themselves on common problems in internal medicine. The first edition of this book appeared in 1974. Since the third edition in 1992, John Francis, one of the original authors, has died prematurely. He was an outstanding physician and teacher. He played a considerable role in the previous editions. We are now a team of four reflecting the increasing specialisation over the recent years. We have extensively revised all the chapters. There are new chapters on Tiredness and fatigue, Stroke, and Movement disorders.

London 2003

Eric Beck
Robert Souhami
Michael Hanna
Diana Holdright

Contents

1

Palpitations

WHAT ARE PALPITATIONS?

Patients and doctors often differ in their understanding of medical terms. This is particularly true when we talk about 'palpitations'. *Doctors* use the term to decribe an awareness of the heartbeat due to an abnormality of the heart rhythm, ranging from simple ectopic beats to important and long-lasting tachycardias. *Patients* use the term to describe many different symptoms which may not even be cardiac in origin. For example, breathlessness may be described by some patients as palpitations. Often patients are simply aware of their pulse, particularly when it is fast, for example when they are anxious or frightened. Patients are sometimes concerned that they can hear the normal heartbeat when lying on one side in bed, typically when the ear is pressed into the pillow.

A simplified approach

Many medical students express anxiety about understanding the complexities of cardiac rhythm disturbance. The interpretation of arrhythmias is actually very straightforward and logical in nearly all cases, as long as the fundamentals of impulse generation and propagation are remembered. Just occasionally it is impossible to interpret an ECG recording of an arrhythmia without sophisticated electrophysiological studies.

Normally the sinoatrial (SA) node governs cardiac rhythm. The SA node can cause sinus tachycardia and bradycardia which may be physiological and appropriate (e.g. with exercise or during sleep, respectively) or pathological (see Box 1.1). When there is disease of the conduction system, for example with ageing or ischaemia, varying degrees of heart block can develop. However, a slowing of the pulse is not usually felt as palpitations but is more likely to cause breathlessness, tiredness, dizzy spells or blackouts.

In considering the differential diagnosis of palpitations, the focus is therefore on tachycardias. However,

many palpitations are simply **ectopic beats** (Fig. 1.2). Ectopic beats are generally harmless, provided there is no evidence of underlying structural heart disease (e.g. prior myocardial infarction or valvular heart disease) or systemic abnormality such as thyrotoxicosis. In fact, the patient typically does not feel the ectopic beat (because it is premature and associated with a lower stroke volume, since the ventricles have less time to fill) but is actually aware of the first sinus beat that follows. This is because there is a short pause after the ectopic beat during which there is longer for ventricular filling and a greater stroke volume. The patient typically decribes this pause, which occurs after the ectopic, and then a strong beat (in fact, a sinus beat originating normally from the SA node).

Tachycardias

Tachycardias either originate in the atria or the ventricles. There are two important ventricular tachycardias (see Box 1.1), namely ventricular tachycardia and ventricular fibrillation. The latter will never be seen in a conscious patient in the outpatient setting. However, contrary to popular opinion, ventricular tachycardia may be well tolerated. This will be determined quite simply by how well the ventricles can contract and sustain an adequate cardiac output at fast heart rates for a period of time.

Supraventricular tachycardias generate the most diagnostic confusion amongst students and doctors, simply because there are several different types. All you need to determine is where the impulse is being generated. So, in atrial fibrillation the electrical activity in the atria is totally chaotic (the atrial equivalent of ventricular fibrillation) with no single point of generation. The ECG (Fig. 1.3) shows an irregular baseline and no co-ordinated atrial activity (that is, no P wave). The electrical storm reaches the AV node very frequently and with no particular pattern, so generating a variable ventricular contraction resulting in an irregularly irregular pulse. A more organized form of chaos in the atria causes **atrial flutter**, typically at an atrial rate of 300 per minute. This more co-ordinated activity is seen classically as a 'sawtooth' baseline on the ECG (Fig. 1.4). The AV node cannot, except in rare cases or infants, conduct the flutter beats at this high rate and typically blocks every second, third or fourth, giving a ventricular rate (and, therefore, pulse) of 150, 100 or 75 bpm. This is felt as a regular pulse unless the degree of block keeps changing. **Atrial tachycardia** is uncommon. It produces an atrial rate slower than atrial flutter and the P waves generated look neither like a sawtooth nor the normal sinus P wave.

Most confusion is probably associated with the supraventricular re-entrant tachycardias, often loosely termed supraventricular tachycardia or SVT. These tachycardias involve one or more extra or accessory pathways capable of transmitting electrical impulses. Accessory pathways are either located within the AV node itself, producing AV re-entrant tachycardias, or between the atria and ventricles outside the AV node,

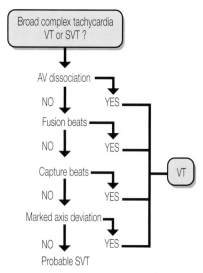

Fig. 1.1 A simple algorithm to distinguish VT from SVT. Remember it is only a guide. If the patient is unwell and hypotensive, he or she should be cardioverted irrespective of whether it is an SVT or VT.

Box 1.1 The causes of tachycardia

Sinus tachycardia
Common causes include fever, anaemia and heart failure. Less common is thyrotoxicosis, which generally presents with other symptoms. Uncommon causes include phaeochromocytoma and carcinoid syndrome.

Supraventricular
(Usually, but not always, narrow complex; paroxysmal or sustained)

- Re-entrant
  AV re-entrant (via an accessory pathway *distinct from* the AV node) – also called pre-excitation e.g. Wolff–Parkinson–White syndrome
  AV nodal re-entrant (AVNRT, via an extra pathway *within* the AV node) – the most common form of SVT
- Atrial flutter
- Atrial fibrillation
- Atrial tachycardia

Ventricular
(Broad complex)

- Ventricular tachycardia
- Torsades de pointes (uncommon, frequently iatrogenic)
- Ventricular fibrillation

Rare tachycardias are intentionally excluded from this box.

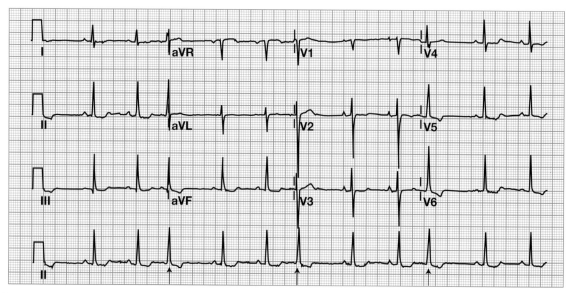

Fig. 1.2 Ectopic beats.

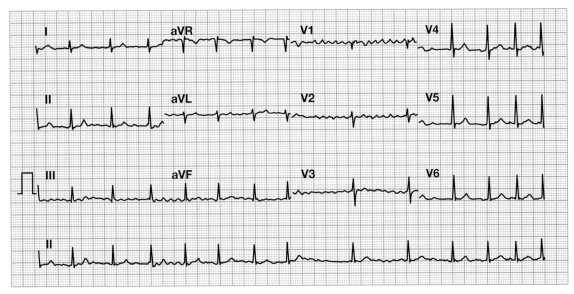

Fig. 1.3 Atrial fibrillation Look carefully at the rhythm strip (lead II). The baseline is irregular and there is no co-ordinated atrial activity. The R–R intervals are completely variable, hence the irregularly irregular pulse.

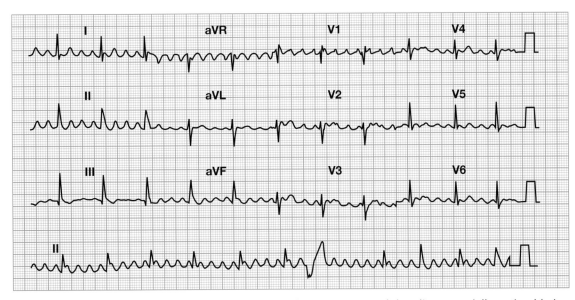

Fig. 1.4 Atrial flutter Note the regular atrial activity producing a saw-tooth baseline, especially noticeable in leads II (note the rhythm strip in particular) and V1.

permitting AV re-entrant tachycardias. The extra or accessory pathway has different conduction properties such that an electrical impulse can travel normally down the AV node, return via the accessory pathway and keep repeating this pathway, producing a rapid re-entrant tachycardia (Fig. 1.5). Sometimes the impulse

can traverse the circuit in the opposite direction. Either way, the end result is a tachycardia, with ventricular rates up to 220 bpm.

Ventricular tachycardia begins either in the specialised ventricular conduction tissue or in the myocardium. The electrical complexes are usually broad

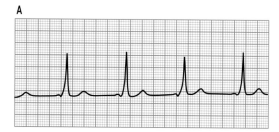

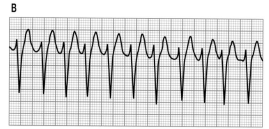

Fig. 1.5 A) Standard lead I of a patient with Wolff–Parkinson–White syndrome. Note the short PR (or PQ) interval and the slurred upstroke of the R wave.

B) Standard lead II of the same patient during an attack of supraventricular tachycardia. Note that the typical features of the WPW syndrome have disappeared.

(>120 msec) and, because the impulse generally begins in an unusual part of the ventricles, the electrical axis is abnormal, for example extreme right/left axis deviation (Fig. 1.6). Atrial activity may be seen, independent of ventricular activity (AV dissociation) or the atria may be depolarised retrogradely by the ventricles (VA association). Fusion beats, where the atrial and ventricular impulses collide to produce a complex midway between the normal sinus beat and the ventricular tachycardia morphology, and capture beats, where the atrial impulse captures the ventricle in the normal way producing a normal-looking QRS, are clues that the tachycardia is ventricular in origin. Non-sustained ventricular tachycardia describes 3 or more beats which is either non-sustained, defined arbitrarily as lasting less than 30 seconds, or sustained, if lasting longer than this.

HISTORY

The most important aspect of the history is to ascertain from the patient precisely what they mean when using the term 'palpitations'. Once the use of the term has become clear the history can be explored in more detail. The history is very frequently the only clinical diagnostic evidence since palpitations are intermittent and it is almost certain that the patient will be symptom-free in the clinic. Examina-

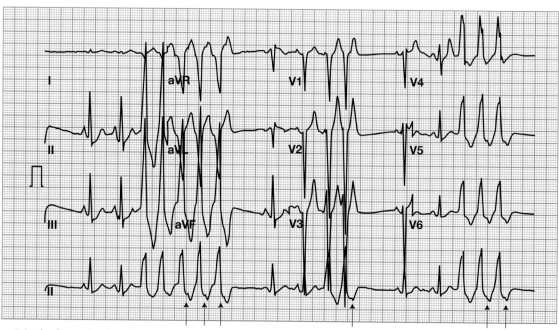

Fig. 1.6 Rhythm strip showing sinus rhythm interspersed with a short run of non-sustained ventricular tachycardia, a ventricular couplet and triplet (from left to right). A–V dissociation is clearly seen (arrows).

tion is often entirely normal, particularly in younger patients.

Some essential features of the history should be established:

Nature and time course of the palpitations. Does the patient experience these as fast or slow? (Generally palpitations are assumed to be fast but occasionally a patient is aware of a slow forceful pulse which may be a sinus bradycardia); are there extra or 'missed' beats and, if sustained, are they regular or irregular? (A useful tip is to ask the patient to tap out the rhythm).

Simple ectopics are usually easy to determine from the history alone. Patients frequently use the terms missed or extra beats, depending on whether they are more aware of the pause or the first post-ectopic beat. They may occur singly or in short runs. In the absence of structural heart disease they are generally benign, so the history should include a careful enquiry for symptoms suggesting possible underlying heart disease.

Paroxysmal atrial fibrillation will often be suggested by the description. Typically the patient decribes sudden bursts of fluttering (like a bird) in the chest (or throat) of variable duration. It is usually fairly rapid. The switch between sinus rhythm and atrial fibrillation is generally felt acutely. Paradoxically, when a patient develops permanent atrial fibrillation it may be better tolerated. **Atrial flutter** is less likely to be paroxysmal in nature and the patient may present with symptoms from sustained atrial flutter, such as breathlessness and fatigue, rather than with palpitations.

A clear onset and offset to rapid regular palpitations is characteristic of **re-entrant tachycardias**. These types of rhythm disturbance typically develop in younger people and a clear-cut history is often obtained. The patient is acutely aware of the start of the tachycardia although the termination is sometimes less clearcut. Re-entrant tachycardias, particularly AVNRT, are generally not associated with the presence of structural heart disease. In contrast, atrial fibrillation and atrial flutter often develop due to stretching of the atria as a consequence of ventricular disease (e.g. prior MI or cardiomyopathy) or valvular heart disease (congenital or acquired). Atrial fibrillation is an important risk factor for stroke and may present in this way.

Ventricular tachycardia as a cause of palpitations is an important rhythm disturbance with serious connotations (Fig. 1.6). With few exceptions it is generally associated with an abnormal ventricle(s). Investigation must therefore focus not only on the rhythm itself but also on the underlying cause. The concern is that short runs of ventricular tachycardia may progress to sustained ventricular tachycardia with the risks of syncope, degeneration to ventricular fibrillation and sudden death.

Precipitating and relieving factors. Has the patient determined what might trigger the attacks and any means of stopping them? Precipitating factors include cigarette smoking, caffeine, alcohol and recreational stimulant drugs. The effect of exercise on an irregular pulse can be of value in differentiating multiple extrasystoles from atrial fibrillation. The patient may either have noticed, or can be exercised to show, that extrasystoles tend to disappear during exercise, whereas the irregular ventricular response to atrial fibrillation becomes more pronounced. Patients may develop techniques that terminate the episodes and this often points to a particular rhythm disturbance, namely supraventricular re-entrant tachycardia. For example, swallowing ice, the Valsalva manoeuvre, pressure on the eyeballs or carotid sinus massage, by causing reflex stimulation of the vagus, may end paroxysms of supraventricular re-entrant tachycardia.

How well are they tolerated? How well a patient 'tolerates' his/her palpitations can be interpreted in different ways. First, there is psychological tolerance. A patient may be frightened that he or she will die suddenly from the palpitations and will therefore tolerate the attacks very poorly from a psychological viewpoint. Physical tolerance depends on two factors, namely the age of the patient and whether or not the heart is structurally normal. Young patients usually have greater reserve and are less likely to decompensate during a prolonged tachycardia.

Older patients and patients with structural heart disease will tolerate prolonged palpitations less well. Pre-existing heart disease may be suggested by other factors in the history. There may be a history to suggest ischaemic heart disease, for example angina or prior myocardial infarction. The patient may have had rheumatic fever or been told that they have a heart murmur. There may have been concerns about the patient's heart in infancy or early childhood. There may be a family history to suggest congenital heart disease. There may be symptoms to suggest ventricular dysfunction such as heart failure.

Associated features. Other symptoms may develop as a result of the tachycardia. Angina may develop during an attack due to a fall in cardiac output and an increase in ventricular end-diastolic pressure. The consequent drop in coronary perfusion may cause myocardial ischaemia even in the absence of coronary artery disease. Prolonged episodes of palpitations may cause breathlessness, light-headedness and, in some cases, acute pulmonary oedema. Polyuria is another feature that should be sought, as the patient may hesitate to volunteer the information thinking it irrelevant. This may come on within a few minutes of the onset of the tachycardia and consists of passing large amounts of dilute urine. It is related to raised atrial pressure and stretching of the atrial wall stimulating the release of atrial naturetic peptide (ANP).

Patients may have symptoms suggestive of an underlying cause such as anaemia or thyrotoxicosis. If palpitations are accompanied by episodes of diarrhoea, flushing, and wheezing, the possibility of carcinoid syndrome must be considered. Phaeochromocytomas are a rare cause but should not be forgotten. The tumour discharges adrenaline or noradrenaline paroxysmally and may produce palpations and other symptoms, such as sweating, tremor, pallor and head-ache. Certain bending, twisting, or rolling movements of the trunk, or, rarely, deep palpation of the abdomen, may also provoke such an attack.

Finally, many different drugs given for non-cardiac conditions may affect the heart. For example, sympa-thomimetic drugs such as those used in the treatment of asthma may cause marked tachycardia. The intro-duction of a potent diuretic may precipitate digoxin toxicity as a result of hypokalaemia even though the digoxin dosage is unaltered. Digoxin must be remem-bered not only as a cause of bradycardia but also some-times as a cause of atrial tachycardia, often with varying degrees of block.

ESTABLISHING THE DIAGNOSIS

Although most patients with palpitations will have an ECG performed, in many cases its chief value will be to reassure the patient that there is no serious cardiac disease present. In sinus tachycardia the his-tory and examination of other systems will often point to the cause. In patients suspected of attacks of paroxysmal tachycardia, it is self-evident that most will be learned by seeing a patient during an attack. Between attacks, the heart and ECG may be com-pletely normal. One exception to this, where the diagnosis can be made between attacks, is the Wolff–Parkinson–White syndrome (WPW), which gives rise to AV re-entrant tachycardias. Here there is a characteristic ECG pattern of apparent shortening of the PR interval (or, more correctly, the PQ interval) caused by a delta wave on the upstroke of the R wave (Fig. 1.5). The delta wave represents premature excitation of ventricular muscle via the accessory pathway, occurring before normal conduction through the AV node. During the re-entrant tachycardia con-duction occurs normally down through the AV node but then *retrogradely* through the accessory pathway, so the delta wave is characteristically lost during tachycardia. Rarely the re-entrant circuit occurs in the opposite direction (anterogradely in the accessory pathway and retrogradely in the AV node) such that

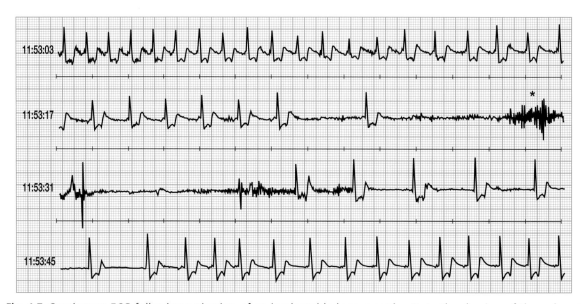

Fig. 1.7 Continuous ECG following activation of an implantable loop recorder. Note the slowing of the pulse at 11:53:17 (h:m:s), culminating in asystole for several seconds. The baseline artefact (*) is probably when the patient collapsed. Some seconds later the pulse starts to return. The patient regained consciousness and a permanent pacemaker was subsequently implanted.

the delta wave persists, producing a broader complex tachycardia.

Difficulty in interpreting the ECG may occur in the differentiation of supraventricular tachycardia with bundle branch block from ventricular tachycardia. These are collectively termed broad complex tachycardias, a purely descriptive term of no diagnostic value. The most important point is that if a patient is compromised, in other words, becoming hypotensive or shocked, the precise ECG diagnosis is not of immediate importance. The patient must be resuscitated and will probably require urgent synchronised cardioversion. As a useful simplification, a broad complex tachycardia in a young normally well person is most probably supraventricular in origin whereas in an older patient, with a greater likelihood of structural heart disease, it may well be ventricular in origin. Remember, do not examine the ECG in isolation but in the context of the clinical situation. Ventricular tachycardia (VT) is a serious occurrence because of the danger that it leads to left ventricular failure and may progress to ventricular fibrillation and cardiac arrest. In broad complex tachycardia where it is unclear whether there is SVT with bundle branch block, or VT, it is better to treat for a presumed VT.

For intermittent symptoms, particularly when short-lived, 24-hour or even 48-hour ambulatory monitoring will be useful. The longer the heart rhythm is monitored, the greater the likelihood of detecting an arrhythmia. Furthermore, the patient may have episodes of arrhythmia that do not give rise to symptoms, so prolonged monitoring gives a more complete picture. There are other monitoring devices, particularly useful when symptoms are infrequent, that the patient can apply during an attack. In very difficult cases where symptoms are rare but disabling, implantable loop recorders can be inserted under local anaesthetic subcutaneously in the anterior chest wall. These devices continuously monitor the heart rhythm and can be activated to store a 40 minute ECG trace when symptoms occur (Fig. 1.7). The information can subsequently be downloaded onto a computer for analysis. Invasive electrophysiological studies (EPS) can be undertaken under local anaesthetic in the catheter laboratory to look very precisely at the electrical activity of the heart. Abnormal rhythms can be 'mapped' and accessory pathways located. These pathways can be ablated using radiofrequency energy and complete cure of conditions such as Wolff–Parkinson–White syndrome can be achieved. Ablation techniques have a developing role in many arrhythmias, not just re-entrant tachycardias, and are increasingly successful.

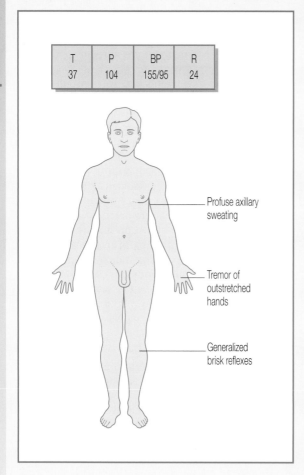

T	P	BP	R
37	104	155/95	24

Profuse axillary sweating

Tremor of outstretched hands

Generalized brisk reflexes

A 39-year-old IT manager was referred to hospital having complained of palpitations for the previous month. He had noticed that following exertion such as climbing stairs at home, he became aware of his heart beating rapidly but regularly. There was often an associated aching pain felt to the left of the sternum. Palpitations and pain would last for about 20 minutes and were accompanied by tremor and sweating of the hands. The symptoms were by no means constant, and tended not to interfere with his work, but rather to occur in the evenings or at weekends when playing with his 8-year-old twin sons. Occasionally they would occur when he was using his home computer.

Six months earlier he had had an inferior myocardial infarction. He had been in hospital for 5 days and there had been no complications. He was discharged on aspirin and a statin (his cholesterol was found to be 8.3 mmol/l). He was not given a betablocker because of a possible history of mild asthma in the past. On discharge from hospital he had been advised to reduce weight and had succeeded to the extent that his weight fell from 80 kg to 71 kg. He had also been advised to stop smoking but had found this difficult despite help from the cardiac rehabilitation team. He had joined a gym but had yet to attend on a regular basis. He had returned to work 3 months prior to his present attendance.

On examination he was anxious. There was a fine tremor of the fingers and profuse axillary sweating. The thyroid was not palpable and no bruit was heard over it. The pulse was 104/min and regular; all the peripheral pulses were palpable. Blood pressure was 155/95. The heart was not clinically enlarged and there were no added sounds or murmurs. All the limb reflexes were very brisk. The optic fundi were normal. No other abnormalities were found on clinical examination or urinalysis.

Chest X-ray showed a normal cardiac silhouette and clear lung fields. ECG showed sinus rhythm. There were Q waves in leads II, III and AVF. The ST segments and T waves had returned to within normal limits compared with 6 months previously.

Questions

1. What are the likely causes of his present symptoms?
2. What investigations would you undertake?
3. What treatment would you recommend?

Discussion

The patient is obviously worried that his present symptoms are a result of his previous myocardial infarction and represent a deterioration in his heart disease. The complications of ischaemic heart disease that have to be considered are angina and left ventricular failure. It is also possible that some form of paroxysmal tachycardia might be occurring.

The pain described does not have the typical features of angina. It comes on after, rather than during, exertion and it lasts too long. It is not in the characteristic site and does not show any radiation. Furthermore, it is not precipitated by a constant amount of physical exertion. Angina can present with many atypical features and may be misinterpreted by the patient and even by the doctor. However, in the majority of patients, close questioning usually helps to clarify the situation.

Significant left ventricular dysfunction as a cause of his symptoms is unlikely. He has had a localized inferior infarct without complication. There has been no cough or breathlessness, there is no gallop rhythm, no murmur to suggest mitral regurgitation and there are no abnormal signs in the lungs. The cardiac silhouette is normal on the chest X-ray.

This patient's palpitations are probably a result of sinus tachycardia. This is suggested by his observation that the pulse is regular. There is no abrupt onset to suggest paroxysmal attacks and, furthermore, the episodes are invariably associated with effort.

A sinus tachycardia is usually caused by overactivity of the sympathetic nervous system. This may be mediated either directly by sympathetic nerves or by circulating catecholamines. These catecholamines may be produced in excess, as in phaeochromocytoma or anxiety, or their action may be potentiated by thyroxine and triodothyronine as in thyrotoxicosis. In all three conditions the resulting stimulation of beta-adrenergic receptors will produce certain similarities in the clinical picture.

Thyrotoxicosis might be suspected in a patient with palpitations, sweating, tremor, brisk reflexes, nervousness, staring eyes, weight loss and increased bowel activity. His weight loss probably represents the results of the dieting advised by his doctors. Furthermore the thyroid gland is not palpable and no bruit is present.

A phaeochromocytoma is also an unlikely diagnosis. There is no evidence of sustained hypertension in the heart size, fundi or ECG. Intermittent paroxysmal discharge from such a tumour may also occur but the pattern of this patient's attacks is not typical.

In addition to these negative points, there are positive features to suggest that this patient's symptoms are due to anxiety. The awareness of his response to exercise is giving rise to anxiety which is enhancing and prolonging this response. Such a situation is readily understandable in a relatively young man with family responsibilities who has sustained a myocardial infarct. Additional anxiety has been created by his inability to stop smoking as recommended by his doctor. The setting of the attacks mainly in the family circle is another indication of the underlying anxiety.

Little further investigation is indicated. The ECG and chest X-ray were helpful, if only for their reassuring effect on the patient. A stress test could be helpful, to exclude ischaemia with exertion or important rhythm disturbance and to reassure the patient. Knowledge of the sleeping pulse rate would be valuable, for in anxiety it is normal, in contrast to the sustained tachycardia of thyrotoxicosis. A serum thyroxine (T4) or TSH estimation would also help to exclude this diagnosis. His blood pressure, raised at the time of examination, should be remeasured after a period of rest as there are no other findings to support a diagnosis of sustained hypertension. If doubt still persists, a non-invasive 24-hour ambulatory blood pressure profile could be obtained. A simple screening test should be done to exclude phaeochromocytoma, such as the estimation of urinary catecholamines.

Treatment of this patient requires empathy with his predicament and the ability to provide effective reassurance. This is frequently best undertaken in concert with the cardiac rehabilitation team, to whom he should be referred once more. Beta-adrenergic blocking drugs such as atenolol can give useful symptomatic relief. It would be helpful to establish with simple lung function tests whether or not he does have evidence of asthma since it is conceivable that he might be able to tolerate a betablocker.

Further investigations, including a stress test, were normal. His wife measured his sleeping pulse on four successive nights and found it to be between 56 and 64 per minute. He attended cardiac rehabilitation for a further 5 sessions and over the next few weeks his symptoms fully resolved.

2

Heart failure

coronary artery disease and hypertension, which frequently co-exist.

Heart failure is common, and incidence increases with age. It is one of the most frequent causes of hospital admission, present in up to 5% of hospitalized patients. Heart failure is, however, a rather ambiguous and unhelpful term and to be given a diagnosis of heart failure is potentially traumatic for the patient. Nevertheless, if the diagnosis is correct, heart failure still carries a grave prognosis.

It is very important to understand that heart failure is not a diagnosis in its own right but a term applied to a constellation of features compatible with pump dysfunction. The doctor must therefore investigate the patient to establish the precise cause of the heart failure, to treat the cause and not simply the manifestations of heart failure. A useful analogy would be to make a diagnosis of anaemia but not to investigate why the patient is anaemic.

What is heart failure? There are many different definitions, most of them reasonable. It is easiest to consider the normal function of the heart. In health the heart is simply a pump, delivering oxygen and nutrients to the tissues. When the heart begins to fail, for whatever reason, the symptoms and signs of heart failure start to develop, partly as a consequence of impaired pump function but also driven by the secondary neurohumoral changes that, in the early stages, are compensatory but with time worsen the clinical situation.

A wide variety of primary cardiac diseases cause heart failure and this may be their initial presentation as well as the terminal event. A number of non-cardiac diseases, in particular severe anaemia and thyrotoxicosis, may produce congestive heart failure as a major complication. Here, treatment of the cardiac failure may be ineffective unless the underlying condition is recognized and treated. Because heart failure is the final pathway of many different pathological mechanisms, the relative importance of various independent but contributory factors may be difficult to determine. Many of these diseases are very common, for example

TYPES OF HEART FAILURE

The following classifications have been used because they illustrate the many different ways that heart failure (or pump dysfunction) can develop or manifest itself. For example, we use the terms right and left heart failure, high or low output failure, congestive or non-congestive heart failure, forward or backward heart failure, compensated and decompensated heart failure, acute and chronic heart failure and systolic and diastolic heart failure.

Right and left heart failure imply ventricular dysfunction that primarily affects one ventricle or the other. For example, a large anterior myocardial infarction will predominantly affect the left ventricle whereas some congenital heart muscle abnormalities may affect the right ventricle with little effect on the left. The two ventricles do not act independently and there is functional interplay between the two ventricles. Some diseases involve the whole heart: for example, acute viral myocarditis, beriberi and many cardiomyopathies. Left ventricular dysfunction will cause left atrial pressure to rise and will manifest with breathlessness and later orthopnoea and paroxysmal nocturnal dyspnoea. Right ventricular dysfunction may cause non-specific symptoms and may be misdiagnosed in the early stages. Tiredness, exhaustion, abdominal discomfort (hepatic congestion and ascites) and ankle oedema are common manifestations.

The term **high output heart failure** implies that some types of heart failure are associated with high output states, for example severe anaemia and AV malformations (which generate large shunts). **Congestive and non-congestive** heart failure describe the presence or lack of oedema (pulmonary and/or peripheral) in association with heart failure. Patients often have a specific pattern of fluid retention. Some may develop significant leg oedema whereas others may tend to collect fluid in the abdominal cavity with little in the way of peripheral oedema.

Forward and backward heart failure are terms less frequently used these days, implying congestion or organ hypoperfusion as the dominant manifestations, respectively. **Compensated heart failure** implies that the symptoms and signs of pump dysfunction are controlled with appropriate treatment and generally the patient has a reasonable exercise tolerance and is not fluid-retaining.

Acute and chronic heart failure are useful terms clinically although they do not shed light on the underlying aetiology. A patient may have chronic heart failure with acute exacerbations. Although the underlying disease process is the same, the presentations are very different. Acute heart failure is typically seen as an emergency, where the patient has severe difficulty in breathing, sitting bolt upright, too breathless to complete sentences, cold, clammy and tachycardic. Chronic heart failure is typically seen in the outpatient setting where a patient has been stabilized on medication and is often oedema-free with a modest exercise capacity.

Perhaps the most useful descriptions are **systolic and diastolic** heart failure since they imply a mechanistic approach to the clinical problem. It must be remembered that relaxation and filling of the ventricles in diastole are as important as the pump action of the heart in systole. Systolic and diastolic abnormalities frequently coexist.

THE PATHOPHYSIOLOGY OF HEART FAILURE
(Fig. 2.1)

The heart is a pump, and its function is to produce an output of blood of a volume and pressure adequate to perfuse the tissues and meet their immediate metabolic needs. The metabolic requirements of most tissues are relatively constant. The perfusion of the gut will vary with the needs of digestion, and that of the skin according to the necessity for heat loss and the maintenance of constant core temperature. The largest variable is the perfusion of the skeletal musculature, which alters greatly with physical activity. Even after there has been a compensatory reduction in blood flow elsewhere, for example to the gut, vigorous exercise will result in a rise in the cardiac output from a resting figure of 5–7 l/min to as high as 20 l/min. This capacity to increase output is the **cardiac reserve**, and in most people results mainly from an increase in heart rate. It will be progressively reduced in heart disease, so that commonly the patient in the earlier stages of illness will only develop symptoms with activities with which the cardiac reserve could previously cope.

Heart failure results from many different mechanisms, including pressure overload (such as systemic hypertension and aortic stenosis), volume overload (such as progressive mitral or aortic regurgitation), myocardial ischaemia (such as prior myocardial infarction and ventricular aneurysm) and primary myocardial disease (such as myocarditis, alcohol abuse and idiopathic dilated cardiomyopathy). Valvular heart disease, pericardial constriction and deposition disorders such as amyloid also give rise to ventricular dysfunction. These and other causes indicate the need for a full evaluation of the patient to determine the precise cause of heart failure.

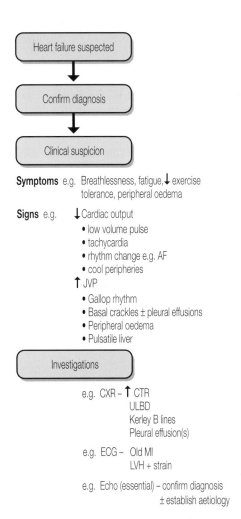

Fig. 2.1 Algorithm illustrating the pathophysiology of heart failure.

When analysing the syndrome of heart failure it is useful to consider the heart as two distinct pumps. The right heart operates against the normally low resistance of the pulmonary circulation, the average pressure in the pulmonary artery being only about 16/7 mmHg, in contrast to 120/80 mmHg for the systemic circulation. This difference in load is reflected in the anatomy of the right ventricle, which is well adapted to deal with an increase in volume but less successful when confronted with pressure. An example of this is an atrial septal defect, where the right ventricle will usually cope for many years with an output much above that of the normal left ventricle. In contrast the thick-walled left ventricle is well adapted to high pressure and can thus cope adequately for a long time with such conditions as systemic hypertension or aortic stenosis. In aortic or mitral regurgitation, the left ventricle is called upon to deal with increased volume of blood. It copes with this less well and once failure has developed, deterioration can be rapid.

Typically heart failure is characterized by ventricular enlargement, except in cases of true diastolic dysfunction, constriction and restriction. As the ventricle enlarges it 'remodels', becoming more spherical in shape, and efficiency falls. Filling pressures rise and, in the early stages, output is maintained according to the Frank–Starling mechanism.

In left heart failure the rising end diastolic pressure in the left atrium is transmitted back to the pulmonary veins and then to the pulmonary capillaries. At this stage the increase in capillary hydrostatic pressure predisposes to pulmonary oedema (Fig. 2.2). The increased accumulation of blood in the lungs makes them less easily expanded, reducing the compliance. The pulmonary artery pressure rises passively and, as a consequence, there is an increased load upon the right heart which may ultimately lead to its failure. Active pulmonary arteriolar vasoconstriction may occur which, while reducing the pulmonary congestion, does so at the expense of increased strain upon the right heart. As cardiac failure develops and cardiac output falls there is an increase in sympathetic activity from the baroreceptors. Heart rate rises and there is peripheral vasoconstriction and constriction of the great veins, thus maintaining blood pressure and increasing venous return. Activation of the renin–angiotensin mechanism causes aldosterone release and salt and water retention, which contributes to oedema.

SYMPTOMS OF HEART FAILURE

The reduction in cardiac output gives rise to some of the most important symptoms. Tiredness, lack of energy and reduced exercise capacity are some of the earliest manifestations. However, these symptoms are non-specific and the patient frequently ascribes them to getting older or putting on weight and so frequently does not seek medical attention for some time.

For diagnosis, perhaps the most useful of the common symptoms of heart failure is breathlessness, which is almost universally experienced. The precise mechanism for dyspnoea in chronic heart failure is still poorly understood. In contrast, in acute pulmonary oedema the patient feels that he or she is drowning,

---

Box 2.1 Common causes of heart failure

Right heart failure	Left heart failure
• Pulmonary hypertension secondary to left heart failure	• Coronary artery disease
• Cor pulmonale	• Hypertension
• Thromboembolic pulmonary hypertension	• Aortic valve disease (stenosis or regurgitation)
• Pulmonary hypertension due to congenital heart disease	• Mitral regurgitation
• Atrial septal defect	• Myocarditis
• Pulmonary valve stenosis	

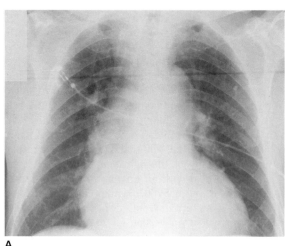 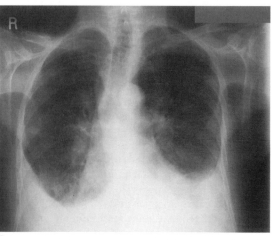

A   B

Fig. 2.2 A) A Chest X-ray showing gross cardiomegaly (↑ CTR) with upper lobe blood diversion (ULBD) and interstitial shadowing.
B) Chest X-ray showing bilateral pleural effusions.

with the production of vast quantities of pink frothy sputum. Sudden impairment of left ventricular function, for example following myocardial infarction or severe prolonged rhythm disturbance, increases left ventricular filling pressure and thus pulmonary venous pressure, causing fluid to accumulate in the lungs. Wheezing may also develop due to bronchospasm developing as a consequence of bronchial mucosal oedema (so-called cardiac asthma).

The respiratory centre will also be stimulated both directly and reflexly by arterial hypoxia and hypercapnia. Dyspnoea of cardiac origin is usually worse when the patient lies flat, so that at night he or she will usually sleep well propped up; in severe cases the patient may resort to sleeping in a chair. This is called orthopnoea and is probably due to a redistribution of blood on lying flat such that a greater proportion is in the lungs, decreasing pulmonary compliance. Attacks of paroxysmal nocturnal dyspnoea may occur. Severe pulmonary oedema often develops on a background of increasing left heart failure with progressive orthopnoea and recurrent attacks of paroxysmal nocturnal dyspnoea. It may also develop without warning, either in association with severe mitral stenosis, or as a result of myocardial infarction. Patients with heart failure have oxygen desaturation at night, often to around 80%. This is caused by periods of apnoea, followed by partial arousal and hyperventilation, so-called Cheyne–Stokes respiration.

Pulmonary vascular congestion predisposes to haemoptysis, which is usually small and may be recurrent. This is especially common in mitral stenosis. Haemoptysis may also result from pulmonary infarction, which can occur in heart failure, usually as a result of deep vein thrombosis, giving rise to pulmonary emboli or from pulmonary venous infarction. Congestion and swelling of the bronchi often give rise to coughing, and cough may occur after exercise when heart failure and pulmonary congestion become more marked. Recurrent attacks of bronchitis will be a common feature in many cases of cor pulmonale, where chronic obstructive pulmonary disease is likely to be the cause, but are also more likely in any situation where the lungs are congested. The wheezing dyspnoea that can result from either congestion and oedema ('cardiac asthma') or bronchitis may lead to the patient's symptoms being misinterpreted as respiratory in origin.

As heart failure progresses systemic venous congestion will finally develop. In part this is due to the expansion of the blood volume that commonly occurs, particularly in association with cor pulmonale (see Ch. 3, p. 19). It is also an important compensatory response maintaining cardiac output by increasing the diastolic filling pressure. The salt and water retention is mediated through the renin–angiotensin mechanism which is activated in heart failure, and augmented by the initiation of diuretic therapy. There is probably also activation of local renin–angiotensin in the tissues. The sympathetic nervous system is also activated in heart failure causing peripheral vasoconstriction, tachycardia and an increased inotropic state of the heart. The cardiac chambers release natriuretic peptides in response to stretch which relax blood vessels and partially oppose the sympathetic and renin–angiotensin systems.

A rise in peripheral venous pressure is a major factor in producing oedema, which will be typically gravitational. It will be most marked in the legs, gradually ascending as the condition worsens. The swelling will be more obvious by the end of the day or after any prolonged period of standing, and will improve or even disappear on lying down. If very severe it may be associated with enlargement of the abdomen due to ascites. If ascites is marked but the peripheral oedema only modest, other causes of oedema, particularly liver disease, must be excluded and the possibility of constrictive pericarditis carefully considered (see Ch. 15). Venous congestion of the liver in heart failure will increase its size and stretch the capsule, giving rise to pain and tenderness. If heart failure has developed rapidly this pain may be severe, sufficient on occasion to falsely suggest a primary intra-abdominal condition. Congestion of the bowel in association with hepatic dysfunction is partly responsible for the poor appetite commonly found in heart failure. This in turn frequently leads to muscle weakness and tissue wasting, termed cardiac cachexia, although weight loss is commonly masked by the accumulating oedema fluid. Rarely, muscle wasting may result from an actual protein-losing enteropathy produced by the failure. Impaired cerebral perfusion may, in the elderly, lead to confusion, restlessness and disorientation. Acute myocardial infarction may sometimes present in this way in old people, chest pain being completely absent.

Specific symptoms related to the cause of heart failure should also be sought, in particular angina, since coronary artery disease remains the most common cause of heart failure in western society. Hypertension, due to better recognition and treatment, is no longer the commonest cause of heart failure.

PHYSICAL EXAMINATION

The physical signs reflect the changes already described. The reduction in cardiac output, although fundamental in producing symptoms, is not always easy to detect clinically. If failure is severe there may be a reduction in blood pressure and a low volume pulse. The skin will be cold and pale in the usual low output state, and there may be peripheral cyanosis. In the much less common situation of high output failure with a hyperkinetic circulation the skin will be warm and the pulse bounding. Central cyanosis, because of a combination of impaired gas exchange, poor perfusion and greater oxygen extraction, must always be looked for centrally in the mucous membranes and tongue, for peripheral cyanosis alone is most commonly due to local factors such as cold. Reduction in renal blood flow may lead to the formation of smaller quantities of more concentrated urine, while there may be some degree of reabsorption of oedema fluid at night, resulting in a loss of the normal diurnal rhythm of urine flow. Body wasting (cardiac cachexia) may be present and, in severe cases, confusion.

Abnormalities of the pulse will usually be the result of associated arrhythmias, especially atrial fibrillation (caused by atrial stretching and dilatation or fibrosis and ischaemia). Hypertension may cause heart failure but a rise in blood pressure may also occur as a consequence of heart failure, perhaps because of impaired perfusion of the brain stem. Hypertension in heart failure should not be regarded as the cause unless there is evidence of end-organ damage, for example hypertensive retinopathy or left ventricular hypertrophy on ECG or more accurately determined echocardiographically.

A grave and important sign of a failing left ventricle is pulsus alternans. Every other beat is weak due to impairment of ventricular contraction, the rate and rhythm being normal. The first heart sound will vary, being louder with the stronger ventricular contractions. The sign is best detected, however, by careful sphygmomanometry. As the occluding pressure is reduced the heart rate will be found to double suddenly once all the beats are transmitted. In most cases of heart failure the heart is enlarged and this can usually be detected clinically. The apex beat will be displaced. Percussion of the heart is clinically difficult and of very limited value.

Pulmonary congestion will give rise to dyspnoea and orthopnoea, and may result in acute pulmonary oedema with the production of large quantities of frothy pink sputum. The increased barrier to diffusion, and ventilation–perfusion mismatch, will increase the hypoxaemia and cyanosis. The usual finding on examination of the lungs is bilateral basal crackles, which may be more widespread if the failure is severe. The percussion note will usually be unimpaired, and stony dullness should always suggest the presence of pleural effusion which may occur in heart failure. If pulmonary infarction has occurred a pleural rub may be heard.

Peripheral venous congestion caused by a rise in right atrial diastolic pressure will be seen as an elevation of the jugular venous pressure, which is a simple manometer of right heart pressure. The patient is best examined lying at an angle of 45° to the horizontal. Gross jugular distension with absence of venous pulsation may result from mediastinal obstruction, but this will usually be obvious from the associated facial oedema and the absence of cardiac signs. If the venous pressure is only a little elevated it can often be made more obvious by sustained compression over the liver – the hepatojugular reflux. If the right ventricle is grossly dilated there may be tricuspid regurgitation with a large systolic or 'cv' wave in the jugular venous pulse and a pulsatile liver.

The liver will frequently be enlarged and is commonly tender, unless cardiac cirrhosis has resulted from longstanding failure. Ascites should be looked for if the abdomen seems protuberant, the characteristic sign being dullness in the flanks which shifts on movement of the patient. It is especially common with constrictive pericarditis. Occasionally there may be a minor degree of splenomegaly, either because of passive congestion or secondary to the cirrhosis, but clinical detection may be difficult if ascites is also present. Peripheral oedema is a major sign of heart failure. It is usually obvious in the legs, but may be confined to the sacrum if the patient has been in bed.

Palpation and auscultation of the praecordium are important aspects of the clinical examination. Dilatation of one or more of the cardiac chambers is often present in failure and there may be secondary mitral and/or tricuspid regurgitation due to stretching of the valve annulus. The loudness of the murmur correlates poorly with its haemodynamic significance. In particular, the murmur of aortic stenosis may be virtually inaudible in patients with severe heart failure due to previously unrecognised but severe aortic stenosis.

Much attention has been paid to the variety of additional heart sounds that may occur in diastole, particularly when a ventricle is under strain or actual failure is present. The third heart sound (S3) is a ventricular sound that occurs during early rapid filling. The precise mechanism is still much debated. It is often present in younger people (e.g. <30 years) with normal hearts. If large quantities of blood flow into a dilated ventricle a pathological third sound is commonly produced. In timing and quality this is identical with the physiological third sound and can only be recognized as pathological from the circumstances under which it occurs. Increased ventricular filling is particularly a feature of disease causing an increase in stroke volume. An abnormal S3 is therefore more likely with left-to-right shunts or regurgitant valves such as severe mitral regurgitation.

The fourth heart sound (S4) occurs as a result of atrial contraction associated with reduced ventricular compliance. It is heard just before the first heart sound, but is absent in atrial fibrillation. Ventricular compliance will be decreased if there is myocardial fibrosis as a result of ischaemic heart disease, and also in rare conditions such as amyloid infiltration of the heart. Compliance is also reduced if there is systolic overload of the ventricle, as a result for example of systemic hypertension or aortic stenosis.

The term gallop rhythm refers to a characteristic cadence of at least three sounds in association with tachycardia. It may be due to a combination of S1, S2 and S3 called 'S3 gallop'. Alternatively a gallop rhythm can be produced by the combination of S1, S2 and S4 called 'S4 gallop'. With rapid heart rates S3 and S4 may occur simultaneously and this can produce a summation gallop, whether or not the individual sounds are abnormal. This is especially likely to occur in hypertensive heart failure.

INVESTIGATION OF CARDIAC FAILURE

Investigations are directed towards confirming the clinical picture, establishing the precise cause and gauging the severity of heart failure.

Blood tests are used to look for potential causes of heart failure: thyroid function tests and serum ACE for sarcoid, immunoelectrophoresis for amyloid and so on, and to assess the severity of heart failure – the serum sodium concentration is a powerful prognostic marker, falling with worsening heart failure. A full blood count is necessary to look for anaemia. Renal function tests are essential since impaired renal perfusion will affect renal function, renal disease can cause heart failure and drugs used in heart failure can worsen renal function. Diabetes mellitus should be sought. Hepatic dysfunction may occur with severe heart failure.

The ECG may of course suggest the cause of the heart failure, such as previous anterior myocardial infarction (deep broad pathological Q waves in the anterior leads), or poorly controlled hypertension (with tall R waves in leads overlying the left ventricle +/– repolarization abnormalities). Atrial fibrillation and frequent ventricular ectopics are common in heart failure and will be demonstrated on the surface ECG.

The chest X-ray is a helpful investigation (Fig. 2.2 A and B). Cardiomegaly can be quantified and chamber enlargement documented. Prominence of the upper lobe veins will indicate a rise in left atrial pressure, while there may be the typical features of pulmonary oedema with perihilar shadowing, Kerley B lines and pleural effusions.

Transthoracic echocardiography is essential in all patients with suspected heart failure since it provides a highly accurate and detailed anatomical and functional assessment of the heart. The size of individual cardiac chambers can be determined and the ejection fraction of the left ventricle can be accurately measured. The heart valves can be assessed to determine whether there is a primary abnormality (for example a bicuspid aortic valve which has stenosed over time) or a secondary change (such as stretching of the mitral valve ring from left ventricular dilatation causing mitral regurgitation). The myocardium may show a characteristic glistening appearance due to amyloid deposition. Pericardial thickening and calcification is readily detected. Extensive assessment of systolic and diastolic function can be made. In some patients good quality images cannot be obtained and it may be appropriate to undertake transoesophageal echocardiography. Biventricular function can also be quantified in the nuclear medicine department using multigated acquisition (MUGA) scans. Coronary artery disease can be assessed either by myocardial perfusion imaging or by coronary angiography in the catheter lab, when detailed assessment of intracardiac pressures, ventricular and valvar function can be made. Cardiopulmonary exercise testing gives a useful objective measure of exercise capacity and maximum oxygen consumption.

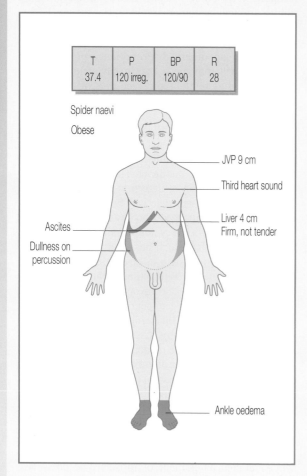

T	P	BP	R
37.4	120 irreg.	120/90	28

Spider naevi

Obese

JVP 9 cm

Third heart sound

Liver 4 cm
Firm, not tender

Ascites

Dullness on percussion

Ankle oedema

A 52-year-old Greek Cypriot businessman presented to his GP because of recent deterioration in his health. Over the previous 12 months he had felt increasingly tired and lacking in energy. His appetite had been worse and he had noticed occasional dyspepsia, particularly after heavy or fatty meals. His bowels had always been constipated and for the last 6 months he had noticed that he was losing bright red blood during and after defaecation. He had no other symptoms but on direct questioning he admitted that he occasionally had left-sided chest pain, which had occurred intermittently over the last 2 years, particularly in association with exercise.

Ten years previously he had suffered from epigastric pain which had occurred in association with meals for about 4 months. He had been told at the time he had a duodenal ulcer and his symptoms had improved with treatment with cimetidine. He smoked 30 cigarettes daily and drank 1½ bottles of brandy weekly. In his family his mother suffered from mild diabetes mellitus, and one brother had had pulmonary tuberculosis as a young man.

Examination showed him to be very obese with a protuberant abdomen. He was a little pale. His pulse and blood pressure were normal. Proctoscopy revealed haemorrhoids. His GP treated him with oral iron and referred him to a surgical Outpatients Department for injection. Here it was thought that the liver was palpable and also that some degree of ascites was present. He was accordingly admitted to a medical ward for further investigation.

On admission (see diagram) his pulse was 120 irregularly irregular; blood pressure 120/90; temperature 37.4; RR 28. He was in no obvious distress and was not orthopnoeic. The apex beat could not be felt. The heart sounds were quiet and a third sound could be heard. The JVP was raised 9 cm. There was dullness on percussion in the flanks and the liver was enlarged 4 cm, firm and not tender. There was a little ankle oedema. A few spider naevi were present over the upper chest but there were no other signs of liver failure.

Initial investigations: Hb 11 g/dl; MCV 73 fl; WBC 6.7 × 10⁹/l; differential normal; ESR 63 mm; blood film showed hypochromia; MSU normal; urea 3.1 mmol/l; electrolytes normal. CXR: some degree of cardiomegaly with clear lung fields. ECG: atrial fibrillation with right bundle branch block.

Questions

1. What are the likely diagnoses?
2. What investigations would you undertake to establish the diagnosis?

Discussion

The diagnosis is by no means obvious in this man. His history is very non-specific and his symptoms could be produced by many different disease processes. A striking feature of the history, however, in view of the signs found on examination, is the absence of any complaint of dyspnoea or orthopnoea. His story of longstanding constipation and the recent passage of bright red blood on the stool is very typical of piles and this is confirmed by the proctoscopy. A digital examination should be made and sigmoidoscopy should be performed as a routine. Blood loss from piles, although usually trivial, can on occasion be marked. It may certainly be sufficient to cause some degree of anaemia and this is especially likely in the elderly, where the diet may be poor and absorption of iron impaired.

It is difficult to evaluate the left chest pain. Despite its association with exercise its site makes it very unlikely to be angina.

A number of points must be considered in his personal history. He is a very heavy cigarette smoker which predisposes him to the development of both coronary artery disease and carcinoma of the bronchus. Furthermore, he admits to drinking several bottles of brandy weekly, which indicates that his alcohol intake is sufficient to cause significant tissue damage. Although the brunt of this insult will fall upon the liver, damage may also occur to the heart. Alcoholic cardiomyopathy is a well-recognized condition. It may occur as a result of deficiency of thiamine or as a result of the direct action of alcohol on the myocardium.

Tuberculosis is common in Cyprus and a family history of this disease is often given by Cypriot immigrants to this country. Pulmonary tuberculosis will not usually present any difficulty in diagnosis once a chest X-ray has been obtained. It should however be remembered that tuberculous pericarditis also occurs and may present with the signs of pericardial constriction many years after the initial infection.

His previous dyspeptic symptoms are difficult to evaluate. Duodenal ulceration has a tendency to recur and he has had recent indigestion. His anaemia may therefore be due to bleeding from the duodenum rather than the haemorrhoids and it is impossible to exclude this possibility without further barium studies or gastroscopy.

The findings on examination reveal a significant rise in the systemic venous pressure and this could explain the hepatomegaly, ascites and peripheral oedema. The firmness and lack of tenderness of the liver suggest that the venous congestion has been present for some time and that cirrhosis is present. This would in turn explain the raised ESR and the presence of a few spider naevi. If alcoholic liver damage were solely responsible for the hepatomegaly and ascites the raised JVP and other cardiac findings would require some further explanation. The cardiac abnormalities consist of atrial fibrillation, a third heart sound, with a raised JVP and the ascites and oedema already discussed. Many of the features of congestive heart failure are therefore present. He is obese and a heavy cigarette smoker and is therefore a candidate for ischaemic heart disease, a common cause of atrial fibrillation and heart failure. Against this interpretation is the absence of any symptoms or signs of left ventricular failure, with only minimal cardiac enlargement. There is, furthermore, no history or X-ray evidence of chronic pulmonary disease.

The combination of peripheral congestion and hepatomegaly and ascites, with the absence of dyspnoea or any evidence of pulmonary congestion, raises the possibility of constrictive pericarditis. The absence of pericardial calcification on a straight chest X-ray does not exclude the diagnosis. The ECG findings are compatible with this diagnosis, although typically there should be low-voltage curves with widespread T-wave inversion. Echocardiography and cardiac catheterization with measurement of intracardiac pressures should confirm the diagnosis. In difficult cases, particularly where the differential diagnosis is restriction, CT or MRI of the heart would be confirmatory.

Alcoholic cardiomyopathy usually produces a picture of biventricular heart failure and dyspnoea is an early and major symptom. Atrial fibrillation and ectopic beats are common and there is usually marked cardiomegaly.

In this patient further investigation confirmed the clinical suspicion of contrictive pericarditis. The aetiology was assumed to be tuberculous and a moderately successful result was obtained from pericardectomy.

3

Peripheral oedema

Oedema results from the accumulation of excess fluid in the interstitial space. It can be caused in a variety of ways, and a simple classification is as follows:

1. *Generalized oedema* due to transudation of salt and water, e.g. hypoproteinaemic syndromes, congestive cardiac failure, acute glomerulonephritis.

2. *Local oedema* due to:
   - increased permeability of small blood vessels, e.g. infection, trauma, burns, allergy.
   - oedema due to lymphatic obstruction, e.g. malignancy, filariasis, chronic infection.
   - oedema due to venous obstruction, e.g. thrombosis, malignant infiltration.

GENERAL PRINCIPLES IN THE FORMATION OF INTERSTITIAL FLUID

In conditions where the small blood vessels are intact, the formation of interstitial fluid is regulated according to the Starling hypothesis (which incorporates 5 factors – capillary hydrostatic pressure, interstitial tissue pressure, plasma oncotic pressure, endothelial permeability and lymphatic function). The arterial hydrostatic pressure, in excess of tissue pressure, tends to cause transudation of salt and water out of capillaries, while the colloid osmotic (oncotic) pressure of the plasma proteins tends to draw fluid back in. There is thus an overall loss of fluid from the capillary at its arterial end, and reabsorption at the venous end. A small amount of protein is present in this transudate. A low colloid osmotic pressure or a raised hydrostatic pressure at the venous end of the capillary will tend to cause oedema. Increasing the tissue pressure (e.g. with an elastic stocking) or raising the colloid osmotic pressure when low (e.g. albumin infusion in cirrhosis) will inhibit oedema formation. Fluid accumulating in the interstitial space passes into thin-walled lymphatic vessels. From here it passes into the general circulation via the main lymphatic channels. Lymph vessels have valves and the passage of lymph is assisted by muscular activity and by negative intrathoracic pressure.

If small blood vessels are themselves damaged directly by thermal injury or infections or allergic reactions, there is loss of fluid from their lumen. Oedema formed in this way has the qualities of an exudate, being rich in protein.

GENERALIZED OEDEMA DUE TO TRANSUDATION OF SALT AND WATER

Among the commonest causes of oedema are heart failure and the hypoproteinaemic states. The mechanisms which are responsible for oedema formation in these conditions are complex and have some similarities.

The control of the extracellular fluid volume, and the formation of oedema

The control of extracellular fluid (ECF) volume is incompletely understood. Since the sodium cation is the most important osmotically active constituent of the ECF, the process mainly concerns the factors that regulate the accumulation of sodium in the body and its excretion by the kidney.

About 85% of all the filtered sodium is reabsorbed in the proximal convoluted tubule. The remaining 15% is variably reabsorbed in the distal tubule, partly with chloride ions and partly in exchange for potassium and hydrogen ions. The regulation of sodium excretion is probably mainly through adjustment of this 15%. In this the role of adrenal steroids is dominant. Aldosterone is the major adrenal mineralocorticoid hormone. The effect of aldosterone is on the distal renal tubule, causing sodium reabsorption and potassium excretion. This effect is blocked by spironolactone. It is not certain if aldosterone has an effect on the proximal tubule. An important stimulus to aldosterone release comes from the renin-angiotensin system. Renin is produced in specialized cells in the juxtaglomerular apparatus. Any fall in ECF volume (for example as a result of haemorrhage or dehydration) results in release of renin into the blood. Here it acts on renin substrate (produced in the liver) to produce angiotensin I which is then converted to angiotensin II in peripheral tissues such as the lung by angiotensin-converting enzyme (ACE). Angiotensin II is the stimulus for aldosterone release. Renal sodium reabsorption then occurs, the blood volume rises and the release of renin diminishes.

The glomerular filtration rate (GFR) exerts a direct effect on sodium excretion. Any factors which tend to decrease GFR (such as a fall in blood pressure for any reason) increase the amount of sodium reabsorbed in the proximal convoluted tubule. In health, marked fluctuations of GFR do not normally occur. Minor fluctuations might still cause significant alterations in sodium excretion.

Distension of the great veins in the chest, or of the atria of the heart causes a water diuresis, probably mediated by inhibition of release of antidiuretic hormone (ADH). Vascular receptors in the cardiac chambers also sense volume change in the circulation, releasing natriuretic peptides such as atrial natriuretic peptide (ANP), which counteracts volume expansion by causing natriuresis.

These processes, that are involved in disorders producing oedema, are now discussed.

Hypoproteinaemic states. The major part of the colloid osmotic pressure of the plasma can be attributed to its albumin content. Hypoalbuminaemia may be due to failure of synthesis, as in protein malnutrition (Kwashiorkor), cirrhosis, and longstanding ill-health from many causes, or to increased loss as in nephrotic syndrome and protein-losing enteropathy. There is a fall in colloid osmotic pressure and when the serum albumin falls below 25 g/l there is transudation of solutes (mainly salt and water) out of capillaries into the intercellular fluid space. When this compartment is expanded by about 10%, clinically evident oedema appears. There is loss of circulating fluid and a fall in plasma volume. Aldosterone is released and sodium and water reabsorption occurs in the kidney. In a normal person this would restore the plasma volume but, as long as hypoproteinaemia continues, fluid thus reabsorbed is again lost into the intercellular space and aldosterone secretion and further salt retention continues with a further increase in oedema.

Heart failure. Many mechanisms are involved in causing oedema in heart failure. In severe heart failure the kidneys respond in a manner similar to that seen in acute severe haemorrhage. Several neural and humoral mechanisms are involved, causing vasoconstriction and maintaining blood pressure and perfusion to vital organs. There are many possible triggers including baroreceptors in the carotid sinus and aortic arch together with atrial, ventricular and juxtaglomerular capillary receptors.

Patients with heart failure have increased sympathetic tone and raised levels of circulating noradrenaline, which correlates with the degree of left ventricular dysfunction and prognosis. Levels of plasma renin and aldosterone are also raised. Sodium and water are retained by the kidneys, thereby expanding the blood volume and predisposing to peripheral and pulmonary oedema. Increased sympathetic activity causes an increase in peripheral vascular resistance. There is constriction of veins which reduces the capacity of the circulation and results in increased filling of the heart. Venous pressure rises and oedema develops, especially in dependent regions. Whether oedema is pulmonary or systemic partly depends on where the rise in capillary pressure occurs. Left heart failure and pulmonary oedema will result from conditions such as ischaemic heart disease, hypertension, aortic and mitral valve disease. Right heart failure also has many causes, for example chronic lung disease, thromboembolic disease and secondary to left heart failure. In pulmonary disease, an elevated pCO_2 contributes to the formation of peripheral oedema by increasing capillary permeability.

Acute glomerulonephritis. The oedema has the property of a transudate, not an exudate. Considerable sodium retention occurs in this condition as a result of the greatly decreased GFR. It is probable that this is the major mechanism accounting for the hypertension and peripheral oedema.

Idiopathic oedema. This condition affects women in early middle age. The oedema is dependent and fluctuates with position and also with the menstrual cycle. The cause is unknown, and paradoxically the condition may be worsened by excessive diuretic therapy. The condition is not usually difficult to diagnose since no other signs of disease are present.

Clinical presentation

Peripheral oedema accumulates in dependent regions and areas where the skin is lax. Swelling of the ankles is usually the earliest sign. In hypoproteinaemic states and in glomerulonephritis there is often oedema of the face and hands, most marked after lying down. The patient with heart failure, on the other hand, is breathless and sleeps propped up; sacral oedema is therefore common. Ascites may occur in all of these conditions, but it is especially likely to do so in cirrhosis of the liver where there is portal hypertension as well as hypoalbuminaemia. Ascites is also likely to occur in constrictive pericarditis. In this condition the venous pressure is markedly elevated and may rise further, rather than fall, on inspiration (Kussmaul's sign).

Hypoproteinaemia will be diagnosed by estimation of the serum proteins. The patient with nephrotic syndrome will have heavy proteinuria. The features of cirrhosis may be present. Intestinal causes of hypoproteinaemia may require tests for malabsorption and small bowel radiology for precise diagnosis.

Acute glomerulonephritis will be suspected by its acute onset, the presence of hypertension and the

> **Box 3.1** Investigation of peripheral oedema
>
> **Generalized oedema**
>
> - Chest X-ray – signs of heart failure, cardiomegaly
> - Plasma albumin – low in nephrotic syndrome, cirrhosis, malnutrition (in the Western world this is likely to be due to chronic disease, especially cancer)
> - Blood urea and electrolytes – diminished GFR in renal disease or in severe cardiac failure
>
> **Localized oedema**
>
> - Chest X-ray – SVCO
> - Pelvic ultrasound or CT scan – pelvic tumours or lymphatic enlargement
> - Lymphangiography – abnormal lymphatic architecture, lymph nodes replaced by tumour
> - Doppler ultrasound or venography – to confirm diagnosis of venous obstruction

finding of protein and red cells in the urine of a patient with oliguria.

Iatrogenic fluid overload occurs mainly in elderly patients, in those with impaired renal function, or in post-operative patients who have difficulty in handling a water load. If a patient on intravenous fluids becomes oedematous the reason is normally that too much fluid has been given too quickly to a patient who may have impaired cardiac or renal function or who has hypoalbuminaemia due to poor nutrition as a result of illness.

OEDEMA DUE TO INCREASED PERMEABILITY OF SMALL VESSELS

Clinically, this form of oedema does not usually present a diagnostic problem, the cause of the subcutaneous swelling accompanying cellulitis or skin ulceration, for example, being obvious. Occasionally various kinds of allergic vasculitis such as erythema nodosum can be accompanied by considerable oedema, and be mistaken for cellulitis.

A form of allergic oedema which may cause some diagnostic confusion is angio-oedema. In this condition there is an exudation of fluid into the subcutaneous tissues especially involving the face, lips and eyelids, although any part of the body may be affected. The tongue may swell and palatal and laryngeal oedema occasionally occur. Urticaria is not usually present, and a history of allergy is often lacking. A hereditary form occurs in which severe abdominal pain may accompany an attack and laryngeal oedema may be severe, and even fatal. This form of the disorder is due to an inherited deficiency of the inhibitor of the activated first component of complement. A low serum comple-

ment is usually found. Angio-oedema may be mistaken for acute glomerulonephritis or the nephrotic syndrome, in both of which there may be facial oedema. The abrupt onset and associated symptoms, and the lack of evidence of renal disease, serve to distinguish these conditions.

OEDEMA DUE TO LYMPHATIC OBSTRUCTION

Lymph vessels have a large collateral circulation, so that any block has to extend over a wide area for oedema to appear. Secondary cancer in lymph nodes may cause oedema in this way but usually the block has been made more extensive by dissection of nodes and radiotherapy, for example in the treatment of carcinoma of the breast. In some tropical countries filariasis is endemic. In affected patients chronic lymphatic obstruction may develop over the years. This is due to the widespread fibrosis in lymphatic channels caused by the adult worm, together with associated secondary infection. An additional feature may be involvement of the retroperitoneal lymphatic system causing leakage of milky lymph into the urine (chyluria).

The oedema of lymphatic obstruction has certain characteristic features. The affected region becomes brawny and thickened, and after oedema has been present for some time may not pit on pressure. The oedema has a very high protein content – up to 40 g/l. This is due to the slow accumulation of protein over a long period of time. Rarely an angiosarcoma may develop in a limb with longstanding lymphoedema such as that which sometimes occurs in the arm following treatment for breast cancer.

OEDEMA DUE TO VENOUS OCCLUSION

The major cause of venous obstruction is deep venous thrombosis, which is a very common cause of leg oedema. If the block is in the inferior vena cava, both legs may swell. Other signs of venous thrombosis and obstruction are often present: dilated superficial veins with delayed emptying, enlarged collateral veins which are especially evident in superior vena cava obstruction, a bluish discoloration of the limb and tenderness along the line of the veins. Veins may be occluded by an adjacent or surrounding neoplasm and by secondary cancer in lymph nodes. There may be evidence of a cause of local compression, such as pelvic or abdominal mass, or a remote cause for venous thrombosis such as malignancy elsewhere causing thrombophlebitis migrans, or polycythaemia. The oedema due to venous occlusion may cause difficulty in diagnosis if the patient is seen after the acute episode has subsided and if the swelling is bilateral.

A particularly important cause of oedema due to venous obstruction is the syndrome of superior vena cava obstruction (SVCO). This condition is almost always caused by a tumour in the superior mediastinum. The commonest cause is lung cancer but lymphomas, thymomas and germ cell tumours are other causes. The patient's face becomes swollen, especially around the eyelids, a dusky discoloration of the skin develops and the neck veins may be hugely distended.

Dilated veins are usually visible over the shoulder and anterior chest. There are distended cutaneous venules typically seen round the lower rib cage under the breasts.

The chest X-ray commonly shows a mediastinal mass, but on occasions this may be difficult to see if there is a small but infiltrating carcinoma. The true position is then revealed by a CT or MR scan of the upper mediastinum.

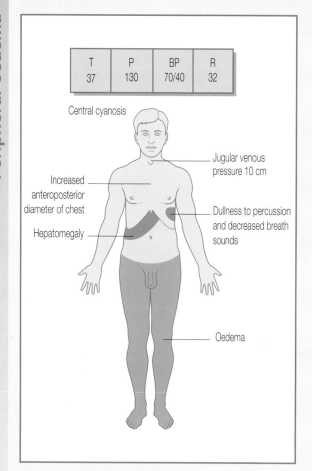

T	P	BP	R
37	130	70/40	32

Central cyanosis

Jugular venous pressure 10 cm

Increased anteroposterior diameter of chest

Dullness to percussion and decreased breath sounds

Hepatomegaly

Oedema

A 60-year-old retired train driver was admitted as an emergency complaining of severe breathlessness, gradually worsening over the preceding week. He had become severely breathless at night and had had to sleep propped up. Over the next few days both legs had become greatly swollen.

He had had a chronic productive cough for 15 years, worse in the winter when he had often been off work with acute bronchitis. In the preceding 12 months he had noticed swelling of both ankles towards the end of the day and increasing shortness of breath on exertion. Over the previous 3 months before admission he had had several episodes of haemoptysis, coughing up small quantities of fresh blood. He had never had chest pain. Before his recent deterioration he had noticed that he had lost about 3 kg in weight. He had smoked 30 cigarettes a day for 40 years and was a moderate beer drinker.

On examination he was dyspnoeic and cyanosed: pulse 130 scarcely palpable, regular with a very small volume; blood pressure 70/40. The jugular venous pressure was greatly elevated. The heart sounds were faint and the apex beat was not palpable. There was oedema of both legs up to the groin, and scrotal oedema. He was barrel-chested. The trachea was central and there was no finger clubbing. There was dullness to percussion with absent breath sounds at the left base extending into the axilla. In the abdomen, the liver was enlarged 8 cm below the costal margin and was tender, firm and with a smooth outline. There was no ascites.

Questions

1. What do you consider to be the possible causes of his sudden deterioration?
2. What investigations should be urgently undertaken?
3. What treatment would you undertake immediately?

Discussion

The history is of chronic bronchitis in a cigarette smoker. The ankle swelling over the preceding 12 months suggests the onset of cor pulmonale. The 3-month history of weight loss and haemoptysis raises the possibility of the development of a bronchial carcinoma. There is a recent sudden deterioration with gross oedema, breathlessness, raised venous pressure and hypotension.

The signs in the chest are those of a pleural effusion. This would not entirely account for his recent deterioration. A myocardial infarction is a possible cause, but there is no history of chest pain, and this diagnosis does not fit in with the pattern of his previous illness. Pulmonary embolism must certainly be excluded. The swelling of the legs came after the onset of breathlessness which is not the typical sequence of events when deep venous thrombosis in the legs gives rise to pulmonary embolism. However it by no means excludes such a diagnosis and signs of venous thrombosis may follow the occurrence of the embolism. Similarly an embolus from thrombus in a pelvic vein or the inferior vena cava could explain his recent deterioration, hypotension and pleural effusion.

Superior vena cava obstruction, which is usually due to carcinoma of the bronchus, would give rise to raised jugular venous pressure but would not account for the oedema of the legs. Pericardial tamponade is a very likely diagnosis, and would account for the raised venous pressure, hypotension and rapid feeble pulse. There may be pulsus paradoxus, detectable by careful sphygmomanometry. In this patient, with a long history of smoking, haemoptysis and weight loss, pericardial tamponade due to malignant infiltration from a bronchogenic carcinoma is highly probable. A carcinoma of the bronchus could also account for the pleural effusion.

Although any cause of hypoproteinaemia might result in oedema and a pleural effusion, this is very unlikely to be the cause in this case. Cirrhosis of the liver, nephrotic syndrome and malabsorption would not explain the hypotension, breathlessness and raised venous pressure, nor would these diagnoses account for his previous illness.

The most useful investigations in the immediate diagnosis would be a chest X-ray, ECG and echocardiogram. A chest X-ray may show a carcinoma of the bronchus and an enlarged cardiac silhouette from heart failure or tamponade. It could also provide evidence of left heart failure, or diminished vascular markings in the case of a large pulmonary embolus. It will confirm the presence of a pleural effusion. An ECG may show evidence of myocardial infarction or the right ventricular strain pattern of pulmonary embolism. In pericardial effusion there may be small voltages throughout. Echocardiography will clinch the diagnosis, showing an echo-free space surrounding the heart, causing right atrial +/− ventricular diastolic collapse.

Other routine investigations such as a full blood count, plasma protein estimation and sputum cytology are not of immediate value. Aspiration and biopsy of the pleural effusion would be unhelpful in immediate management but could be of great value in diagnosis. A bloodstained pleural effusion is strongly suggestive of malignancy, but may occur in a minority of patients with pulmonary infarction (30% of cases). Examination of the fluid for malignant cells may give the diagnosis, as may the pleural biopsy.

Pericardial tamponade necessitates emergency aspiration and drainage, which will provide immediate relief and a dramatic improvement in the patient's vital signs and general clinical condition. Cytological examination of the fluid may demonstrate malignant cells.

> This man had a bronchial carcinoma infiltrating the pericardium, causing a haemorrhagic effusion. Aspiration brought temporary relief, but he died several days later.

4

Central chest pain

All thoracic and many extrathoracic structures may give rise to central chest pain. These include muscles and joints of the chest wall, pleura, pericardium, lungs, heart, oesophagus, great vessels, stomach and gall-bladder. In practice the first question to be answered is usually whether or not the pain is cardiac.

ISCHAEMIC HEART DISEASE

Ischaemic heart disease is one of the commonest causes of death in men and women in the western world. Coronary atherosclerosis may present as stable angina, unstable angina, acute myocardial infarction and its sequelae, namely heart failure, palpitations and sudden cardiac death. Terminology has changed in recent years in an attempt to reduce the number of different terms applied to the varying manifestations of coronary disease, such as Q wave and non-Q wave infarction, crescendo angina and unstable angina. Instead, the term 'acute coronary syndrome' is used as an umbrella term to cover all forms of unstable angina and myocardial infarction, but excluding stable angina. One of the reasons behind this, beyond the need for a simpler classification system, is to dispel the myth that unstable angina and non-Q wave myocardial infarction have a more benign course than does transmural or Q-wave myocardial infarction; they do not. In all three conditions the pathology within the coronary artery is the same, namely plaque rupture with superimposed platelet activation and thrombus formation, but the extent of myocardial necrosis (ranging from none to a large area of infarction) will vary, depending on the degree of coronary artery occlusion and whether there is spontaneous or drug-mediated fibrinolysis.

Angina and infarction pain have certain common characteristics, although the symptoms of infarction are generally far more intense. The first point to make is that angina is not really a pain at all. A careful history shows that angina can be described in many ways (pressure, discomfort, crushing, squeezing, aching) but very rarely will the patient use the word pain. Despite this, doctors continue to call angina a pain and this can create confusion – just occasionally a patient will deny having chest pain on direct questioning. The doctor may then assume, erroneously, that the patient does not have angina at all.

Angina is typically situated in the centre of the chest and may radiate to the neck and jaw (even, at times, mimicking toothache) and to the arms, usually the left. Patients describe a pressure, heaviness or tightness within the chest, as if someone is sitting on them. Sometimes, however, the symptom is most atypical, for example an ache in the wrist with exertion – the key here is that the symptom is brought on by exercise, a feature of stable angina. Symptoms are more frequently atypical in the elderly, in diabetics and in women.

By definition, stable angina is brought on by stress (physical or mental) and rapidly relieved by rest. When the pattern changes and symptoms come unexpectedly, such as with minimal effort or at rest or at night, this signifies the development of unstable symptoms and the risk of myocardial infarction. These patients should be evaluated in the same way as patients with acute myocardial infarction since they are at significant risk of progressing to infarction. Symptoms that persist for more than 15 minutes herald the risk of infarction and require emergency treatment.

Myocardial infarction generally develops unexpectedly, the incidence peaking in the morning and late afternoon. In retrospect, the patient may have been aware that the pattern of his/her angina had changed in the preceding days or weeks. However, myocardial infarction is often the *first* manifestation of coronary artery disease. The patient may have no past history to help in assessment and, equally, the patient may have no reason to suppose that the symptoms are cardiac in origin. With acute infarction there is frequently intense sweating, malaise and nausea and the chest symptoms are generally most severe.

The past history may be helpful if the patient is known to have coronary artery disease. Other manifestations of cardiovascular disease should be sought, such as previous TIA or stroke and claudication. The lower incidence of coronary artery disease in women before the menopause, compared with men of the same age, disappears after oophorectomy. A full cardiovascular risk profile should be established, including a family history of premature coronary artery disease, the possibility of familial hyperlipidaemia (patients are now far more aware of the importance of cholesterol and may have had a cholesterol check as part of a screening programme or insurance medical), smoking history, the presence of diabetes mellitus or hypertension and general lifestyle (diet, exercise, alcohol intake).

Although there are no physical signs of angina or of uncomplicated infarction, there may be evidence of predisposing factors and underlying causes. These include **obesity**, **hyperlipidaemia** as shown by arcus senilis in young men, xanthelasmata and tendon xanthomata. **Hypertension** may not be present when the blood pressure is taken following infarction, but evidence of it may be found in the fundi or on ECG. In **aortic valve disease**, particularly stenosis, angina may develop in the absence of coronary artery disease due to increased ventricular muscle mass and relative underperfusion of the hypertrophied myocardium. **Hyperthyroidism** due to a nodular goitre or adenoma in the elderly may lack many of the features of thyrotoxicosis and can present as angina (masked thyrotoxicosis). A particularly dangerous situation is over-rapid replacement therapy with thyroxine in a newly diagnosed case of myxoedema because myxoedema predisposes to ischaemic heart disease. Development of **anaemia** may unmask co-existing myocardial ischaemia. A sudden **arrhythmia** such as supraventricular tachycardia, atrial flutter or fibrillation, or complete heart block may cause an abrupt reduction in cardiac output and cause isch-aemic pain.

The most useful bedside tests are the ECG (Figs 4.1, 4.2) and a rapid troponin (T or I) assay, now available in many casualty departments.

In stable angina the ECG is frequently normal unless the patient has suffered previous myocardial infarction or there may be ECG changes of left ventricular hypertrophy in a patient with undiagnosed or poorly controlled hypertension, for example. A stress test (treadmill or bicycle) in which graded exercise is carried out following a predetermined protocol (e.g. Bruce protocol) will be helpful, to clarify the diagnosis and begin risk stratification. This may provoke the chest pain and/or ECG changes. Myocardial perfusion imaging (using thallium or technetium radionuclides) and stress echocardiography are suitable alternatives. Coronary angiography will define the coronary anatomy precisely.

The ECG changes associated with full thickness myocardial infarction (ST elevation, loss of R wave and the development of pathological Q waves and T wave inversion) take time to evolve and an early ECG may be normal. Posterior infarction may be difficult to diag-nose from the ECG and may be interpreted wrongly as anterior ischaemia. ECG changes vary in unstable angina from an apparently normal ECG to minor T wave changes to widespread ST and T wave changes, generally evolving over time. Troponin testing in patients with suspicious chest pain but with nondiag-nostic ECGs is particularly helpful since the troponin assays are highly accurate, detecting even very minor degrees of myocardial necrosis. A 'negative' troponin assay puts the patient in a good prognostic group. Patients with positive troponin tests (which may take 12 hours to become positive) should be admitted to CCU and be treated for presumed unstable angina with aspirin, low molecular weight heparin, betablockers and nitrates, together with serial ECGs and cardiac

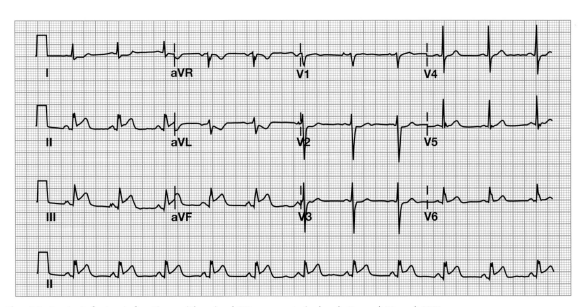

Fig. 4.1 Acute inferior infarction with raised ST segments in leads II, and III and AVF.

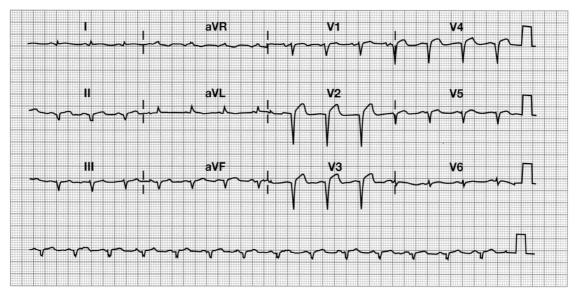

Fig. 4.2 Recent extensive anterior infarction with QS waves and ST elevation in leads V2–V4.

enzyme measurements to look for evidence of progression to acute infarction necessitating fibrinolysis, or in some cases primary angioplasty. There is an increasing emphasis on early coronary angiography in unstable angina patients, to select those cases where angioplasty (PTCA) or bypass surgery should be considered. Some interventional centres prefer to offer primary PTCA rather than fibrinolysis to patients with acute infarction, particularly in some parts of Europe and the US. Similarly, there are marked regional and national variations in the role of cardiac catheterization following myocardial infarction.

PERICARDITIS

Acute pericarditis from any cause may closely mimic myocardial infarction. One feature of the pain is that it may be worse on inspiration. This is sometimes due to associated pleural inflammation. Unlike myocardial infarction the pain may be modified by position, with relief on leaning forwards. The pathognomonic sign of pericarditis is a pericardial friction rub, which is qualitatively different from a murmur, being superficial, scratchy and having three phases if in sinus rhythm. One should be alert to the possibility of an associated pericardial effusion causing tamponade. The signs which would suggest this are pulsus paradoxus and a raised jugular venous pressure. A difficulty may be the transient pericardial friction rub which is occasionally heard in the first few days following myocardial infarction. In pericarditis the ECG will show ST elevation in the presence of upright T

waves and the absence of pathological Q waves (Fig. 4.3). In contrast, following myocardial infarction T waves are initially upright, becoming inverted within 48 hours and, in addition, pathological Q waves are generally present, since the rub signifies a sizeable infarction.

THORACIC AORTIC ANEURYSM

A dissecting thoracic aortic aneurysm classically gives rise to a tearing sensation radiating to the back. Usually there are accompanying signs which vary according to the site of dissection. A tear in the aortic root and ascending aorta may cause acute aortic regurgitation, tamponade and myocardial ischaemia. A tear in the arch may cause neurological signs such as hemiparesis and disappearance or inequality of pulses. Shock may supervene as a consequence of myocardial ischaemia or tamponade, rupture through the aortic wall or severe pain. A pleural effusion, particularly left-sided, may develop. Although atherosclerosis with hypertension is the commonest aetiology, it may occur in younger patients with the Marfan syndrome. A tall patient with arachnodactyly, lens dislocation, high arched palate and hyperextensible joints will suggest this possibility. There may be a family history.

In aortic dissection the characteristic appearance on chest X-ray is of widening of the mediastinum +/– a pleural effusion (Fig. 4.4). Diagnosis may be made by spiral CT, MRI (Fig. 4.5A and B) or echocardiography (transthoracic and transoesophageal).

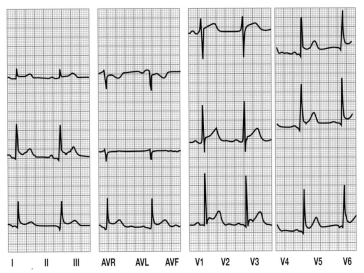

| I | II | III | AVR | AVL | AVF | V1 | V2 | V3 | V4 | V5 | V6 |

Fig. 4.3 Acute pericarditis. The ST segments are concave and raised. This is seen in most leads, in contrast to the regional changes of acute ischaemia.

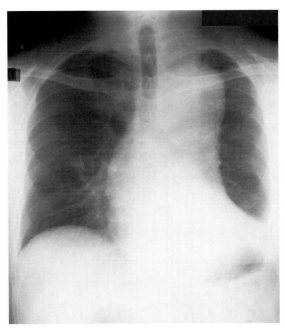

Fig. 4.4 Chest X-ray showing gross widening of the superior mediastinum, prominence of the ascending aorta and a small left pleural effusion in a young hypertensive man who presented with acute dissection of the descending thoracic aorta.

PULMONARY EMBOLISM AND INFARCTION

Pulmonary embolism may cause an acute occlusion of the pulmonary artery or a major branch. This typi-

cally causes sudden central chest pain, hypotension, dyspnoea, cyanosis, and right heart strain with failure. It has to be differentiated from myocardial infarction. A dramatic onset, the absence of signs in the chest and the possible presence of deep venous thrombosis will point to the diagnosis. However, the textbook description of the ECG in acute pulmonary embolism (S wave in lead I, Q wave and T wave inversion in lead III–SI QIII TIII, and features of right heart strain) are variable. Sometimes only widespread T wave inversion or T wave inversion in leads VI–4, representing right heart strain and ischaemia, are seen (Fig. 4.6). This may easily be misinterpreted as unstable angina. In pulmonary infarction smaller vessels are occluded. There are fewer haemodynamic changes and the clinical picture is of pleurisy and haemoptysis (see Ch. 7).

The same causes predispose to embolism and infarction as they both usually follow deep venous thrombosis. The embolus is composed of freshly formed thrombus which may break off before there are local signs of leg or calf tenderness and swelling. For this reason the physician should be alert to early signs of thrombosis such as an unexplained slight rise in temperature in a patient bedridden as a result of injury, operation or myocardial infarction. Other factors predisposing to venous thrombosis are varicose veins and the contraceptive pill. Should the condition recur without an obvious underlying cause the possibility of anti-phospholipid antibodies predisposing to thrombosis should be excluded.

In pulmonary embolism there may be little abnormality on chest X-ray apart from the difficult sign of

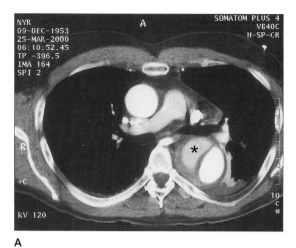

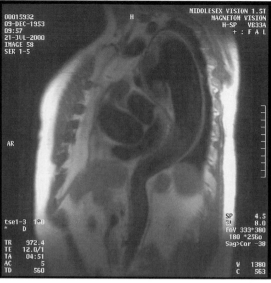

Fig. 4.5 MRI scan (**A** transverse with contrast and **B** sagittal without contrast) showing massive aneurysmal dilatation of the descending thoracic aorta, originating just beyond the left subclavian artery. There is a large anterior dissection flap (*) and a contained rupture within which is thrombus.

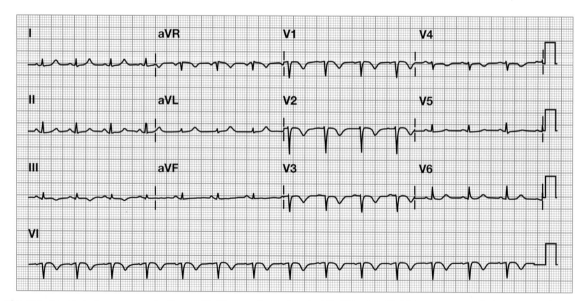

Fig. 4.6 Acute pulmonary embolism with T wave inversion in V1–V4, also III. This was wrongly interpreted as unstable angina with anterior ischaemia. Subsequent coronary angiography was normal but a lung ventilation–perfusion scan showed multiple areas of mismatch, confirming widespread pulmonary emboli.

oligaemia of part of a lung field. In pulmonary infarction, by contrast, there may be a wedge-shaped infarct or linear atelectasis, with elevation of the hemidiaphragm and a pleural reaction. Isotope lung scanning, spiral CT or MRI are valuable investigations.

SPONTANEOUS PNEUMOTHORAX

Sudden pain and dyspnoea, sometimes after a bout of coughing or straining, are the characteristic features of this condition, which can occur at any age. Dyspnoea may be disproportionate to the degree of lung collapse. Any underlying chronic chest disease will make the patient's distress greater. If there is associated cough the positive pressure of coughing may be transmitted to the pleural cavity and sometimes result in a tension pneumothorax, which may impair venous return and thereby cause cardiac embarrassment. Mediastinal shift to the opposite side shown by displacement of the apex beat or trachea may then occur, as well as hyper-resonance on percussion and diminution of breath sounds. A chest X-ray is essential (Fig. 4.7). A small pneumothorax can easily be missed and a film should be taken in expiration as well as the standard inspiratory film if the diagnosis is suspected. In a partial left pneumothorax a click or crunch may be heard with each heart beat, particularly when the patient lies on his left side.

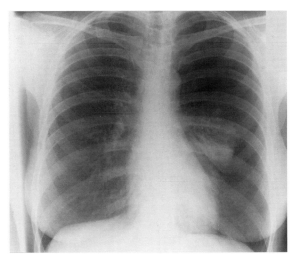

Fig. 4.7 Chest X-ray showing a left pneumothorax with collapse of the left lung but no mediastinal shift.

OESOPHAGEAL PAIN

Gastro-oesophageal reflux disease (GORD), sometimes associated with a sliding hiatus hernia, may cause a wide variety of chest pains which at times may mimic cardiac ischaemic pain. Heartburn should easily be recognized. It occurs after meals or lying flat or bending, with relief on sitting or standing up, belching and taking antacids. If there is associated oesophagitis, pain on swallowing hot or cold liquids, citrus juices or spirits may occur. Upper GI endoscopy and radiological examination with barium studies are useful investigations. The presence of *H. pylori* should be sought and eradication therapy prescribed if found. In more difficult cases ambulatory oesophageal pH and pressure measurements may help. A two-week therapeutic trial of a proton pump inhibitor will relieve symptoms of GORD even in the absence of radiological or endoscopic abnormality.

Oesophageal spasm may occur in relation to gastro-oesophageal reflux, and may also be responsible for the pain. Relief of chest pain by nitrates does not prove it to be cardiac, since oesophageal spasm may also respond.

SPINAL PAIN

Degenerative changes in the lower cervical or upper thoracic spine may give rise to pain which is referred to the anterior chest. A history of pain on exertion may suggest angina, especially as there may be root pain radiating to the arm; however, with care, it can be demonstrated that the pain can be clinically reproduced by certain movements. Above the age of 50 most cervical spine X-rays reveal degenerative changes irrespective of the presence or absence of symptoms, and the interpretation of abnormal findings, even in oblique views showing the outlet foramina, can be difficult. Rarely, neoplastic deposits, vertebral collapse from osteoporosis or osteomalacia, or a paravertebral abscess may cause central chest pain. Herpes zoster can cause chest pain, usually in a root distribution, and there may be diagnostic difficulty before the rash appears.

ATYPICAL CHEST PAIN

There is a group of patients with chest pain which fits no particular disease entity and no abnormality can be found despite careful investigation. These patients should be reassured and told that their prognosis is excellent. It is also important to indicate to the patient that he/she is not malingering since, when no cause is found, some patients feel doctors disbelieve their symptoms.

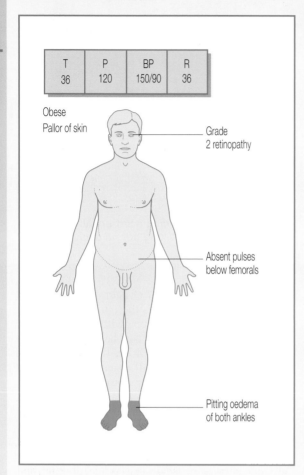

T	P	BP	R
36	120	150/90	36

Obese
Pallor of skin

Grade
2 retinopathy

Absent pulses
below femorals

Pitting oedema
of both ankles

A 52-year-old interior decorator was admitted to hospital complaining of severe central chest pain radiating to the back. This had come on suddenly as he went to bed after a late evening meal. At the onset of the pain he had a bout of coughing, but produced no sputum. He took a proprietary antacid that he kept by his bedside which made him belch, but did not relieve his pain. The pain persisted over the next hour until the emergency doctor arrived, and was associated with considerable breathlessness, together with cough productive of mucoid sputum containing flecks of blood.

He had been well until 6 years previously when he had developed bronchial asthma for which there was no obvious precipitating cause. Bronchodilators had been ineffective in controlling his wheezing and he had been treated since its onset with prednisolone, requiring a maintenance dose of 12.5 mg daily. He had gained 25 lb in weight and for the previous year had suffered indigestion particularly after fried food. Three months previously he had told his general practitioner that he had morning headaches and he had been found to be hypertensive (BP 180/125). Since then, he had been taking nifedipine with relief of his headaches.

On examination in hospital he was overweight with truncal obesity and striae in the flanks. He was distressed, pale and sweating. He was unable to lie flat and was tachypnoeic with poor movement of the chest wall. The trachea was central. There was loud generalized wheezing, more marked during expiration. The pulse was 120/min and regular, and BP was 150/90. The femoral pulses were palpable but distal pulses were difficult to palpate. Heart sounds were normal and no murmurs were heard. Fundoscopy showed narrowing and tortuosity of the retinal arteries with arteriovenous nipping. The JVP was not raised. There was slight pitting oedema of both ankles. The remainder of the examination did not reveal any abnormality.

Questions

1. What are the possible causes of the chest pain?
2. What immediate investigations would you undertake?
3. What would be your immediate treatment?

Discussion

This patient is a severe asthmatic, in that he requires a considerable dose of steroids to suppress his symptoms. Although he had a cough at the onset of his present illness, one cannot attribute his condition to asthma alone as this does not explain his chest pain. None the less the possibility that the chest pain is a complication of asthma or steroid therapy must be considered.

The most likely diagnosis is that of myocardial infarction. Hypertension and obesity resulting from steroid therapy would be predisposing factors. The site, onset and persistence of the pain are all in keeping with this diagnosis. Although infarction pain usually radiates to the shoulders, arms and neck, radiation to the back may sometimes occur. The development of breathlessness and orthopnoea, with wheezing and blood-flecked sputum, suggests that left ventricular failure and pulmonary oedema have developed.

Spontaneous pneumothorax cannot be ruled out as the typical physical signs may not be obvious in an obese and distressed patient, and the occurrence of a pneumothorax following a bout of coughing is not uncommon. Pleural adhesions from past infections may prevent complete collapse of the lung and continued coughing could result in positive pressure developing in the pleural space. Both asthma and steroid therapy are considered to be factors predisposing to spontaneous pneumothorax.

A probable additional complication of steroid therapy in this patient is his dyspepsia. The pain of gastro-oesophageal reflux can closely mimic cardiac pain and radiate to the back. Antacids and belching usually give relief. One would not expect considerable breathlessness to be precipitated by oesophagitis.

The presence of pain in the back raises the possibility of a collapsed dorsal vertebra, resulting from osteoporosis induced by steroid therapy. Localized tenderness and aggravation of the pain by movement of the spine would then be expected, but are absent in this patient.

The pain associated with dissecting aneurysm of the aorta characteristically radiates to the back and often moves to the loin as the dissection progresses. Unequal, absent or delayed pulses of the major arteries may be found and neurological signs frequently result from occlusion of major branches of the aortic arch. Preservation of the femoral pulses with reduced distal pulses is not a feature of dissection. This can be explained in this patient by the presence of left ventricular failure, reduced cardiac output, peripheral vasoconstriction and the likelihood of peripheral vascular disease.

The possibility of polyarteritis nodosa must always be considered when a patient presents with late onset asthma. Asthma may be the only symptom present for some years before involvement of other systems such as the kidneys, and, rarely, the heart where it may cause myocardial infarction.

Pulmonary embolism must always be considered in the differential diagnosis of sudden severe central chest pain. The absence of signs of a deep vein thrombosis does not exclude the diagnosis. When haemoptysis occurs it is more likely to be due to a peripheral lung infarct causing pleuritic pain than to a massive embolism occluding the pulmonary artery or one of its major branches. In any event, signs of acute right, rather than left, heart failure would be expected, with elevation of the JVP. His mild ankle oedema, if long standing, is more likely to be due to nifedipine.

The essential immediate investigations in this patient are an ECG and chest X-ray. The ECG would obviously be of great value in diagnosing myocardial infarction. If there are no diagnostic changes on the ECG it should be repeated 1 hour later. A rapid troponin assay would determine if there was myocardial necrosis but, similarly, if the patient presents early it may be normal and should be repeated several hours later. The value of the chest X-ray will be in excluding a pneumothorax for which films in both inspiration and expiration are necessary. Furthermore, signs of left ventricular failure and pulmonary oedema might be seen. These include engorgement of the upper lobe veins, basal septal (Kerley B) lines, and perihilar haze ('bat's wing' shadow). The chest X-ray can be normal in dissecting aneurysm but may show widening of the mediastinum.

The most likely diagnosis in this patient is myocardial infarction causing pulmonary oedema, for which conventional treatment would be aspirin, oxygen therapy, intravenous opiates, nitrates, judicious use of diuretics and, of course, a fibrinolytic. Beta blockade is contraindicated due to his asthma and the development of pulmonary oedema. In addition the stress induced by the condition of the patient may fail to evoke an appropriate adrenocortical response due to adrenal suppression by steroid therapy. He should, therefore, be given intravenous hydrocortisone.

The development of pulmonary oedema is a bad prognostic sign, implying extensive infarction. The differential diagnosis should include acute severe mitral regurgitation following chordal or papillary muscle rupture or a ventricular septal defect, although these conditions generally take time to develop after a myocardial infarct.

Flecks of blood in the sputum are not a contraindication to fibrinolytic therapy, although of course there is always a bleeding risk, but the benefits in extensive infarction are great. If there was a contraindication to fibrinolytic therapy, primary PTCA should be considered where facilities exist, particularly if the patient develops cardiogenic shock.

> The ECG confirmed the presence of an acute anteroseptal myocardial infarction. The chest X-ray showed the features of pulmonary oedema.

5

Shock

The term 'shock' is used to describe a clinical state. Although the word is difficult to define precisely and is often used inaccurately, it remains useful because it characterizes a syndrome which is generally well recognized, and because there are mechanisms common to all causes underlying the disorder. A more formal definition is 'acute circulatory failure with inadequate or inappropriately distributed tissue perfusion resulting in generalized cellular hypoxia'.

A shocked patient is pale and sweating with cold and often cyanosed peripheries. The blood pressure is low, the pulse is rapid and the peripheral veins are collapsed. There may be restlessness and mental confusion. A patient in this state would be generally regarded as being in shock. This is a life-threatening condition requiring emergency treatment.

THE PATHOPHYSIOLOGY OF SHOCK

Haemorrhagic shock

The shock which results from haemorrhage has been widely studied, and is the easiest model for understanding the circulatory abnormalities in a shocked patient (Fig. 5.1). In haemorrhagic shock, there is first a reduction in blood volume. Since the venous system contains the largest part of the circulating blood, the fall in blood volume causes a fall in venous pressure and a reduction in venous return to the heart. The cardiac output, which is dependent on venous return, falls, the stroke volume diminishes and the blood pressure falls. The fall in blood pressure threatens the cerebral circulation and various circulatory reflexes are activated to counteract this. These originate in the carotid sinus and aortic arch, and result in intense stimulation of the sympathetic nervous system, causing release of catecholamines with tachycardia and arteriolar vasoconstriction. The vasoconstriction is most marked in the skin and gut. The blood pressure is thus maintained, at least in the initial stages, but at the price of hypoxia in the vasoconstricted areas.

If the circulating blood volume is not rapidly restored, the function of vital organs will begin to deteriorate. Subsequent reperfusion may worsen organ function and multiorgan failure may develop. Tissue damage in the splanchnic bed can be so great that fluid and blood are lost from the capillary network and further hypovolaemia results. The therapy of prolonged haemorrhagic shock has to take into account this disturbance in the microcirculation. Pressor agents will increase arteriolar vasoconstriction and worsen the situation, while drugs which block alpha-receptors – provided adequate fluid replacement is achieved – cause splanchnic vasodilatation and can improve survival.

Irreversible shock due to haemorrhage alone is uncommon in humans. In cases of haemorrhage where shock is irreversible, other complicating factors such as tissue injury, burns and sepsis are usually present, all contributing to hypovolaemic shock. Other mechanisms then contribute to the pathophysiology of the condition.

Pump failure. Although primary pump failure is the major mechanism in cardiogenic shock, some degree of heart failure is also found in other shock states. Direct depression of myocardial function occurs in the toxaemia of septic shock. Impaired coronary perfusion due to prolonged hypotension causes myocardial dysfunction from ischaemia, particularly if there is pre-existing coronary artery disease.

Increased peripheral vasoconstriction. This leads to tissue hypoxia and contributes to mental confusion, bacteraemia (from gut-derived organisms) and oliguria. This process is exacerbated by arteriovenous shunting of blood past the capillary bed.

Hypoxia. This leads to lactic acidosis and further depression of myocardial function.

Cardiogenic shock

Here the drop in blood pressure is primarily due to the failure of the heart as a pump, for example following a large myocardial infarction. The arteriolar vasoconstriction that follows is mediated through the same mechanism as in haemorrhagic shock and the same disturbance in small blood vessels in the splanchnic circulation can result. The fall in blood pressure is of particular importance to the damaged heart, because the heart is unique in that the coronary circulation fills in diastole and if the diastolic pressure is very low, there may not be enough pressure for adequate coronary perfusion. Maintenance of diastolic pressure is there-

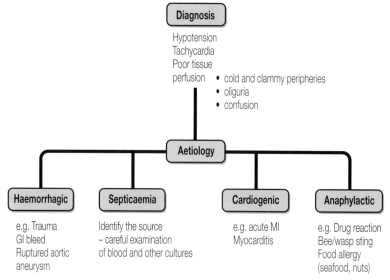

Fig. 5.1 Differential diagnosis of shock.

fore of prime importance in keeping an effective circulation through the coronary arteries to an already damaged myocardium. For this reason an objective of treatment is to achieve an adequate 'mean' or 'driving' pressure, and not to reach a particular systolic blood pressure when, in fact, the mean perfusion pressure is inadequate.

Septic shock

Septic shock is also characterized by low blood pressure and cardiac output, sometimes accompanied by intense peripheral vasoconstriction and reduced tissue perfusion. Two-thirds of cases are caused by Gram-negative septicaemia. Lipid-A of endotoxin damages capillary walls and endothelial damage may be accompanied by thrombocytopenia and disseminated intravascular coagulation (DIC – see Ch. 19). The endotoxin causes arteriolar vasoconstriction and pooling of blood in veins. The venous pressure falls and as a result there is a profound fall in cardiac output. Blood volume is not reduced at first, but later on there is reduction in blood volume due to loss of fluid from hypoxic capillaries.

The picture of shock in Gram-negative septicaemia is modified when it occurs in patients with hepatic cirrhosis. These patients are especially prone to this complication and often have a cardiac output greater than normal. The presence of bacteraemic shock may not result in reduction in cardiac output below the normal range. In shock caused by Gram-positive bacteraemia the picture may be identical with that produced by Gram-negative organisms.

In some patients septic shock is accompanied by vasodilatation and increased capillary permeability leading to hypovolaemia. Endothelial damage in pulmonary capillaries leads to 'shock lung' with diffuse consolidation on chest X-ray and impaired gas exchange with progressive hypoxia. All forms of septic shock are commoner in immunocompromised patients and in patients undergoing instrumentation, operation or with indwelling intravenous lines.

Anaphylactic shock

Anaphylaxis is a life-threatening condition that is becoming more common, particularly in children and young adults. Anaphylaxis manifests in many different ways and can be mild, moderate or severe. Features include erythema, general pruritus, urticaria, angio-oedema, laryngeal oedema, bronchospasm, rhinitis, conjunctivitis, vomiting, abdominal pain and collapse. Anaphylaxis develops due to an interaction of an allergen with specific IgE antibodies, causing mast cell activation with the release of vasoactive mediators, including histamine. These compounds cause capillary leak (manifesting as urticaria, angio-oedema and hypotension), mucosal oedema (causing laryngeal oedema, rhinitis and asthma) and smooth muscle contraction (causing asthma and abdominal pain). **Anaphylactoid** reactions are caused by mast cell activation but without the involvement of IgE antibodies. The clinical manifestations are identical.

Common causes are foods (especially peanuts and shellfish), bee and wasp stings, drugs (such as penicillin and intravenous contrast media) and latex rubber.

Shock predominates when the allergen is injected systemically, such as with bee stings and intravenous drugs, although shock can develop if the allergic reaction is severe, irrespective of the portal of entry.

Consequences of shock

Whatever the cause of shock, a variety of secondary changes may accompany it. Tissue hypoxia occurs, and with it local acidosis and the liberation of metabolites. There is subsequent systemic acidosis, the severity of which depends on the degree of stagnation of blood flow. Either hypoxia, acidosis or metabolites finally relax the precapillary sphincters so that more blood flows into the capillary bed. This results in further hypovolaemia and the formation of tissue oedema.

Renal blood flow is low as a result of hypotension and glomerular filtration rate falls. Oliguria is therefore a common accompaniment of shock. If renal blood flow falls to very low levels, acute tubular necrosis may occur. Before this stage there is a rising blood urea and excretion of urine of low specific gravity.

Hypoglycaemia may occur in the late stages of shock, probably due to failure of hepatic production of glucose.

THE DIAGNOSIS OF THE CAUSE OF SHOCK
(see Fig. 5.1)

The cause of haemorrhagic shock is often self-evident, but gastrointestinal bleeding may be concealed and must be excluded in any shocked patient where the cause is not apparent. A past history of peptic ulceration should be sought and rectal examination may reveal melaena. A less obvious source of occult haemorrhage is retroperitoneal bleeding, either following abdominal surgery or spontaneously from an aortic aneurysm. Often the blood tracks along the large vessels and appears later as areas of bruising in the thighs and sacral region.

Bacteraemic shock is often overlooked. This is a common cause of shock, and must also be excluded in any patient where no other obvious source is present. A previous history suggestive of infection is often present, such as cholecystitis, pyelonephritis, cholangitis or pneumonia. Ischaemia of the bowel due to vascular thrombosis, volvulus or strangulated hernia are other predisposing causes. Any form of peritonitis, especially faecal peritonitis, may be complicated by endotoxin shock. A careful examination of the abdomen is therefore essential, including rectal examination and listening for bowel sounds. Gram-negative septicaemia may also occur after major abdominal surgery, and here the differentiation between bleeding and endotoxin shock may be especially difficult. Gram-negative shock may occasionally occur following the relatively minor procedures of cystoscopy and termination of pregnancy.

Cardiogenic shock may occur in the context of myocardial infarction when the diagnosis is straightforward. However, elderly patients may present with the complications of myocardial infarction rather than with the characteristic chest pain. Shock may be the presenting feature of such a case, and an ECG must always be performed.

Anaphylactic shock is suggested by the clinical picture. There is usually a clear history of exposure to antigen, for example an intravenous injection of penicillin or contrast media. The patient feels an itching burning sensation within a few minutes. Bronchoconstriction then develops with cyanosis, and there may be laryngeal oedema and stridor. The blood pressure falls and the patient may rapidly die.

INVESTIGATIONS

An ECG is essential. The chest X-ray may show pulmonary oedema in myocardial infarction, or an unsuspected pneumonia in an elderly patient. A straight X-ray of the abdomen may show gas under the diaphragm if there has been perforation of a viscus, or fluid levels in intestinal obstruction from volvulus or mesenteric thrombosis.

Blood cultures are essential if there is any possibility of bacteraemic shock. Cultures of sputum and urine should be taken if appropriate. Plasma urea and electrolytes and arterial blood gases with determination of the acid–base status are essential. The urine output must be carefully monitored and sent for measurement of electrolytes and osmolality. Hypoglycaemia can closely resemble shock, and plasma glucose should always be estimated.

TREATMENT OF SHOCK

One of the most important aspects of the treatment of shock is careful and accurate monitoring of intravascular volume and tissue and organ perfusion. Patients with a low cardiac output may maintain a reasonable blood pressure by vasoconstriction such that measurement of blood pressure alone is inadequate and may be misleading. Intra-arterial monitoring provides continuous measurement of blood pressure and allows regular sampling for gas and acid–base analysis. Central venous access provides an estimate of filling pressure. The response to inotropes, pressors and fluid can be assessed by the relative change in CVP with these manouevres. Pulmonary artery (Swan–Ganz) catheters can be used to determine left ventricular filling (via the pulmonary capillary wedge pressure, PCWP), although this is a matter of considerable controversy, since some studies have shown a worse outcome with their use than without. Oesophageal Doppler probes are a useful and safer alternative, permitting continuous measurement of cardiac output and myocardial function.

Tissue perfusion is assessed clinically (skin colour, capillary refill, sweating), by the core–peripheral temperature gradient, by urine output (which should be measured hourly using a urinary catheter) and by acid–base status (acidosis occurring through cellular hypoxia, anaerobic glycolysis and lactic acid production).

Volume replacement

Most causes of shock are associated with depletion of circulating blood volume. This is reflected in hypotension, collapsed veins and a tachycardia. It is essential that blood volume is restored, aiming for a mean arterial pressure of at least 60 mmHg, and preferably 80 mmHg. Blood volume is restored with colloid, crystalloid or blood and blood products, depending on the cause of the hypovolaemia. A fluid challenge of 100–300 ml should not cause a rise of CVP or PCWP of more than 3–4 mm Hg. If volume depletion has been a major contributory factor to the shock the blood pressure rises, and the pulse rate falls, the extremities become warm and the veins fill. Urine flow increases. If fluid replacement is too rapid or too great, especially if the patient is elderly or has heart disease the CVP or PCWP will rise rapidly and pulmonary oedema may develop.

Vasoactive and inotropic agents

When signs of shock persist despite adequate fluid replacement, inotropic and vasoactive agents can be used to improve cardiac output and blood pressure. At low dose, dopamine enhances renal blood flow; at higher doses it is more positively inotropic but also causes increasing vasoconstriction. Dobutamine is a positive inotrope, but also causes a degree of peripheral vasoconstriction. Noradrenaline infusion is often very effective at raising blood pressure in septic shock. Although it causes intense vasoconstriction, its use is often accompanied by restoration of urine output as the blood pressure rises.

Persistent cardiogenic shock may require intra-aortic balloon counterpulsation. In the case of shock following extensive myocardial infarction, emergency coronary angioplasty (PTCA) should be considered where facilities permit. In anaphylactic shock, adrenaline should be given intramuscularly, and if necessary intravenously; an antihistamine and hydrocortisone should be given, both intravenously. Antibiotics are an essential part of the treatment of septic shock. The choice of antibiotics(s) depends on the likely or known infectious agent. The key to successful antibiotic therapy lies in taking appropriate cultures before treatment is started. Corticosteroids are sometimes given (e.g. high dose hydrocortisone) in bacteraemic shock although it is not clear whether or not prognosis is altered.

Mechanical ventilation

Low cardiac output in shock results in tissue hypoxia. Gas exchange is frequently impaired in the lungs. In many cases, particularly of septicaemic shock, the adult respiratory distress syndrome (ARDS – 'shock lung') develops. Hypoxaemia, deteriorating mental state, exhaustion and retention of secretions may all lead to the need for either assisted respiration using CPAP or formal ventilation, which abolishes or minimises the work of breathing, reduces oxygen consumption and improves gas exchange.

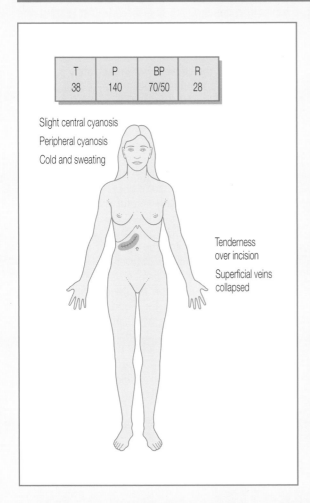

T	P	BP	R
38	140	70/50	28

Slight central cyanosis
Peripheral cyanosis
Cold and sweating

Tenderness
over incision

Superficial veins
collapsed

On examination on admission she was unwell and was pyrexial (38.2°C). Her blood pressure was 140/90 and she had a sinus tachycardia of 125 bpm. The heart and lungs were normal. There was extreme tenderness in the right upper quadrant of the abdomen. At laparotomy a gangrenous gall bladder was removed which contained several stones. There was some free fluid in the abdomen, but no other abnormalities. Exploration of the common bile duct was negative.

Following the operation she made an uneventful recovery at first. However 2 days later she complained of nausea and of feeling unwell. These symptoms had come on over a period of a few hours. She had not had pain, cough or shortness of breath.

On examination (see diagram) she looked very ill: she was pyrexial (38°C); blood pressure 70/50; pulse 140; respiration 28/min. She was cold and sweating. There was marked peripheral cyanosis and slight central cyanosis. The jugular venous pressure was not raised and superficial veins were collapsed. The heart and lungs were normal. In the abdomen, there was residual tenderness over the region of the laparotomy. Bowel sounds were present. Rectal examination was normal. A urinary catheter was passed and 100 ml of residual urine obtained which contained a trace of protein but no red cells or white cells.

A 65-year-old woman was admitted to hospital with a 5-day history of fever, rigors and severe right upper abdominal pain. She had noticed dark urine over the same period and had lost her appetite. Previously she had always been well.

Questions

1. What do you consider to be the probable diagnosis?
2. What investigations do you think are essential for immediate management?
3. What would your immediate management be?

This patient has become shocked in the early post-operative period, and the differential diagnosis must include intra-abdominal bleeding and Gram-negative septicaemia. The latter diagnosis is made more probable by the operation having been performed for an infective cause. Pulmonary embolism is less likely so soon after the operation; the patient has not complained of chest pain or dyspnoea and the venous pressure is not elevated. Myocardial infarction should certainly be considered although the absence of chest pain makes this diagnosis less probable. Biliary peritonitis and pancreatitis are unlikely because she has not complained of pain, there is no abdominal tenderness and bowel sounds are present.

Investigations will include haemoglobin and white cell count. The presence of anaemia strengthens the probability of bleeding but its absence does not exclude it. A neutrophilia suggests an infective cause. Tests for disseminated intravascular coagulation should be performed including fibrin degradation products, platelet count, and prothrombin time and examination of the blood film for fragmented red cells.

An ECG is essential since this may show changes suggestive of pulmonary embolism or myocardial infarction. A chest X-ray may show an area of diminished vascularity of the lung suggestive of pulmonary embolism, or changes of pulmonary infarction. The appearances of pulmonary oedema due to myocardial infarction may be present.

Measurement of central venous pressure is essential both in diagnosis and in management. A raised venous pressure may be found in pulmonary embolism, while haemorrhage and septicaemic shock are both accompanied by low venous pressure. During treatment, careful observation of the venous pressure will lessen the risks of fluid overload.

The urine should be cultured, and a centrifuged specimen examined under the microscope. Although there is nothing in the history and physical examination to suggest urinary infection, this must be excluded in any patient where the diagnosis of septicaemic shock is possible and where the cause is not immediately apparent. The blood urea and urinary sodium, urea, and osmolality should be measured. These measurements will probably not be of immediate value in management, but will be useful if the patient becomes oliguric, when it may be difficult to decide whether intrinsic renal damage is present. Blood cultures are essential. Cultures should also be taken from the drainage tube site.

Treatment must be started at once. Intravenous fluids must be swiftly given with careful monitoring of the haemodynamic response. If the patient has uncomplicated haemorrhagic shock, the blood pressure will rise with blood transfusion and the signs of peripheral circulatory failure will disappear. Irreversible haemorrhagic shock is rare. Volume replacement is essential in septicaemic shock, and must be combined with antibiotic treatment without waiting for blood culture results. In the patient described here, where the shock might be due to haemorrhage alone, it would be reasonable to transfuse the patient quickly and if there was no obvious clinical improvement after 1–2 hours, to start antibiotic treatment as well. Bactericidal antibiotics covering a wide range of bacteria must be given.

> The patient had an *E. coli* septicaemia and was treated with intravenous fluids and antibiotics, beginning before the results of blood culture were obtained. Her venous pressure rose, as did the blood pressure, without further deterioration. Her tachycardia resolved. She was oliguric for a further 12 hours but this normalized, helped by low dose dopamine.

6

Breathlessness and cyanosis

A breathless patient may not be cyanosed but a cyanosed patient is almost invariably breathless. How do we define breathlessness and cyanosis?

BREATHLESSNESS

Breathlessness is a common symptom of many respiratory and cardiac diseases. Musculoskeletal, neurological and other system abnormalities, for example anaemia, can also give rise to breathlessness. It is important to ask the patient precisely what he/she means, since some patients use the term to describe chest pain or palpitations. Breathlessness is a subjective feeling of difficulty in breathing. It can also be defined as the unpleasant sensation that increased respiratory effort is needed. Some include in the definition any condition in which increased respiratory effort is present, without it necessarily being unpleasant. In practice most physicians exclude the hyperpnoea which occurs in metabolic acidosis and the tachypnoea which occurs in acute anxiety. However, hyperpnoea may itself cause distress and the distinction is often arbitrary.

The underlying mechanism

The mechanism by which the sensation of breathlessness is produced is not well understood. Perhaps the easiest condition to understand is acute pulmonary oedema, in which pulmonary venous congestion causes pulmonary oedema and hypoxia which are potent stimuli to breathlessness. The orthopnoea of left heart failure is caused by increased venous return when lying flat, which increases pulmonary venous congestion, leading to a fall in pulmonary compliance and bronchial mucosal oedema. The exertional breathlessness of chronic heart failure is more difficult to explain. It cannot be explained by disturbance in blood gas tensions alone, since many breathless patients do not have hypercapnia or hypoxia. Surprisingly, there is no direct relationship between breathlessness and pulmonary venous congestion in chronic heart failure. Mechanisms other than changes in blood gases and pH include stimulation of intrapulmonary and respiratory muscle receptors and an awareness of the level of ventilation.

CLASSIFICATION OF BREATHLESSNESS

There are many ways of classifying breathlessness. A useful practical classification system is based on the pattern of onset and progression. This is shown in Box 6.1. The main pulmonary changes which give rise to a sensation of breathlessness are airways obstruction, decreased lung volume and decreased elasticity of the lung. The most important cardiovascular abnormalities are elevation of left atrial pressure and pulmonary embolism.

Breathlessness of rapid onset

The diagnosis of the patient who complains of the rapid onset of breathlessness can be difficult. In the history, the most important features are the rapidity of onset, the presence and nature of any pain and the past medical history.

Severe breathlessness occurring abruptly is very suggestive of pneumothorax or pulmonary embolism. In the former, there may be a history of sharp chest pain felt on the side of the pneumothorax. A large pneumothorax may cause mediastinal shift. Pulmonary embolism usually occurs in patients who have a predisposing cause and there is little difficulty in distinguishing it from pneumothorax on history and physical signs. In massive embolism there may be crushing chest pain, probably due to acute heart strain and myocardial ischaemia. On examination there is commonly hypotension, cyanosis and a gallop rhythm. There is usually no clinically detectable abnormality in the lungs in the early stages. Anxiety, hypoxia and stimulation of stretch receptors in the pulmonary arteries contribute to the sensation of breathlessness. Sudden breathlessness or stridor, especially in children, may be due to an inhaled foreign body. Signs of lobar collapse may be present, but physical examination may be of little help and a chest X-ray is essential.

Severe breathlessness coming on over 1–2 hours is most likely to be due to asthma or left heart failure. The latter may be due to myocardial infarction, aortic or mitral valve disease or sudden rhythm disturbance. Asthma is usually easily distinguished from left heart failure by the history of previous attacks, by the absence of a history of chest pain and the absence of cardiac murmurs. The differential diagnosis may however be difficult at times, especially if left heart

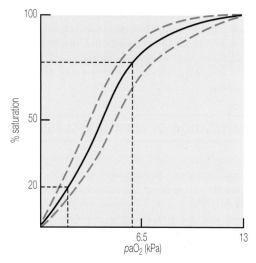

Fig. 6.1 Oxygen dissociation curve. The haemoglobin is 100% saturated when the PaO_2 is above 12.0 kPa. When the PaO_2 falls below 7.0 kPa cyanosis is usually visible. When the curve is shifted to the right more oxygen is liberated for a fall in PaO_2. The converse is true when the curve is shifted to the left.

failure gives rise to wheeze. Pneumonia, particularly in a patient with chronic bronchitis, may cause severe breathlessness. Usually the presence of pleuritic pain, cough with purulent sputum and signs of consolidation make the diagnosis straightforward.

Pericardial tamponade may cause difficulty in diagnosis. There is often a clear history of an antecedent febrile illness, together with central chest pain typically relieved by sitting forward. However, tamponade can occasionally come on rapidly and silently, particularly when due to involvement of the pericardium by malignant tumour, the commonest being carcinoma of the bronchus. The patient with tamponade usually has a low blood pressure, pulsus paradoxus and a raised jugular venous pressure. These features on history and examination usually serve to distinguish the condition from left ventricular failure and pulmonary embolism.

Hyperventilation due to metabolic acidosis may occasionally give rise to the sensation of breathlessness, but more often this is a relatively minor accompaniment of a self-evident illness such as diabetic ketoacidosis. Renal failure should be excluded by measurement of blood urea and electrolytes and the urine examined.

Drugs and poisons may make the patient hyperventilate, for example salicylate, due to a direct effect on the respiratory centre causing a respiratory alkalosis, followed by a metabolic acidosis. Methanol and ethylene glycol cause a profound metabolic acidosis.

Psychogenic breathlessness may also be of a rapid onset but usually has features which are unlike organic

Box 6.1 Classification of dyspnoea by its clinical presentation

Breathlessness of rapid onset

1. Pulmonary
   - Acute bronchitis
   - Pneumonia
   - Pneumothorax
   - Asthma
   - Inhaled foreign body

2. Cardiovascular
   - Acute left heart failure
   - Pulmonary embolism
   - Pericardial tamponade
   - High altitude

3. Psychogenic

4. Metabolic
   - Diabetic ketoacidosis
   - Uraemia
   - Poisons

Breathlessness progressing over several weeks

1. Pulmonary
   - Pleural effusion
   - Tumour (including lymphangitis carcinomatosa)
   - Pulmonary infiltrations and fibrosis
   - Tuberculosis

2. Cardiovascular
   - Heart failure
   - Anaemia
   - Recurrent pulmonary embolism

3. Neuromuscular
   - Myasthenia gravis

Breathlessness which is slowly progressing

1. Pulmonary
   - Chronic bronchitis
   - Emphysema
   - Pneumoconiosis
   - Diffuse pulmonary fibrosis

2. Cardiovascular
   - Heart failure
   - Recurrent pulmonary embolism

3. Mechanical
   - Gross obesity
   - Ankylosing spondylitis
   - Scleroderma

disease. The patient may complain of not being able to take a satisfactory breath in or of a sensation of being suffocated. There may be obvious hyperventilation, more marked during examination, and symptoms of tetany may occur. Breathlessness may occur after exertion rather than during it. The patient often does not seem to be in any distress at all. It is important to remember that psychogenic breathlessness, due to anxiety, may be present in a patient who has organic disease of mild degree, for example ischaemic heart disease or pulmonary tuberculosis, and that this may be responsible for the initiation of the symptoms.

Breathlessness progressing over several weeks

A pleural effusion may present in this way. Malignant effusions may be very large, and often present as breathlessness. Primary carcinoma of the lung is the commonest cause, but secondary tumours, lymphomas and pleural mesothelioma may be responsible. A large pleural effusion will be accompanied by clearcut physical signs (see Ch. 8). Pulmonary neoplasms may cause breathlessness by obstruction of a main bronchus, by secondary pleural effusion or by widespread lymphatic infiltration. Both pleural effusion and tumour are easily diagnosed by physical examination together with a chest X-ray.

Diffuse pulmonary fibrosis is a more difficult problem. The physical signs and radiological appearances can be very slight early on in the disease, although breathlessness may already be a prominent feature. The diagnosis is easier if there is a disease present known to be associated with pulmonary fibrosis, such as sarcoidosis. Some help will usually be gained from pulmonary function tests (see below).

Chronic heart failure causes breathlessness, initially only with significant exercise but, as the disease progresses, exercise tolerance falls until ultimately symptoms are present at rest. The diagnosis can be missed. Similarly many patients are given a diagnosis of heart failure when, in fact, the heart is normal and an alternative cause must be sought. Cardiac causes of breathlessness may be revealed by careful clinical examination, in particular listening for abnormal heart sounds and murmurs. A chest X-ray will usually show cardiac enlargement and possibly signs of left heart failure such as distension of upper lobe pulmonary veins or Kerley B lines (see Ch. 2).

Any cause of anaemia may give rise to breathlessness, and this is especially likely to occur if any other predisposing cause is present, for example ischaemic heart disease.

Recurrent pulmonary embolism can be extremely difficult to diagnose. There may be a history of deep venous thrombosis of calf or pelvic veins, of recent pregnancy or of taking the contraceptive pill. The symptoms of pulmonary infarction, pleuritic chest pain and haemoptysis may be absent in a patient presenting with breathlessness due to pulmonary hypertension from thromboembolism. The patient may complain of exertional dizziness or, worryingly, syncope. This is not always the case however and this diagnosis must be kept in mind in any patient with breathlessness while the cause remains uncertain. Physical examination may reveal an enlarged heart with a left parasternal heave. The second sound in the pulmonary area may be accentuated and an ejection click after the first sound is sometimes present. No abnormality is found in the lungs in most cases.

A chest X-ray may show enlargement of the cardiac shadow. The clinical and radiological signs of pulmonary hypertension do not occur until a significant proportion of the pulmonary vascular tree has been obliterated. The changes of right ventricular hypertrophy and strain may be seen on the ECG. A lung scan (perfusion +/− ventilation) will usually be helpful even in the absence of physical signs, and in the presence of the frequently normal chest X-ray. Spiral CT or MRI with contrast will show occlusion of major pulmonary vessels.

Breathlessness which is slowly progressing

Chronic lung disease of any kind normally presents in this way. Chronic bronchitis and emphysema, widespread bronchiectasis, diffuse pulmonary fibrosis, pulmonary thromboembolism, pneumoconiosis and tuberculosis will generally be suggested by typical features of history and by radiological appearances. However, the physical signs and radiological appearances of emphysema may not be marked, and some patients with emphysema have little cough or wheeze but have a main complaint of breathlessness. Appropriate lung function tests, particularly the measurement of diffusing capacity, are indicated.

Diffuse pulmonary fibrosis can cause breathlessness over a long period of time without abnormal physical signs being present. Points to note on examination are the presence of cyanosis, and the amplitude of the chest movements which are typically restricted. Clubbing of the fingers and fine basal crackles are often present. An accentuated right ventricular impulse and loud second sound in the pulmonary area indicate right ventricular enlargement and pulmonary hypertension. This may follow thromboembolic disease or destructive disease of the lung from any cause.

CYANOSIS

Cyanosis is caused by the presence of an excess of deoxygenated haemoglobin which is visible in the small vessels of the skin and mucous membranes. Hypoxia means that there is insufficient oxygen available for the normal metabolic requirements of the tissues. The term hypoxaemia is used when the partial pressure of oxygen in the blood is reduced. If this reduction is of sufficient severity, cyanosis results. It is useful to describe cyanosis as central or peripheral, as different mechanisms may be responsible for these two appearances.

Central cyanosis is a bluish discoloration of the lips, tongue and conjunctivae. It is due to desaturation of arterial haemoglobin. Peripheral cyanosis is a bluish discoloration of the skin of the hands or feet and of the nail beds. It is always present when there is central cyanosis, but may occur without there being central cyanosis if there is diminished or slowed blood flow through the peripheries. Whereas peripheral cyanosis may be a purely local phenomenon, central cyanosis means that there has been a failure of oxygenation of blood in the lungs, and that hypoxaemia is present. A rare exception is methaemoglobinaemia.

The underlying mechanism

The saturation of haemoglobin with oxygen refers to the amount of oxygen the haemoglobin is carrying as a percentage of its total carrying capacity. The haemoglobin is normally fully saturated at a paO_2 of 12 kPa. As the paO_2 falls below 12 kPa a most important change occurs in the saturation of haemoglobin. At first there is a gradual but slight decrease in saturation, but below a paO_2 of about 7–8 kPa the saturation of haemoglobin falls sharply for a relatively small fall in paO_2, explaining the shape of the oxygen dissociation curve (Fig. 6.1). Cyanosis develops as the oxygen saturation falls. However, the clinical detection of cyanosis is difficult and crude. The often repeated statement that 5 g reduced haemoglobin is required for cyanosis to be manifest is incorrect. It may be detectable at an oxygen saturation of 90%, which is equivalent to only 1.5 g reduced haemoglobin if the total haemoglobin is 15 g, but it may not become clinically obvious until it falls to around 80% (a paO_2 of about 7 kPa). It is difficult to detect cyanosis in a severely anaemic person and conversely cyanosis is more obvious for a given paO_2 when it occurs in a polycythaemic patient.

Although the degree of saturation of haemoglobin with oxygen is what determines the presence of cyanosis, desaturation is not the only cause of hypoxia. In Box 6.2 the causes of hypoxia are classified. Anaemia causes tissue hypoxia because there is diminished oxygen carrying capacity of the blood, even though the haemoglobin is fully saturated. The causes and diagnosis of anaemia are dealt with in Ch. 18.

THE PRODUCTION OF CYANOSIS IN PULMONARY DISEASE

There are several reasons why patients with lung disease become cyanosed. The most important is an

---

Box 6.2 The causes of tissue hypoxia

Failure of oxygenation of blood in the lungs

1. Pulmonary causes
   - Ventilation–perfusion mismatch
     chronic bronchitis and emphysema
     multiple emboli
     pneumonia
     asthma
     pulmonary fibrosis
   - Loss of surface area for diffusion
     emphysema
     pulmonary infarction
     pulmonary fibrosis
   - Severe hypoventilation
     chronic bronchitis
     severe asthma
     primary alveolar hypoventilation
   - Alveolar–capillary diffusion defect
     left heart failure (pulmonary oedema)
     diffuse pulmonary fibrosis
     lymphangitis carcinomatosa

2. Cardiac causes
   - Right-to-left shunt
   - Cardiac failure

3. Low inspired pO_2
   - High altitude

Diminished oxygen-carrying capacity of blood

   - Anaemia
   - Methaemoglobinaemia
   - Sulphaemoglobinaemia

Inadequate release of oxygen in tissues

1. *Poor perfusion of tissues*
   - Shock
   - Peripheral vascular disease
   - Cold

2. Decreased red cell 2,3-DPG (systemic acidosis)

Failure of uptake by tissues

   - Tissue poisons, for example cyanide

---

abnormality of the relationship between ventilation and perfusion of alveoli (V/Q abnormality). In a normal alveolus, CO_2 diffuses out of the pulmonary arterial blood and is exhaled. Oxygen crosses the alveolar wall by diffusion and is sufficient in quantity to oxygenate all the blood perfusing that alveolus. If there is alveolar hypoventilation with normal perfusion, or normal alveolar ventilation with shunting, there will be a failure of oxygenation and desaturated blood will reach the systemic circulation. Normal oxygenation in other parts of the lung cannot compensate for this. (The events are shown in Fig. 6.2.) On the other hand,

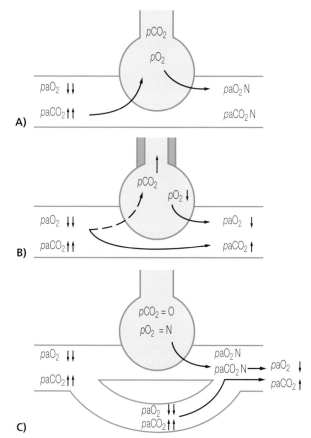

Fig. 6.2 In patients with V/Q abnormalities the final blood gas concentrations will be determined by the relative proportions of these three situations.

A) Deoxygenated blood with a high $paCO_2$ perfuses the alveolus which contains air with no CO_2 and high pO_2. Normal diffusion occurs and the efferent blood is fully oxygenated with a lower $paCO_2$ (N = normal).

B) Deoxygenated blood with a high $paCO_2$ perfuses the underventilated alveolus which contains air with a subnormal pO_2 and a raised pCO_2 due to obstruction of air flow. The CO_2 cannot be adequately eliminated. If there are enough normally ventilated alveoli to allow CO_2 to be eliminated on subsequent circulations, the $paCO_2$ will not rise overall. On the other hand, the hypoxaemia cannot be corrected by an increased uptake in other alveoli and the patient may be cyanosed.

C) There is normal ventilation but diminished perfusion with intrapulmonary shunting. The shunt allows deoxygenated blood with increased CO_2 to bypass the alveolus. As in B, cyanosis may occur but CO_2 can be eliminated in other normal alveoli on subsequent circulation.

localized areas of alveolar hypoventilation will not cause a rise in $paCO_2$ in the pulmonary venous blood since the remaining alveoli are normally ventilated and any tendency towards CO_2 retention is rectified. Abnormalities of the ventilation–perfusion relationship occur patchily throughout the lungs in chronic bronchitis, emphysema, pulmonary fibrosis and in severe asthmatic attacks. In acute massive pulmonary embolism, blood is diverted from the obstructed pulmonary artery through other vessels and overperfusion of the remaining lung results, causing cyanosis.

In lobar pneumonia the affected alveoli are full of exudate, and the perfusing blood is not oxygenated, again causing cyanosis. The severity of the infection and the degree of mental confusion correlates closely with the degree of desaturation.

Oxygen diffuses less readily than CO_2 and if there is a loss of surface area for gas transfer, hypoxia will be a more prominent feature than hypercapnia. A loss in surface area occurs after pneumonectomy, in emphysema, diffuse pulmonary fibrosis and multiple pulmonary infarction.

Diffusion of oxygen is also impaired in pulmonary oedema, and this accounts in part for the cyanosis often seen in this condition. In left heart failure, however, the blood flow through the lungs is not normal, and overperfusion of relatively underventilated areas, such as the upper lobes, occurs and contributes to the cyanosis. Although the hypoxia in diffuse pulmonary fibrosis is often ascribed to a diffusion defect ('alveolar-capillary block'), this is probably not an important factor. There is considerable disturbance of the ventilation–perfusion balance in affected areas of the lung, and conventional tests such as carbon monoxide transfer for 'diffusion' defects do not distinguish between these two mechanisms.

Generalized hypoventilation of all alveoli also causes hypoxaemia. This is a less important cause of hypoxaemia than the other mechanisms. A reduction in ventilation from 5 l/min to 3 l/min will lower pao_2 from 12 to 8 kPa (90–60 mmHg) at which point the haemoglobin will still be 85% saturated. However, alveolar hypoventilation is the most important cause of hypercapnia, and in the example quoted the $paCO_2$ will have risen from 5.3 to 9.3 kPa (40–70 mmHg). Dangerous hypercapnia is thus present without the patient being cyanosed. Ventilation–perfusion abnormalities and loss of surface area for diffusion do not affect elimination of CO_2 as mentioned above.

Occasionally major vascular shunts occur in the lungs and cause cyanosis. These include vascular tumours and fistulae.

THE PRODUCTION OF CYANOSIS IN HEART DISEASE

If a major right-to-left intracardiac shunt exists, cyanosis is of course inevitable, and the condition is easily distinguished from pulmonary disease. Diagnosis of the cause of the shunt depends on clinical examination and investigation. The shunt may be at any level:

a) In the great vessels: patent ductus arteriosus or aortopulmonary window with reversed shunts, transposition of the great vessels.

b) In the ventricles: ventricular septal defect with reversed shunt, Fallot's tetralogy, single ventricle.

c) In the atria: atrial septal defect with reversed shunt. Anomalous pulmonary venous drainage.

In cardiac failure the cyanosis is due to a combination of redistribution of blood flow and impaired diffusion as already described. Many patients with raised venous pressure and peripheral oedema are suffering from cardiac failure secondary to chronic respiratory disease, especially chronic bronchitis and emphysema (cor pulmonale). In these patients left heart failure may not be present, and cyanosis can be attributed to the lung disease.

DIAGNOSING THE CAUSE OF CENTRAL CYANOSIS

In the vast majority of cyanosed patients the cause is clear from the history and clinical examination. Tissue hypoxia may itself give rise to symptoms and signs irrespective of the underlying cause. The elderly in particular tolerate hypoxaemia poorly, especially if there is an impaired circulation due to atherosclerosis. Hypoxia of the tissues causes fatigue and exhaustion. In hypoxaemia, underlying arterial disease may result in specific symptoms developing: angina, symptoms of heart failure, intermittent claudication and, in chronic cases, symptoms of dementia. These symptoms may occur regardless of the cause of hypoxaemia and do not help to make the diagnosis.

The great majority of cyanosed patients are suffering from respiratory or cardiac disease. The history in patients with pulmonary disease will usually be of breathlessness on exertion, cough and sputum. An exception is in thromboembolic pulmonary hypertension in which the onset may be insidious, without cough or sputum. Heart failure will present with the usual symptoms. Cor pulmonale is a common cause of cyanosis, and the hypoxaemia caused by the chronic respiratory disease is one of the factors which exacerbates heart failure, by the direct effect of myocardial hypoxia, and by causing pulmonary arteriolar vasoconstriction.

Examination may show signs of chronic obstructive airways disease: widespread wheeze, use of accessory respiratory muscles, increased anteroposterior diameter of the chest with reduced expansion, and decreased liver and cardiac dullness. Clubbing of the fingers and basal crackles may occur in diffuse pulmonary fibrosis. Left heart failure may be present as shown by bibasilar crackles and a gallop rhythm, together with the signs of a cause of left heart failure such as myocardial infarction, mitral or aortic valve disease or hypertension. When there is a right-to-left intracardiac shunt present there may be clubbing of the fingers and physical signs of right ventricular enlargement and pulmonary hypertension. A murmur associated with an atrial or ventricular septal defect or patent ductus may be present.

INVESTIGATION OF A PATIENT WITH BREATHLESSNESS WITH OR WITHOUT CYANOSIS

Chest X-ray

A chest X-ray is the most helpful investigation. It may show enlargement of the heart, pulmonary infiltration, pleural effusion, tumours, collapse or consolidation. In fibrosing alveolitis the X-ray may be normal at the outset, later showing a mottled appearance more marked in the lower zones, with areas of translucency. There is an overall loss of lung volume with elevation of the diaphragm. In emphysema, the classical changes are low flat diaphragms with a narrow heart shadow. The ribs are horizontal and there are diminished peripheral lung markings. Bullae may be present. Small pneumothoraces can easily be missed and if this diagnosis is suspected, films should be obtained in full expiration as well as full inspiration.

12-lead ECG

An ECG will often provide clues to the diagnosis. Congenital heart disease causing cyanosis is never associated with a normal ECG. Changes in axis, evidence of cardiac chamber enlargement with or without strain, conduction abnormalities and rhythm change will be easily recognized. Examples are right atrial and ventricular hypertrophy in cor pulmonale and in right-to-left intracardiac shunts and right bundle branch block and axis shift with an atrial septal defect.

Echocardiography

Transthoracic with or without transoesophageal echocardiography is an invaluable test in patients with suspected heart disease. Structural abnormalities are readily detected and the secondary physiological effects can be accurately quantified. Septal defects and more complex congenital heart disease can be diagnosed in most cases without the need to resort to cardiac catheterization with invasive pressure measurement and shunt calculations. Acquired valvular, myocardial and pericardial disease can be documented. Patients may have co-existing lung disease which also contributes to their breathlessness but also may result in a poor echo 'window' due to hyperinflation of the chest. In these patients echocardiography is technically challenging and, at times, simply impossible.

Lung function tests

Spirometry is a valuable investigation. A reduced forced vital capacity (FVC) is found in any condition which restricts lung excursion. Reduction of lung volume has this effect and occurs in recurrent pulmonary infarction, large pleural effusions and after pneumonectomy. Restriction of expansion of the lung also occurs in pulmonary fibrosis from any cause, when the muscles of respiration are weak as in myasthenia gravis, and when there is an external restriction to full respiratory movements such as is caused by the rigid thoracic cage in ankylosing spondylitis. Airways obstruction from any cause will also reduce FVC. The ratio of forced expiratory volume in one second (FEV_1) to FVC is a better measure of airways obstruction. In asthma, for example, the FVC may be only slightly reduced, but the FEV_1 greatly so. This is called an obstructive ventilatory defect (Fig. 6.3). Therefore spirometry should always be repeated after inhalation of a potent bronchodilator to assess the degree of reversibility. The conditions reducing FVC but without causing airways obstruction will inevitably give rise to a reduction in FEV_1 but the ratio of FEV_1/FVC will be normal (Fig. 6.4).

Another simple, but less accurate, measure of airways obstruction is the peak expiratory flow rate (PEFR). In diffuse pulmonary fibrosis a restrictive ventilatory defect may be detected when clinical examination has been unhelpful. On the other hand normal spirometry, even when corrected for age, sex and height, does not exclude organic disease.

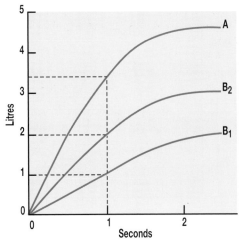

Fig. 6.3 A = Normal spirogram. FEV_1/FVC = 3.4/4.6 = 74%. B = Obstructive ventilatory defect, before (B_1) and after (B_2) bronchodilator inhalation. The airways obstruction is partially reversed. B_1 FEV_1/FVC = 1.1/2.0 = 55%. B_2 FEV_1/FVC = 2.0/3.0 = 66%.

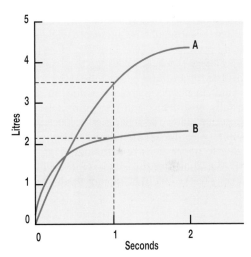

Fig. 6.4 A = Normal spirogram. FEV_1/FVC = 3.5/4.4 = 80%. B = Restrictive ventilatory defect. FEV_1/FVC = 2.1/2.3 = 90%.

Estimating the transfer factor (diffusing capacity) may be of value. It is usually the earliest functional abnormality in diffuse pulmonary fibrosis. Any disease where there is a great loss of alveolar surface area (such as in emphysema) or where there is a restriction of the free diffusion of oxygen (such as in pulmonary oedema) will cause a low transfer factor. The test is unreliable in the presence of airways obstruction. Tests of pulmonary compliance (or of elasticity) are occasionally helpful in the diagnosis of diseases such as

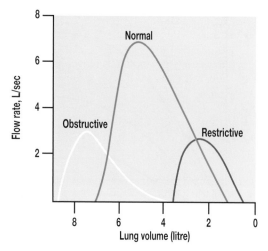

Fig. 6.5 Flow/volume curves in obstructive and restrictive lung disease. The three curves represent a maximal forced expiration in normals and in obstructive and restrictive lung disease.

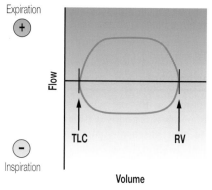

Fig. 6.6 Flow/volume loop in a patient with fixed upper airways obstruction. There is flow limitation and flattening of both inspiratory and expiratory limbs. TLC, total lung capacity; RV, residual volume.

diffuse pulmonary fibrosis, where the compliance is decreased because of the increased rigidity of the lungs.

Flow/volume loops, plotting the rate of flow against the total volume of air moved, in both expiration and inspiration are of value in analysing more fully obstructive and restrictive defects and in addition may allow the separation of obstruction due to lower airways disease from the less common obstruction due to upper airways pathology (Figs 6.5, 6.6). Indeed the characteristic shape of the flow/volume curve may be the first indication of the true site of the lesion.

Blood gases

Arterial blood gas analysis is of great help in certain circumstances. In recurrent pulmonary embolism there is shunting of deoxygenated pulmonary arterial blood. This may give rise to a low paO_2 if the process is widespread. The $paCO_2$ is normal or low since the patient hyperventilates slightly in response to the low paO_2. On exercise the patient hyperventilates greatly but becomes even more hypoxic, and this is a valuable diagnostic test in distinguishing these patients from those with hysterical overbreathing who have a normal paO_2 on exertion. Hypercapnia does not occur in pulmonary thromboembolic disease because of the greater solubility of CO_2 allowing free diffusion across the alveolar–capillary membrane. In diffuse pulmonary fibrosis there is also a low paO_2 but this tends to occur later in the disease. Early on there is a fall in paO_2 on exercise, with an accompanying hyperventilation and fall in $paCO_2$. If the $paCO_2$ is raised, then alveolar hypoventilation is occurring and this is usually due to chronic bronchitis and emphysema. When there is mixed cardiac and pulmonary disease there is no easy way of deciding their relative contributions.

If a patient with breathlessness has no abnormality on physical examination and all investigations are normal, then the physician can be fairly confident that no organic disease is likely to be present. Whether these patients should have their symptom labelled 'psychogenic' is another matter. Some will go on to develop obvious organic disease with the passage of time.

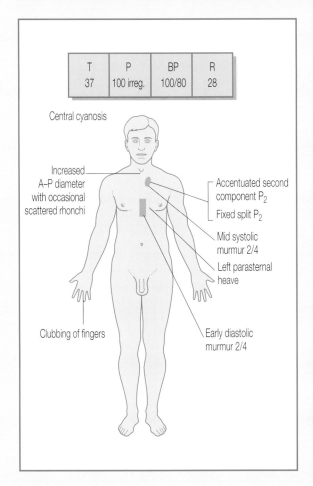

T	P	BP	R
37	100 irreg.	100/80	28

Central cyanosis

Increased A–P diameter with occasional scattered rhonchi

Accentuated second component P$_2$

Fixed split P$_2$

Mid systolic murmur 2/4

Left parasternal heave

Clubbing of fingers

Early diastolic murmur 2/4

A 50-year-old electronics specialist presented with a history of increasing shortness of breath of 2 years' duration. He had noticed a decline in his exercise tolerance over the preceding 5 years, but this had not become severe until 2 years previously, since when even moderate exertion had proved difficult. He was able to walk as far as he wished on the flat, but had to stop on any slight incline and after 12 stairs. He had smoked 20 cigarettes a day for 30 years, and had had a morning cough productive of mucoid sputum for many years. There was no history of swelling of the ankles.

In the past he had always been well. However, he had been turned down for service in the army at the age of 18, when a heart murmur had been noticed. This was not investigated in detail at that time, except for a chest X-ray which was reported as normal.

On examination he was cyanosed both centrally and peripherally. The pulse was 100/min and irregularly irregular. Blood pressure 100/80. There was no evidence of cardiac failure. The apex beat was not displaced, but there was a prominent left parasternal heave. The second sound in the pulmonary area showed a marked fixed split, with accentuation of the pulmonary component. There was a moderately loud ejection murmur heard over the pulmonary area, while a diastolic murmur could be heard down the left sternal border. The trachea was central and there was slight clubbing of the fingers. The anteroposterior diameter of the thorax was increased, and respiratory movements were restricted. There was occasional wheeze on auscultation of the lungs. The rest of the physical examination was normal.

Questions

1. What are the likely causes of cyanosis in this case?
2. How would you distinguish between them?

Discussion

This patient has been a heavy cigarette smoker for many years, and has signs suggestive of chronic bronchitis and emphysema. In addition he has a cardiac lesion with an arrhythmia which is probably atrial fibrillation. The signs point to a diagnosis of pulmonary hypertension. Pulmonary hypertension of this severity is unlikely to have developed as a result of chronic bronchitis without there being a past history of heart failure in addition, and without signs of CO_2 retention being present, such as tremor, warm hands and a full-volume pulse. The physical signs, fixed splitting of the second heart sound, and systolic and diastolic murmurs in the pulmonary area, strongly suggest a diagnosis of an atrial septal defect (ASD). It is not uncommon for atrial septal defects to present in middle age at a time when pulmonary hypertension develops and the shunt begins to reverse, which may cause cyanosis and clubbing. The fact that a cardiac murmur had been noticed 32 years previously supports this diagnosis. The physical signs are not likely to be due to mitral stenosis, although tight mitral stenosis can be present without a mitral diastolic murmur being audible. There is however no opening snap, there is fixed splitting of the second sound, and the murmurs of increased pulmonary blood flow and pulmonary regurgitation due to the longstanding pulmonary hypertension.

This patient has both cardiac and pulmonary causes of breathlessness and cyanosis, and investigation is necessary to decide the role which each plays in his condition. A chest X-ray would be helpful. It will usually show low flat diaphragms in emphysema, and may show any other pulmonary disease which might contribute to breathlessness such as bronchiectasis or pulmonary fibrosis. The heart will be enlarged and the pulmonary arteries prominent. If there is an ASD there will be pulmonary plethora. Cardiac and pulmonary artery enlargement with 'pruning' of peripheral pulmonary vessels could be attributed to severe chronic bronchitis and emphysema. If this were the case, CO_2 retention should be present, and spirometry would show a severe ventilatory defect.

An ECG would confirm the rhythm to be atrial fibrillation, with loss of the characteristic changes of the P wave seen in pulmonary hypertension (tall peaked P waves due to right atrial hypertrophy, seen in the right precordial and inferior leads). Pulmonary hypertension, from whatever cause, results in a dominant R wave and T inversion in right precordial leads and a dominant S wave in left precordial leads. The QRS may be widened and, in the case of an ASD, shows right bundle branch block. A classical secundum ASD produces right axis deviation in contrast to the left axis shift seen with a primum defect, which would present far earlier in life.

An echocardiogram would show right-sided chamber enlargement in pulmonary hypertension, cor pulmonale and ASD. Flow across an ASD could be seen with colour Doppler. Tricuspid regurgitation is almost invariably present in pulmonary hypertension and allows indirect measurement of pulmonary artery pressure. Any co-existing left heart abnormality should be detectable.

Estimation of $paCO_2$ and paO_2 and spirometry are useful investigations. The paO_2 will be low since the patient is cyanosed, but no conclusions about the cause of cyanosis can be drawn from the degree of desaturation. It will indicate the severity of either the pulmonary or cardiac lesion. If the $paCO_2$ is normal or low then the diagnosis of ASD is strongly supported. If there were great elevation of $paCO_2$ there is clearly severe pulmonary disease although this would not rule out an ASD being present as well. Spirometry will show reduction of FVC and a proportionately greater reduction of FEV_1 in severe chronic bronchitis and emphysema. Modest reductions of FEV_1 and FVC are not associated with hypoxaemia or hypercapnia.

This man had mild chronic bronchitis and emphysema and an ASD with a reversed shunt. Investigations showed $paCO_2$ 5.32 kPa, paO_2 6.4 kPa, FEV_1/FVC = 2.2/3.6 l. After 100% oxygen the paO_2 was 7.0 kPa. The 12-lead ECG showed right bundle branch block, right axis deviation and atrial fibrillation and echocardiography confirmed the presence of an ASD with shunt reversal.

7

Haemoptysis

This common symptom usually brings the patient quickly to a doctor. It is generally recognized by the patient that it may be the initial presentation of serious disease and needs adequate investigation and explanation. This can usually be done as an outpatient, as haemoptysis itself is rarely large or persistent enough to endanger the patient. However, if associated with other sudden severe symptoms such as dyspnoea, raising the possibility of pulmonary embolism, admission and rapid investigation to disprove the diagnosis is a medical emergency.

A very large number of conditions can cause haemoptysis. In forming a framework for its differential diagnosis it is important to think in anatomical and pathophysiological terms:

- Airways
- Lung parenchyma
- Lung vascular system and the heart
- Bleeding disorders.

Associated symptoms and physical signs may then guide further investigation beyond the chest X-ray with which each patient will, inevitably, start. It can be a very early symptom of disease, so that if initial investigation is negative follow-up of the patient is needed for at least a further 6 months, with repeated chest X-rays. Even with full initial investigation and careful follow-up, in most patients with haemoptysis where initial investigation has not revealed the cause, no further abnormality will develop and the haemoptysis will settle spontaneously. Some of these patients have chronic bronchitis.

It must first be established that the patient's complaint is truly the coughing up of blood from the lungs. This is not usually difficult, particularly as haemoptysis is commonly associated with other symptoms such as cough or sputum which will point to disease of the lungs. A common description of true haemoptysis is of blood suddenly 'coming into the back of the throat'. It is of particular importance to differentiate this from vomiting of blood. There is the occasional patient who is unable to describe his symptom clearly and considerable confusion results, and in such cases one may unavoidably be forced to investigate both alternative sources of bleeding!

Another problem is to recognize bleeding from the upper respiratory tract, nose or from the mouth. It is obligatory to examine these areas and obvious lesions such as ulcers, naevi or carcinoma may be seen. Sometimes the patient confuses bleeding from unhealthy gums with haemoptysis, although usually the relation of such bleeding to teeth cleaning and the appearance of the gums resolves the problem. The deliberate production of a little blood, for example by biting the cheek, is not difficult and very occasionally this symptom may be a feature of malingering. The diagnosis is always difficult to prove and even if suspected should not prevent the simpler investigations being carried out.

CLINICAL HISTORY

The symptom of haemoptysis must first be established. One should enquire whether the blood is bright red in colour, how much has been produced and whether it is associated with sputum. A history of recent trauma should be sought. Indirect damage as from blast injury, as well as the more obvious direct damage, as may occur in a game of rugby football, may present shortly afterwards as haemoptysis. The duration of the symptom is important as the causes of small infrequent haemoptyses over many years tend to be different from those of a single large recent bleed.

The other main respiratory symptoms should be carefully asked for: cough, sputum, chest pain, shortness of breath, and wheeze. These may point to the underlying cause. Thus cough and purulent sputum suggest infection, while pleuritic chest pain in association with haemoptysis always raises the possibility of pulmonary infarction. Tuberculosis commonly presents with haemoptysis, which can be of any degree. Other more general symptoms may be present, and the physician must ask if there has been fever, night sweats, weight loss, and bleeding into other sites, such as skin, urine or bowel to suggest a systemic vasculitis.

The past medical history may be important. Chest disease in childhood, followed by recurrent cough and sputum suggests bronchiectasis, which may subsequently give rise to bleeding at any age. In some cases small haemoptyses are the major feature and there is little in the way of purulent sputum, so called bronchiectasis sicca. There are a number of cardiac causes of haemoptysis. Rheumatic fever in childhood may cause mitral stenosis in which recurrent haemo-

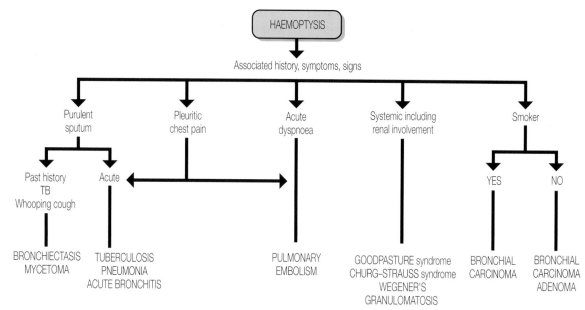

Fig. 7.1 A guide to the diagnosis of haemoptysis.

ptyses are common. Any cause of left ventricular or left atrial failure can give rise to haemoptyses.

Pulmonary embolism from deep-vein thrombosis has a tendency to be recurrent and a past history of venous thrombosis or pulmonary embolism is very important. The deep venous thrombosis in a leg or pelvic vein which is the source of embolus is often clinically silent. A history of any factor known to predispose to venous thrombosis, such as childbirth, the contraceptive pill, a recent operation or injury, or any other form of immobilization, is of obvious importance.

In the family history there may be some bleeding tendency such as haemorrhagic telangiectasia or a disorder of coagulation. A history of pulmonary tuberculosis or of respiratory symptoms suggesting such a diagnosis may be obtained in a member of the family or a close associate.

In children an important condition is inhalation of a foreign body. This will lead to bronchial obstruction and collapse, and can cause haemoptysis. In adults a detailed smoking history is essential. It is surprising how often the heavy smoker who stopped his habit only days previously will say he is a non-smoker and not mention his previous smoking.

PHYSICAL EXAMINATION

The general appearance may suggest some serious disease such as disseminated malignancy, but the majority of patients complaining of haemoptysis

appear in good health. One may observe the typical mitral facies, while sometimes a carcinoma of the bronchus has already produced mediastinal obstruction with oedema and swelling of the face and neck, and engorgement of the veins draining into the superior vena cava. There may be purpura as a result of a generalized bleeding disorder. Clubbing is an important sign in both carcinoma and chronic suppurative lung disease, and may also be seen in advanced pulmonary tuberculosis. Hypertrophic pulmonary osteoarthropathy may occur, with clubbing, usually as a result of an underlying non-small cell bronchial carcinoma, and may be misdiagnosed as arthritis.

The pulse may be small and irregular due to atrial fibrillation in mitral stenosis. In severe hypertension nose bleeds may occur and can masquerade as haemoptysis. The fundi should be examined for hypertensive changes and could also show haemorrhages due to a bleeding disorder. The mouth, gums and throat must be examined.

The most important signs are likely to be in the chest. Bronchitis, bronchiectasis or pneumonia may give their typical signs, while evidence of apical disease suggests tuberculosis. Collapse of a lobe or lung in a child suggests an inhaled foreign body, while in an adult it is more likely to be due to carcinoma or adenoma. A localized wheeze may be present over the underlying obstruction. A pleural rub may be due to infection but is also a common feature of infarction. Localized tenderness of the chest wall will suggest a fractured rib, especially if the pain is made worse on 'springing' the chest. The signs in the heart of possible relevance would be those of mitral stenosis or other causes of left heart failure. In tight mitral stenosis the murmur may be absent. The legs must be examined for evidence of deep venous thrombosis. In addition to tenderness and oedema one should also look carefully for increased filling of the superficial veins, with increased warmth.

INVESTIGATION

By far the most important aid in diagnosis is the chest X-ray. In the majority of cases where any firm diagnosis is reached it can be made on the clinical findings and chest X-ray alone. Tuberculosis, carcinoma, pneumonia, lung abscess and aneurysm will usually be obvious, while bronchiectasis and pulmonary infarction can often be suspected. Fractured ribs may also be seen, although these can often be surprisingly difficult to demonstrate on X-ray, and on occasion an isotope bone scan can be of the greatest value in clearly demonstrating them. The cardiac outline may suggest mitral stenosis or there may be cardiac enlargement due to left ventricular failure from any cause. If there is any suspicion of valvular disease, then echocardiography is essential.

Sputum cytology is of value in the diagnosis of carcinoma, and may allow a firm diagnosis to be made even though the chest radiograph is normal. Examination of the sputum for acid-fast bacilli is unlikely to be positive in the presence of a completely normal chest X-ray. A more common problem is the patient with haemoptyses who has apical fibrosis, probably due to old healed tuberculosis. The occurrence of haemoptyses does not necessarily imply that the disease is active, and serial chest X-rays will usually be needed to answer this question. The area of damaged lung may be the site of bronchiectasis or there may be a cavity containing a mycetoma. On chest X-ray the mycetoma may give a characteristic appearance of a solid ball within a cavity surrounded by a crescent-shaped air shadow. The sputum may show aspergilli. The sputum must be examined and cultured for tuberculosis as a routine in all cases of haemoptysis. Routine microscopy and culture of the sputum for other pathogens will rarely be of value, except in the diagnosis of *Klebsiella* pneumonia which is commonly associated with haemoptyses.

An ECG may show right heart strain, suggesting pulmonary embolism (see Fig. 4.6, p. 28). Atrial fibrillation may be present, suggesting the sequence of clot formation in the right atrium leading to pulmonary embolism and thus haemoptysis. If a pleural effusion is present it should be aspirated and the pleura biopsied. The effusion caused by a pulmonary infarct often contains an excess of eosinophils, while pleural biopsy may show tuberculosis or carcinoma when these involve the pleura (see Ch. 8).

Bronchoscopy is of the greatest value if either foreign body or neoplasm is suspected. It will enable a more precise diagnosis to be made and most foreign bodies can be removed. Tumours can be biopsied and the rarely occurring adenoma may be diagnosed. Often it will be obvious that the carcinoma is inoperable, so that thoracotomy can be avoided. Even if no tumour is seen, bronchial secretions can be aspirated for cytology and culture. Bronchography and tomography has been superseded by computed tomography (CT) and high resolution computed tomography (HRCT) as the method of choice in the diagnosis of bronchiectasis.

In any patient where pulmonary embolus is suspected, a radioisotope lung scan should be done as soon

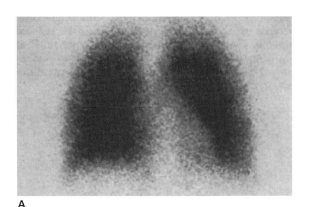
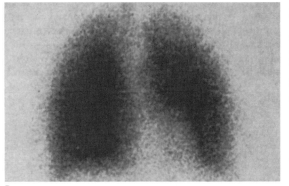

A   B

Fig. 7.2 Lung scans.

A) Normal perfusion scan showing homogeneous distribution of technetium.

B) Normal ventilation scan in the same patient showing homogeneous distribution of inhaled krypton.

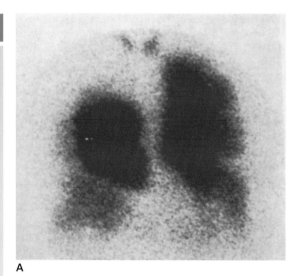 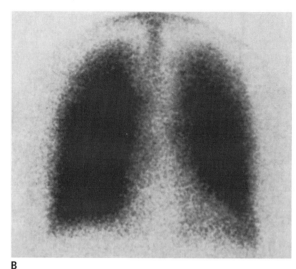

A   B

Fig. 7.3 Lung scans.

A) Abnormal perfusion scan showing multiple areas of diminished perfusion in a patient with multiple pulmonary emboli.

B) Ventilation scan in the same patient showing normal distribution of inhaled krypton. This disparity between ventilation and perfusion is typical of pulmonary embolism.

as possible. Gross defects of perfusion may be seen due to single or multiple emboli, even in the presence of a completely normal chest X-ray. Ideally a ventilation lung scan should also be done at the same time, but this is not always available. In pulmonary embolism, when ventilation and perfusion scans are performed at the same time, areas of underperfused but normally ventilated lung may be revealed (see Fig. 7.3). When the chest X-ray is abnormal and only a perfusion scan is available, it is difficult to distinguish between pulmonary embolism and other lung diseases. A normal ventilation–perfusion scan usually excludes pulmonary embolism and a clearly abnormal one carries a high probability. The difficulty arises with those deemed 'intermediate' probability. Here, Doppler flow studies or venography of the leg veins should be done and, if positive, the patient treated as for pulmonary

embolism. If this test is negative but high clinical suspicion remains, pulmonary angiography would be the final arbiter but is rarely undertaken. (It will also reveal the rare condition of pulmonary angioma.) Increased levels of D-dimer, a product of proteolysis of dot fibrin mediated by plasmin, have been found in many patients with proven pulmonary embolism and may further help to resolve difficult diagnoses.

In a considerable number of patients all investigations prove negative, the cause is never found, and the bleeding settles spontaneously. In some cases, occasional haemoptyses continue, often because of some degree of bronchiectasis, but fortunately these haemoptyses are usually small. If all the simple tests are negative, pulmonary emboli should be reconsidered as in this potentially fatal condition effective treatment is possible.

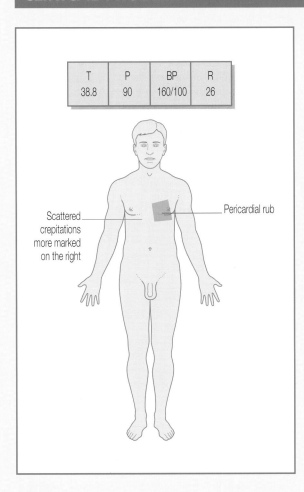

Scattered crepitations more marked on the right

Pericardial rub

T	P	BP	R
38.8	90	160/100	26

A 47-year-old schoolteacher presented to his general practitioner with the complaint that for the previous few weeks he had been coughing up small quantities of blood. Over the same period of time he had noticed some cough with a moderate quantity of yellow sputum, and had felt increasingly unwell. On direct questioning he admitted to progressive shortness of breath over the preceding month, so that he was unable to climb the three flights of stairs to his flat without stopping. After exertion he had noticed a tendency to wheeze, and this symptom only gradually settled with rest. Throughout this time his appetite had been poor and he had lost about 5 kg in weight. He smoked 10 cigarettes daily and drank only moderate quantities of alcohol. He had been well in the past with no previous chest problems or other illness. In his family, his father had suffered from chronic bronchitis for a number of years.

On examination, he looked ill but was not cyanosed or dyspnoeic at rest. Temperature 38.8°C. Pulse 95/regular. Blood pressure 150/90. In the chest, there were scattered crepitations present in most areas, together with some prolongation of expiration. The initial chest X-ray was reported as showing bilateral basal consolidation, more marked on the right.

He was treated with amoxycillin, salbutamol and choline theophyllinate, but showed little improvement. A week later he was still feverish and continuing to have small haemoptyses. He was admitted to hospital.

In addition to his presenting symptoms he was now complaining of central chest pain which was worse on deep breathing. He had also noticed aching in the knees and elbows, with some stiffness but no swelling.

On examination, T 38.8°C, BP 160/100, P 90 (see diagram). On auscultation the crepitations were more marked, particularly over the right lower lobe. In the cardiovascular system there was now an obvious pericardial rub, but no signs of tamponade. The fundi were normal. There was no evidence of arthritis. On routine testing the urine revealed a trace of protein and a weakly positive test for blood.

QUESTIONS

1. What do you consider to be the more likely diagnoses?
2. What further investigations are indicated?

Discussion

Recurrent haemoptyses always deserve full investigation. It is unlikely that they will occur due to simple bacterial infection alone and the chest X-ray of this patient is open to many other interpretations. Haemoptysis may occur in an acute attack of bronchitis, but is unusual, and would not be expected to continue for a number of weeks. Thus despite the presence of cough, sputum and fever, this is unlikely to be the diagnosis. The wheeze and shortness of breath might suggest asthma and yellow sputum containing large numbers of eosinophils may be produced in this condition. A little blood staining in association with the rusty sputum of pneumococcal lobar pneumonia can occur, but the pattern of the illness in this patient, its slowly progressive time course and the mild fever, do not support this diagnosis. Blood-stained sputum is a common feature of *Klebsiella* pneumonia but again such an illness is more acute, the patients are mostly older and debilitated and the changes are usually in the upper lobes.

The symptoms of fever, haemoptysis and weight loss also suggest a tuberculous infection, but the chest X-ray appearance would be highly unusual, and the acute pericarditis is not typical of this diagnosis.

At this age, carcinoma of the bronchus is common, and may infiltrate the pericardium and cause acute pericarditis, which commonly progresses to tamponade.

Rarer conditions that can give rise to an illness of this type are the systemic vasculitides which are now classified by the size of artery affected, clinical features and serological findings. Classical polyarteritis nodosa (PAN) affects medium-size arteries of muscle, nerve, skin and abdomen, including renal, and may cause hypertension. Pulmonary consolidation or infiltrates with chest pain are recognized. The diagnosis may be made by renal angiography or (affected) muscle biopsy. Small vessel disease occurs in microscopic polyangiitis (MPA), Wegener's granulomatosis (WG) and Churg–Strauss syndrome (CSS). WG patients may have a preceding history of chronic upper respiratory tract illness (sinusitis, otitis media, recurrent rhinitis) before renal involvement (focal segmental necrotizing glomerulonephritis) and cavitating lung lesions develop. In CSS allergic rhinitis and nasal polyposis may long precede late onset asthma associated with pulmonary infiltrates and eosinophilia. Nodular-papular rash and mononeuritis are common and the latter provides a means of diagnosis by sural nerve biopsy showing vasculitis of the vasa nervorum. Cardiac involvement is also frequent and a common cause of death. Whereas histological diagnosis from granuloma (WG) or nerve (CSS) biopsy was not always positive the detection of anti-neutrophil cytoplasmic antibodies (ANCA) has been a significant advance. In WG C-ANCA and in CSS P-ANCA are typically positive. The likelihood of systemic disease is increased by the presence of the pericarditis although a pleuropericardial friction rub is not uncommon in pyogenic infections of the left lung. There is nothing in the history or examination to suggest pulmonary emboli.

Investigation must obviously include a full blood count and ESR. The chest X-ray should be repeated and the pericarditis confirmed electrocardiographically. The sputum should be examined for acid-fast bacilli and malignant cells, and for eosinophils.

Renal disease is a common feature of systemic vasculitides and is suggested by the slight rise in blood pressure and the trace of protein and blood in the urine. It should be excluded by full examination of the urine and measurement of the blood urea and creatinine.

Investigation of this man showed a mild degree of anaemia, with a neutrophil leucocytosis and a very high ESR. There was also eosinophilia. The sputum contained eosinophils rather than pus cells. No acid-fast bacilli or malignant cells were present in the sputum. There was moderate proteinuria together with microscopic haematuria. The blood urea was normal. The gamma globulin was markedly raised on serum electrophoresis, but the ANF test was negative. The ECG showed widespread S-T elevation consistent with pericarditis. The anti-neutrophil cytoplasmic antibody test (P-ANCA) was positive, confirming the diagnosis of Churg–Strauss syndrome.

8

Pleural effusion

Pleural effusion is a sign of underlying disease and is not a diagnosis in itself. It may, however, be the earliest sign of disease or a prominent feature of a disorder where other signs and symptoms are not helpful in diagnosis. The symptoms are breathlessness, the severity of which depends on the size of the effusion, and chest discomfort. The differential diagnosis of the cause of a pleural effusion is a common problem in general medical practice.

PHYSICAL SIGNS

The effusion, which is an accumulation of fluid in the pleural space, must have a volume of about 500 ml before it can be reliably detected on physical examination. The most characteristic finding is stony dullness on percussion, with absent or diminished breath sounds, and decreased voice sounds and vocal fremitus. The dullness extends horizontally into the axilla and this is a point of differentiation of effusion from lower lobe consolidation or collapse. Above the effusion, a small area of bronchial breathing is often present. If the effusion is large there may be shift of the mediastinum away from the effusion with displacement of the apex beat and trachea. These are signs of fluid in the pleural cavity, but fluid may also accumulate in the interlobar fissure or above the diaphragm (infrapulmonary effusion) and here cause no detectable physical signs.

RADIOLOGICAL APPEARANCES

The smallest effusions are shown on a chest X-ray as filling-in of the normal costophrenic angle, often described by radiologists as a pleural reaction. Larger effusions have a concave upper surface and the shadow extends further upwards in the axilla. This appearance, often described as fluid 'rising' in the axilla, is due to the fluid being seen edge on. A common misconception, which arises from this appearance, is that the impairment of percussion note also should rise in the axilla. Infrapulmonary effusions have a similar radiological appearance to a raised hemidiaphragm, but when the patient lies on one side, the fluid moves in position unless it is encysted. Interlobar effusions appear as an opacity in the lung fields which may simulate a pulmonary tumour. When a large pleural effusion is present, the hemithorax may be completely obscured. An important practical point is that the upper limit of a pleural effusion is often underestimated on a chest X-ray compared with the physical signs. When deciding on the level at which to aspirate an effusion, the extent of dullness to percussion is often the better guide. Small or loculated effusions may be better detected by ultrasound, which can be used to guide needle aspiration and drainage.

THE CAUSES OF PLEURAL EFFUSION

A collection of pleural fluid may be due to exudation or transudation (Box 8.1). Bleeding into the pleural space produces a haemothorax. A chylothorax is due to collection of lymphatic fluid. The distinction is made on the basis of the underlying disease, and on the protein and cell content of the fluid. Exudation is due to inflammation of the pleura and is characterized by a higher protein content than transudates, generally quoted to be more than 30 g/l, although there is some overlap. Transudates are due to the loss of fluid from the pleural capillary bed and are caused by the same conditions that cause oedema elsewhere in the body (see Ch. 3). The fluid is typically straw-coloured and does not clot on standing. A bloody effusion is either traumatic or associated with malignancy. Chyle is milky in appearance.

The glucose content of pleural fluid is normally the same as in plasma, except in rheumatoid arthritis, TB, empyema and some malignancies. The cell count in a transudate is generally low, <1000/mm^3, comprising lymphocytes, polymorphs and mesothelial cells. Higher cell counts are found in exudates but are not of diagnostic value.

Pleural exudates

The majority of pleural effusions are exudates, and usually they occur as a complication of pulmonary disease which has already been diagnosed. The following are the main causes to be considered:

Pulmonary infarction. This condition often presents considerable difficulty in diagnosis. One of its common accompaniments is a pleural effusion, which is usually

Box 8.1 Causes of pleural effusion

Transudates

- heart failure
- cirrhosis
- nephrotic syndrome
- peritoneal dialysis

Exudates

- infection – e.g. pneumonia, TB
- neoplasia – primary or secondary malignancy
- pulmonary infarct
- collagen vascular disease

Haemothorax

- traumatic

Chylothorax

- lymphoma, carcinoma, trauma

small, and which may be the only physical sign that infarction has occurred. It is often said that the effusion is haemorrhagic, and although this is sometimes the case, especially soon after the infarction, it is more commonly straw-coloured. The effusion contains neutrophils and lymphocytes and occasionally large numbers of eosinophils. Aspiration and examination of the fluid can never confirm the diagnosis of a pulmonary infarction. This will usually be based on evidence of a source of embolism elsewhere, such as deep venous thrombosis in the legs or pelvis. Examination of the fluid is helpful in cases where the effusion is the only sign of disease and the differentiation between infarction and malignant or tuberculosis effusion must be made.

Pneumonia. Pleural effusion may complicate bacterial pneumonia, although it is rare in viral pneumonia. Post-pneumonic effusions may become the seat of pyogenic infection resulting in an empyema. Usually, the effusion develops after a patient with bacterial pneumonia has already been started on antibiotics. If an empyema develops, the patient's condition will deteriorate, with increasing fever. In such a case the fluid must be aspirated completely and is usually straw-coloured with numerous neutrophils. The fluid must always be cultured, although it is often sterile. Complete aspiration of the effusion, together with appropriate antibiotic therapy, is usually curative. A bacterial pneumonia, particularly if complicated by pleural effusion, may be the first sign of an underlying bronchial neoplasm. In such cases the fluid must be examined for malignant cells and a pleural biopsy performed. The suspicion of an underlying carcinoma is strengthened

when an apparently straightforward post-pneumonic effusion recurs repeatedly after aspiration.

Malignancy. The commonest cause of a malignant pleural effusion is a primary carcinoma of the bronchus involving the pleura. This may be the first evidence of the tumour. The effusion is often large, causing a shift of the mediastinum, and may accumulate very rapidly, causing dyspnoea. If there is underlying collapse of the lung due to the tumour, the mediastinum may paradoxically be shifted to the side of the effusion. The bronchial carcinoma has usually been previously diagnosed, and other signs due to the primary tumour or its metastatic spread will commonly be present. Aspiration reveals fluid which is usually bloodstained, but may be straw-coloured. It often reaccumulates rapidly after aspiration. This is a feature of pleural effusion which always suggests malignancy. There may be malignant cells in the effusion but their absence does not exclude the diagnosis. A pleural biopsy is valuable if the diagnosis has not been established previously.

Other pulmonary tumours may cause pleural effusions. Metastatic tumours may involve the pleura at a time when the primary site is unknown. Similarly an effusion may be the first indication of recurrent tumour after the primary has been excised. The effusion may be bilateral, and metastases may be visible in the lung fields. Malignant lymphoma may involve the pleura and the chest X-ray may show other features suggestive of this diagnosis such as enlarged hilar and mediastinal nodes. Cytology may suggest the nature of the underlying neoplasm. Breast cancer may spread to the pleura via the lymphatic system. Pleural effusion secondary to ovarian or gastrointestinal malignancy generally occurs by haematogenous spread. Primary malignant tumours of the pleura are still uncommon, but pleural mesothelioma is being seen much more often as a result of people being exposed to asbestos dust 30 years ago. Other radiological signs of asbestosis, such as fibrosis in the lower zones and calcified pleural plaques, may be present.

Tuberculosis. Tuberculous pleural effusions are caused by a combination of direct tuberculous infection of the pleural space, and a state of hypersensitivity to the tubercle bacillus. Effusions may accompany primary infections in young children, but are uncommon. In these patients, the effusion is often accompanied by radiological signs suggestive of the diagnosis, such as a primary focus or enlarged hilar nodes. The pleural aspirate often contains tubercle bacilli. In adolescents pleural effusion may be the sole sign of the disease, although they may go on to develop further signs of the infection if left untreated. In adults infection of the pleural space with tubercle bacilli is uncommon, but can occur as a complication of established pulmonary disease such as tuberculous bronchopneumonia, or following rupture of a cavity into the pleural space.

The effusion can be very large, and acid-fast bacilli may be seen in the centrifuged deposit after aspiration. Culture of the fluid for the bacillus must be carried out, and repeated culture increases the chance of success. It is in the diagnosis of tuberculous pleural effusion, that pleural biopsy, repeated if necessary, is of the greater value. The Mantoux test is always positive in these patients since the effusions are in part due to hypersensitivity.

Connective tissue disease. Rheumatoid arthritis may be accompanied by pulmonary complications and these are commoner in men. The commonest complication is pleural effusion, and although this usually develops in a patient with established disease, it may be the presenting feature. Pleural effusions are more common in patients with subcutaneous nodules and high titres of rheumatoid factor. On aspiration the fluid is clear, with a high protein content. A low glucose concentration may be found. Biopsy is needed if tuberculosis or malignancy are possible causes of the effusion. In rheumatoid arthritis biopsy usually shows chronic inflammation without distinguishing features, although sometimes appearances similar to rheumatoid granulomata are found. Pleurisy with a small effusion also occurs in systemic lupus erythematosus.

Other causes. A pleural effusion may arise as a result of disease below the diaphragm, such as a subphrenic or hepatic abscess. Although the diagnostic signs of the primary disorder will usually be present, difficulty may arise in the diagnosis of subphrenic abscess. The patient may complain of shoulder-tip pain with no signs other than fever and a pleural effusion.

Acute pancreatitis may be accompanied by a pleural effusion. The mechanism of its formation is obscure, but it is usually bloodstained and has a high concentration of amylase.

Actinomycosis is exceedingly rare as a cause of pleural effusion, but it may present in this way.

Pleural transudates

The general principles underlying the formation of pleural fluid are the same as those in the formation of interstitial fluid elsewhere in the body. The main causes of pleural transudates are:

Heart failure. This is the commonest cause, and other signs of heart failure will usually be present. The effusions are usually small and bilateral. When unilateral the effusion is usually right-sided and can be very large.

The chest X-ray will show other features of heart failure such as enlargement of the heart shadow and upper lobe venous distension (see Fig. 2.2A and B, p. 12). Pleural effusion may occur in constrictive pericarditis and this diagnosis will be strongly suggested by calcification in the pericardium.

Hypoproteinaemic states. Cirrhosis of the liver, nephrotic syndrome and malabsorption syndrome are the commonest causes of hypoproteinaemia. There is usually considerable salt and water retention as well. All of these conditions may be accompanied by pleural effusion, but the underlying disease is usually obvious, and the plasma albumin concentration is low.

Chylous pleural effusions

Perforation of the thoracic duct leads to the accumulation of lymph in the pleural space and a chylous pleural effusion (chylothorax). Most cases are the result of trauma or of surgery, but chylothorax can also be caused by malignant infiltration of the thoracic duct by primary or secondary tumours and lymphomas. The signs are those of a large pleural effusion, which reaccumulates rapidly after aspiration. The fluid has a milky appearance and the protein content is high. Repeated aspiration leads to lymphopenia and profound protein loss.

INVESTIGATION OF A PLEURAL EFFUSION

Many pleural effusions have causes which are clinically self-evident, and little further investigation is required. A great deal of information will be obtained by routine investigations such as full blood count, chest X-ray and sputum culture and cytology.

There remains the not uncommon clinical problem where a patient has a pleural effusion without clinical evidence of any underlying disease, and examination of the sputum and chest X-ray have not contributed to the diagnosis. In these patients, aspiration of the pleural fluid is essential.

Biopsy of the pleura and aspiration are usually performed at the same time. The fluid should not be aspirated too quickly, and about 500 ml fluid can be withdrawn without risk to the patient.

Bloodstained effusions suggest malignancy, although pulmonary infarction is occasionally a cause. Clear watery fluid is found in transudates, which are usually bilateral, and purulent fluid in an established empyema. The protein content of the effusion helps to distinguish transudates from exudates, although this is seldom a point at issue.

Bacteriological culture for pyogenic organisms is always essential, but a positive culture does not rule out malignancy as a cause of the underlying disease. Culture for tubercle bacilli is mandatory whenever an effusion is aspirated for diagnostic purposes.

The cells in the effusion should be examined. Numerous neutrophils suggest pyogenic infection, while large numbers of lymphocytes may indicate TB or lymphoma. Of interest is the finding of large numbers of eosinophils in some pleural aspirates which, although not diagnostic, tend to be associated with benign inflammation.

The chest X-ray should always be repeated after aspiration to see if any underlying abnormality has thereby been revealed.

These investigations will normally have been successful in discovering the cause. Occasionally further investigation may be necessary, especially if it is felt that there is an underlying carcinoma. In these cases CT scanning, fibreoptic bronchoscopy and image-guided biopsy may be necessary.

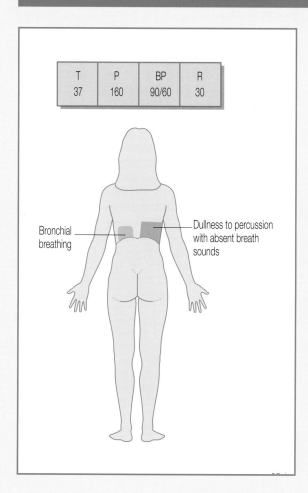

T	P	BP	R
37	160	90/60	30

Bronchial breathing

Dullness to percussion with absent breath sounds

A 55-year-old woman had suffered from asthma for 10 years and had required oral steroids for 7 years. During this time she had had recurrent upper abdominal pain, which was relieved by alkalis and occasional courses of ranitidine. For 2 months before admission she had been feeling unwell, tiring easily, with a cough which troubled her during the day but which was unproductive of sputum. She was a non-smoker. One week before admission her asthma worsened, and she increased her prednisolone to 40 mg/day. This produced improvement and she had reduced the dose to 20 mg/day by the time of admission. Two hours before admission she had developed sudden severe upper abdominal pain, and collapsed in the train station on the way home.

On examination she was very ill: blood pressure 90/60, temperature 37°C, pulse 160/min. In the chest there was generalized expiratory wheeze, and dullness to percussion at the right base posteriorly, extending into the axilla. There was general abdominal rigidity with diffuse tenderness. Bowel sounds were absent. Before laparotomy, she was given hydrocortisone, which was continued post-operatively. At operation there was free fluid in the abdomen, and a small perforation of a posterior duodenal ulcer. The perforation was sutured.

She made a good initial post-operative recovery, but on the third post-operative day she developed a pyrexia of 39°C which persisted. She was found to have dullness at the right base with absent breath sounds and an area of bronchial breathing at the left base. She was treated with amoxycillin and erythromycin, initially intravenously, for 7 days, with improvement of the signs at the left base but without any effect on those at the right. A chest X-ray at this time showed a right pleural effusion, patchy shadowing at the left base, air under the diaphragm, and a calcified hilar lymph node.

Questions

1. What are the most probable reasons for her right pleural effusion?
2. What are the investigations which would be most helpful in diagnosis?
3. What would be your immediate management of this case?

Discussion

This asthmatic patient has taken a high dose of steroids for many years, and has suffered from a perforated ulcer which is a hazard of this form of treatment. It is probably significant that it followed an increase in the dose. She had been feeling unwell for several weeks prior to the acute emergency, and at the time of admission already had signs of a right-sided pleural effusion. The likely cause of this patient's effusion is pulmonary tuberculosis or malignant disease, either primary of the lung or due to secondary deposits. Malignant pleural effusion may be the initial presentation of an occult primary carcinoma, and carcinoma of the breast is a possibility even though the breasts may appear clinically normal.

Although subphrenic abscess may follow perforation of a duodenal ulcer, and pulmonary embolism may follow any operation, these do not account for her previous ill-health and the signs of pleural effusion before surgery. A previous pyogenic infection may have caused a pleural effusion but this is an unlikely cause of chronic mild ill-health. On the other hand, tuberculosis is an important complication of long-term steroid therapy which may unmask a previously quiescent focus. Such a focus is suggested by the hilar calcification. There is nothing to suggest heart failure as a cause of the effusion.

The most important investigation is aspiration of the pleural effusion with pleural biopsy. The fluid must be cultured for acid-fast bacilli as well as pyogenic organisms. It should also be examined for malignant cells. If these investigations are negative, and if the effusion persists, the aspiration and biopsy should be repeated. Radioisotope lung scan may be of considerable value in the diagnosis of pulmonary embolism. This is not a likely diagnosis in this case, and it could be misleading in this patient who has abnormalities in both lungs clinically and radiologically. The sputum must be examined for tubercle bacilli, and malignant cells. A full blood count will be done, but is unlikely to be of diagnostic help. The Mantoux test ought to be positive in view of the hilar calcification, and could be strongly positive if there is active disease, but might be suppressed in a patient on steroids. It is therefore of no value in diagnosis.

The best immediate management of this case would be to continue her steroids because she is recovering from a stressful operation and has been on this treatment for 7 years. Physiotherapy and continuation of antibiotics will be needed for her left basal pneumonia which is already improving. Her pleural effusion will not need treatment until its cause has been found.

Aspiration of the effusion revealed a turbid fluid with numerous lymphocytes. A biopsy revealed tuberculosis. Culture of the fluid grew tubercle bacilli sensitive to all first-line drugs. One year after treatment she was quite well and chest X-ray showed residual right-sided pleural thickening.

9

Dysphagia

The symptom of difficulty in swallowing often results in an automatic request for a barium swallow and endoscopy. Although both these investigations may prove necessary, a surprising degree of precision in diagnosis can often be achieved by careful history-taking. The ability to ask the right questions requires some knowledge of the underlying physiology of swallowing and the ways in which different disease processes interfere with it. Not only will a diagnosis based on history enable the appropriate confirmatory test to be undertaken, but it may also lead to earlier diagnosis and treatment. Generally speaking, physical examination will be of secondary importance to the history, but may show evidence of disease in other parts of the body such as the central nervous system.

PHYSIOLOGY OF SWALLOWING

Solids are first masticated, which requires sound teeth, efficient bite, adequate lubrication with saliva and an absence of painful lesions of the tongue and mouth. Swallowing begins with the soft palate meeting the base of the tongue to enclose the bolus. By a piston-like action of the tongue the bolus is then propelled backwards into the pharynx while the soft palate moves backwards and upwards to close off the nasopharynx. Failure of the latter mechanism leads to regurgitation through the nose. As the bolus moves backwards so the epiglottis is tilted over the glottis, the larynx rising to meet it, resulting in closure of the airway and inhibition of respiration. Failure of this mechanism will lead to inhalation of food or liquid at the time of swallowing. This is in contrast to inhalation occurring later, due to regurgitation of food some time after a meal or at night. A slight delay occurs as the upper oesophageal sphincter (cricopharyngeus muscle) then relaxes. Normally this sphincter is closed with a high resting pressure of about 30 mmHg (see Fig. 9.1). Inco-ordination

of relaxation is said to be an aetiological factor in the formation of a pharyngeal pouch as the high pressures generated in the pharynx during swallowing cannot be transmitted onwards into the oesophagus. Instead, there is bulging at the site of dehiscence in the posterior pharyngeal wall. This failure of relaxation may be visualized by pooling of barium in the valleculae and pyriform fossae.

Following relaxation the cricopharyngeus immediately contracts, producing a pressure twice that of its resting value. This ensures that the primary oesophageal peristaltic wave, which generates a pressure of 30 mmHg, cannot cause reflux. With the momentum gained from pharyngeal contraction and peristalsis the bolus takes approximately 9 seconds to reach the lower oesophagus and is greatly assisted by gravity. Hence, to detect the earliest defects in peristalsis, as in systemic sclerosis, an anti-gravity barium swallow is essential.

Whereas primary peristalsis is initiated by the voluntary act of swallowing, secondary oesophageal peristalsis occurs as an unconscious reflex in response to distension of the oesophagus by any remaining food particles. Although there is probably no true anatomical lower oesophageal sphincter, there is an area of relatively high pressure (about 15 mmHg) in the lower 7 cm of the oesophagus. This physiological sphincter lies partly above the diaphragm and partly in the 4 cm below it. The subdiaphragmatic portion, to which is transmitted the positive intra-abdominal pressure, is crucial in preventing gastro-oesophageal reflux, since any rise in intra-abdominal pressure affects intragastric and intraoesophageal pressures equally. One or two seconds after primary peristalsis starts, the gastro-oesophageal sphincter begins to relax to allow the bolus to enter the stomach. However, the pressure does not fall to the intragastric level (5 mmHg), otherwise reflux could occur since there is a negative pressure at rest in the intrathoracic oesophagus. Failure of relaxation at this site is the cause of the symptoms of achalasia. The hydrostatic pressure of food and liquid accumulating in the lower oesophagus can finally overcome the tone of the sphincter in achalasia.

CAUSES OF DYSPHAGIA

It is logical to consider causes of dysphagia from above downwards. Emphasis will be on the points in the history, examination and investigations which allow the various causes to be differentiated (Fig. 9.2).

Psychogenic

The patient is usually a woman suffering from anxiety, often with a hysterical personality. The complaint is of

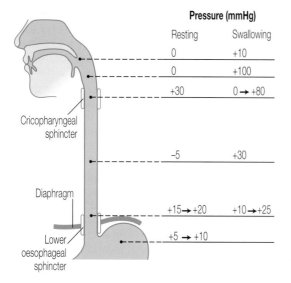

	Pressure (mmHg)	
	Resting	Swallowing
	0	+10
	0	+100
	+30	0 → +80
	−5	+30
	+15 → +20	+10 → +25
	+5 → +10	

Cricopharyngeal sphincter

Diaphragm

Lower oesophageal sphincter

Fig. 9.1 Representative pressures at rest and swallowing.

an inability to swallow rather than any discomfort during swallowing. Dryness of the mouth, associated with emotion, may exacerbate the condition. Sometimes attention may have been drawn for the first time to a small goitre, the patient then becoming aware of a 'lump in the neck'. This, in turn, engenders fear, which expresses itself as inability to swallow. It should be remembered that dysphagia due to goitre is exceptional, though it can occur with sudden haemorrhage into a cyst in a multinodular goitre.

Sjögren's syndrome

The features originally described were dryness of the eyes (keratoconjunctivitis sicca) and mouth (xerostomia), salivary gland enlargement, and arthritis of the rheumatoid type. It is called secondary Sjögren's syndrome when associated with other connective tissue diseases such as rheumatoid arthritis, systemic lupus erythematosus and systemic sclerosis or autoimmune diseases such as primary biliary cirrhosis, chronic

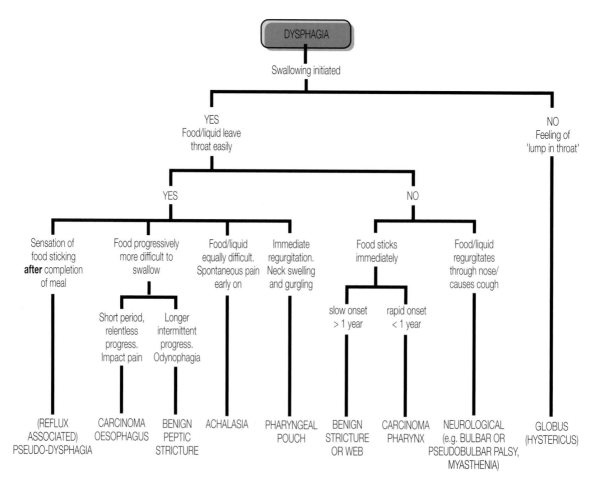

Fig. 9.2 A guide to the diagnosis of dysphagia.

active hepatitis, myasthenia gravis and thyroiditis. However, ocular and oral involvement (the 'sicca' syndrome) may be the sole manifestation and is designated primary Sjögren's syndrome. Dryness of the mouth, sufficiently severe to interfere with chewing and swallowing, will be present with a red tender tongue, cracked lips and swollen salivary glands. The dryness and grittiness of the eyes due to lack of tear formation by the involved lacrimal glands can be demonstrated by the Schirmer test. In this test one end of a strip of blotting paper is placed under the lower eyelid and fails to become moistened.

Inflammatory and neoplastic conditions in the mouth

Most painful conditions of the mouth and tongue are usually self-evident from the history and examination. The premalignant condition of leucoplakia and its sequel, carcinoma of the tongue, will interfere with swallowing. Glossitis may be associated with various nutritional deficiencies, lack of iron being the most important. Infections, such as tonsillitis, peritonsillar abscess, pharyngitis, and severe caries can all cause pain. Although the recently edentulous patient may not actually complain of dysphagia, considerable weight loss, obviously due to decreased food intake, can occur.

Mechanical causes

A foreign body (fishbones are notorious) may lodge in the tonsillar bed or pyriform fossa. Although the pain impairs swallowing, the original event may have been unnoticed. A much more dubious cause of dysphagia is the protrusion of lower cervical intervertebral discs onto the posterior oesophagus. As with the attribution of other symptoms to cervical spondylosis, the diagnosis should not be lightly made, as radiological changes in the neck are common from middle age onwards and are generally asymptomatic.

Neuromuscular causes

In most instances dysphagia will be only one part of a more widespread neurological disturbance which, considered as a whole, will indicate the underlying disease. The neurological control of swallowing is complex. There is no clearly defined anatomical centre controlling swallowing, but the medulla oblongata is of great importance in this respect and is also concerned with interrelated actions such as chewing, licking, gagging, coughing, sneezing, vomiting, belching and breathing. These activities are influenced by afferent impulses from the cerebral cortex, glosso-pharyngeal nerves and various branches of the vagus. The motor outflow is via

the cranial nerve nuclei (V, VII, IX, ambiguus, X, XI and XII) and the upper three cervical segments. In cerebellar disorders, coordination of swallowing, and of speech, with breathing is no longer automatic, and failure of the glottis to close at the right moment may cause choking.

The various bulbar causes of dysphagia include infections such as diphtheria and poliomyelitis. Other causes are the malformation of syringobulbia, which may be associated with platybasia and the Arnold–Chiari malformation, the bulbar palsy of motor neurone disease, the pseudobulbar palsy of bilateral strokes, and the variable weakness of myasthenia gravis. In this type of dysphagia, difficulty arises when liquids, and to a lesser extent solids, leave the throat to enter the gullet. There is no problem usually in initiating swallowing, but fluid will immediately either regurgitate through the nose, or cause coughing by entering the larynx. This contrasts with the few seconds delay between swallowing and coughing when the patient has an oesophagotracheal fistula.

Pharyngeal pouch

Although food and liquid are swallowed easily, they may be regurgitated immediately or on bending over or turning the head. A bulging in the neck may be noticed which may gurgle on drinking. The patients are often elderly and the chief hazard is of recurrent aspiration pneumonia. Confirmation of the diagnosis is by barium swallow.

Sideropenic dysphagia

In this condition of many synonyms (Plummer–Vinson, Paterson–Brown–Kelly), epithelial changes due to iron deficiency sometimes cause glossitis but, more importantly, affect the upper oesophagus. Here there may be a web of fine membrane affecting only the anterior wall or encircling the oesophagus. The complaint is of solids, but not liquids, sticking in the throat immediately on swallowing (i.e. without awareness of an interval). A delay between swallowing and the sensation of sticking indicates an obstruction lower in the oesophagus since passage of the bolus down the oesophagus may take up to 10 seconds, whereas emptying of the pharynx is virtually instantaneous. A general point is that localization of obstruction is more accurately made by timing impact rather than by taking the level indicated by the patient. The latter is notoriously unreliable as the sensation may often be felt some distance above the true site. The patient with a web will usually give a surprisingly long history of months or years because symptoms may only occur with a particularly large bolus and therefore may be intermittent.

Associated with the web, the patient, generally a middle-aged woman, may have spoon-shaped nails (koilonychia), glossitis, cheilitis, splenomegaly and a hypochromic anaemia. The association between web and carcinoma at the same site is no longer thought to be strong. Generally malignant strictures, which are rare in the upper oesophagus, have a short and progressive history. Confirmation of the diagnosis of a web is by the characteristic findings on barium swallow and oesophagoscopy, and by the associated haematological abnormalities.

External pressure

These are very unusual causes of dysphagia, occurring at mid-oesophageal level and rarely amounting to total obstruction. Vascular causes are aneurysm of the arch of the aorta or an aberrant right subclavian artery arising from the left side of the aorta passing posterior to the oesophagus and causing an indentation on barium swallow (dysphagia lusoria). Mediastinal nodes involved with secondary malignancy, usually from the bronchus, generally produce other symptoms and signs before such a mobile structure as the oesophagus is compressed. Inflamed nodes, usually due to tuberculosis, may become adherent and produce a traction diverticulum, although this seldom causes dysphagia.

Systemic sclerosis

Although lower oesophageal involvement can often be demonstrated, symptoms are relatively rare and mild. However, heartburn and acid regurgitation are common and may be severe. Impairment of peristalsis, with failure of the gastro-oesophageal physiological sphincter to close, occurs early in the disease. It contributes to gastro-oesophageal reflux disease (GORD) rather than dysphagia because of the role of gravity in swallowing. The defect can best be shown by an antigravity barium swallow. Later in the disease, narrowing of the lower oesophagus with slight dilatation above it is seen, usually due to a peptic stricture resulting from the longstanding associated reflux oesophagitis. Evidence of the disease elsewhere such as scleroderma of the hands and face, Raynaud's phenomenon, arthritis, pulmonary and renal involvement may be present, in addition to disordered small bowel peristalsis causing diarrhoea and the stagnant loop syndrome. Often it is these other clinical features that suggest the diagnosis and lead to a barium swallow.

Achalasia

This disease is often diagnosed only after much delay, and cardiomyotomy (Heller's operation) is frequently considered too late in its natural history. This is regrettable because little can be done to help a patient who has reached the stage of mega-oesophagus to lead a normal life again. The disease is due to an idiopathic degeneration of the ganglion cells of Auerbach's plexus, although an identical lesion is seen in Brazil in Chagas' disease caused by the neurotoxin of *Trypanosoma cruzi*.

In the early stages of denervation the muscle is hypersensitive to endogenous and exogenous cholinergic substances which result in spasm, causing dysphagia and pain. Although swallowing, particularly of iced drinks, sometimes provokes pain, it also may occur spontaneously but transiently at any time of day or night. Radiation of the pain to the neck, together with its intensity, may erroneously suggest a cardiac cause. Although food and liquid leave the pharynx normally the failure of peristalsis and relaxation of the sphincter will slow their progress. Therefore neither food nor liquid can be taken rapidly in the early stages. When the patient reaches the mega-oesophagus stage, the large capacity of the gullet may make it possible to drink fast while it fills. Indeed, the hydrostatic pressure generated as the mega-oesophagus fills may overcome the sphincter. The patient often learns the value of forcible drinking to facilitate passage of food into the stomach. Unlike a carcinoma, dysphagia for both solids and liquids is often present from the outset and for a long time. The rapid progression from solid to liquid dysphagia is more suggestive of a stenosing lesion. Pain on eating solids is also much more a feature of carcinoma. The diagnosis is usually made by barium swallow which may be greatly enhanced by video fluoroscopy. In cases where doubt remains manometry shows the same features of reduced or absent lower oesophageal peristalsis combined with a failure of relaxation of the lower oesophageal sphincter whose pressure may or may not be increased. In the later stages, plain chest X-ray may show a widened mediastinum with a fluid level, loss of gastric air bubble, and evidence of repeated episodes of aspiration pneumonia from spillover. A barium swallow is still the most important investigation and will show disordered peristalsis and oesophageal dilatation with a funnel-shaped obstruction. Carcinoma occurs in 10% of patients with long-standing achalasia (Fig. 9.3).

Benign oesophageal stricture

Apart from the rare and usually obvious cases due to drinking corrosives, benign strictures are invariably the result of reflux oesophagitis. This, in turn, is usually associated with a sliding hiatus hernia, where the intra-abdominal portion of the oesophagus is pushed into the chest, removing one of the important anti-reflux defences. A history of flatulent dyspepsia, heartburn and regurgitation made worse by bending or lying flat, together with persistent iron deficiency anaemia, may precede dysphagia. Although most peptic strictures occur in the lower oesophagus they may be found as high as mid-oesophagus. Liquids can usually be drunk rapidly but food will stick; however, this is a slowly progressive and, initially, intermittent process with periods of days with trouble-free swallowing. This may be due to variability in reflux of the acid–pepsin juice provoking oesophageal spasm. Such spasm, described radiologically as tertiary contractions or corkscrew oesophagus, may in turn give rise to a pseudodysphagia with a sensation of food sticking, coming some minutes or more after meals. Pain from associated oesophagitis (odynophagia) may be provoked by drinks too hot or too cold, grapefruit juice or alcoholic spirits. The diagnosis is confirmed by barium swallow and oesophagoscopy (Fig. 9.4).

Carcinoma of oesophagus

Carcinoma of the fundus encroaching on the gastro-oesophageal junction may be silent until it produces its own variant of dysphagia. Difficulty in swallowing solids occurs at the beginning of each meal, but after a few pain-producing mouthfuls the rest of the meal passes with relative ease. This can be differentiated from achalasia by the time course, the pain, and the dysphagia for solids alone in the early stages.

The more common lower oesophageal malignant strictures differ from benign strictures by spreading along the oesophagus at the same time as spreading circumferentially (Fig. 9.5).

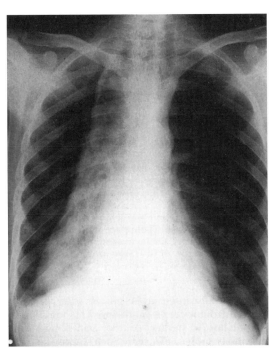

Fig. 9.3 Chest X-ray of a 64-year-old man with a long history of difficulty in swallowing and repeated episodes of right basal pneumonia. Gross widening of the mediastinum, containing gas shadows to the right and left of the trachea and irregular opacification within it adjacent to the right heart border; the right costophrenic angle is blunted. The appearances are those of mega-oesophagus due to longstanding achalasia of the cardia, giving rise to 'spillover' aspiration pneumonia. The patient died of carcinoma of the oesophagus.

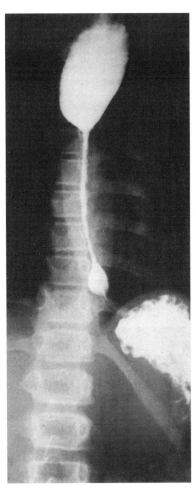

Fig. 9.4 Barium swallow in a young child who, 8 weeks earlier, had drunk bleach, a corrosive agent. A lengthy stricture involving the lower half of the oesophagus with dilatation above it is seen. The surface of the lining of the stricture is slightly irregular because of the accompanying oesophagitis.

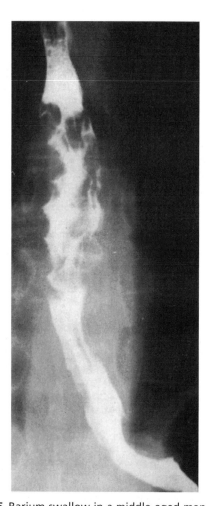

Fig. 9.5 Barium swallow in a middle-aged man with a short history of dysphagia for solids and weight loss. An area of irregularity due to multiple filling defects associated with loss of peristalsis and delay in transit of barium is seen. The cause was a fungating squamous-cell carcinoma of the oesophagus.

Although the history is very much shorter and progresses more rapidly, impaction pain may be most marked at the outset, diminishing with time (unlike a benign stricture). This may be partly spurious, as the patient stops attempting to swallow solids, but also occurs because of replacement of sensitive mucous membrane and peristaltic muscle by tumour above the stricture. Unlike a peptic stricture, dysphagia occurs with each meal from the time of the first symptom. The stage of inability to swallow liquids may be soon reached, and the patient regurgitates.

Longstanding GORD, the commonest cause of benign stricture, may also cause transformation of the lower oesophageal squamous mucosa to a columnar lining (Barrett's oesophagus). In some patients this may further change to a premalignant dysplasia and, subsequently, an adenocarcinoma in the region of the gastro-oesophageal junction. This must always be borne in mind should symptoms suggesting recurrence of stricture occur. Any patient found to have dysplasia on endoscopic biopsy requires regular follow-up.

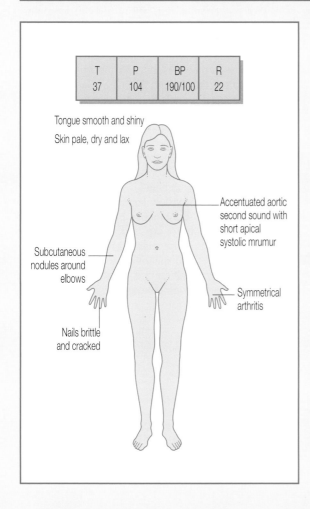

T	P	BP	R
37	104	190/100	22

Tongue smooth and shiny

Skin pale, dry and lax

Accentuated aortic second sound with short apical systolic mrumur

Subcutaneous nodules around elbows

Nails brittle and cracked

Symmetrical arthritis

A 52-year-old widow was referred from a chest clinic with the complaint of intermittent difficulty in swallowing for 3 years. She had noticed that toast and meat especially seemed to stick at the level of the manubrium some seconds after swallowing. At first the symptom occurred only about twice a week, usually at the beginning of a meal. She said that occasionally about 5 minutes after a large meal there was a heavy sensation 'as if something was stuck' at the lower end of the sternum. She had always been able to swallow liquids rapidly, without pain. In the preceding 4 months the difficulty in swallowing had occurred more frequently. Her weight had fallen from 95 kg to 89 kg. There had been no vomiting. For some years she had found that it was uncomfortable to lie on her left side at night.

For the previous 6 months she had noticed increasing breathlessness on exertion, together with tiredness. There was no cough or sputum, but at the end of the day her ankles were sometimes swollen.

She had been attending a rheumatology department for 9 years for rheumatoid arthritis, which had led to marked deformity of her hands. This had initially been treated with salicylates alone, but for the previous 5 years she had also been taking a low dose of prednisone.

On examination she was obese. She was not orthopnoeic. The skin was pale, dry and lax and the nails were brittle and cracked. The tongue was smooth, moist and shiny with loss of papillation. In the cardiovascular system, the pulse was 104/minute, regular and of good volume. Blood pressure was 190/100. The apex beat could not be localized, there was a short systolic murmur in the apical region, and the aortic second sound was accentuated. There was a symmetrical polyarthritis involving the metacarpophalangeal joints of both hands with ulnar deviation, the proximal interphalangeal joints, and the elbows and shoulders. Both ankles and knees were slightly affected. There were subcutaneous nodules around the elbow joints.

The following investigations had been performed in the chest clinic:
Haemoglobin 7.9 g/dl; MCV 72 fl; MCH 24 pg. film shows anisocytosis, microcytosis and hypochromia; WBC 8.7 × 10⁹/1 with normal differential; ESR 32 mm in 1 hour.
Chest X-ray: Cardiothoracic ratio 17 : 30 cm.
Lung fields clear.

Spirometry: $\dfrac{FEV_1}{FVC} = \dfrac{1.6}{2.0}$ litres

Stools positive for occult blood

Questions

1. What are the likely diagnoses?
2. Which other investigations would be helpful in diagnosis?

Discussion

This patient was referred to the chest clinic because of breathlessness. This is due to her anaemia which has the characteristics of iron deficiency. Obesity is a contributory factor and could also account for the mild restrictive ventilatory defect seen on spirometry. Her cardiomegaly is due to the anaemia and mild hypertension.

The cause of the anaemia is probably the occult blood loss. The dysphagia is long-standing while the symptoms of anaemia are recent. This suggests that the anaemia is the result of whatever is producing dysphagia. It is unlikely that she has longstanding iron deficiency causing the dysphagia (so called sideropenic dysphagia).

The most likely cause of the dysphagia is an oeso-phageal stricture. Despite the patient localizing the site of obstruction to the manubrial region it is quite possible that the stricture is at the lower end of the oesoph-agus. The sensation of food sticking within seconds of swallowing, particularly of rough solids, suggests an organic stricture, although there may be some additional element of spasm. The feeling of 'something stuck' at the lower end of the sternum is very likely to be pseu-dodysphagia due to oesophageal spasm due to gastro-oesophageal reflux. This symptom is most likely to occur after meals, when it is thought that the falling level of gastrin causes the gastro-oesophageal sphincter to relax and allow reflux. Reflux may also occur at night because the horizontal position removes the protective effect of gravity, and patients often complain that their symptoms are worse when they lie on their left side. The stricture is most probably benign and due to fibrosis secondary to the peptic oesophagitis. A malignant stricture is unlikely in view of the length of the history. The recent deterio-ration and weight loss is probably due to a worsening of the stricture but could be due to the develop-ment of a carcinoma, which is more likely to occur in a patient with chronic oesophagitis, when it may be an adenocarcinoma arising from a Barrett's lining (gastric columnar epithelium replacing the squamous epithelium).

She has no skin changes of scleroderma and the deforming polyarthritis with typical rheumatoid nodules is against this diagnosis. There is nothing to suggest the diagnosis of Sjögren's syndrome and the dysphagia is not due to a dry mouth. Achalasia is unlikely as she has always been able to swallow liquids rapidly. In addition there has been no spontaneous pain, no evidence of spillover disease in the lungs and nothing to suggest mega-oesophagus, on the chest X-ray.

Barium swallow and meal examination is therefore the best initial investigation. It is usual for it to precede the equally important oesophagoscopy, as the latter may be dangerous if performed as a blind procedure. Oesophagoscopy allows direct inspection of the inflamed oesophagus, visualization of reflux, biopsy of the mucosa and stricture and, if benign, its dilatation.

This patient had a sliding hiatus hernia with gastrooesophageal reflux and a benign stricture. Her anaemia was due to the oesophagitis and aggravated by her rheumatoid arthritis and its treatment.

Haematemesis and melaena

Acute gastrointestinal haemorrhage remains one of the commonest medical emergencies. It is rather disappointing to note that annual mortality figures over the past 15 years have shown little improvement in the figure of 5%–10%. Closer analysis reveals that this, in part, may be due to a changing disease pattern in that more patients are falling into the categories that carry a high risk. Many of these deaths could be deemed unavoidable and such improvement as is now beginning to be seen is not so much attributable to high technology medicine in diagnosis and treatment as careful attention to detail by a team approach involving skilled and experienced physicians, surgeons and nurses. The published data suggest this can best be done in a designated combined medical–surgical gastrointestinal unit.

Old age is the predominant mortality risk factor since it is associated with an increased incidence of other disorders, such as chronic bronchitis and ischaemic heart disease, which give bleeding from peptic ulcer in the over 60s a poorer prognosis (Table 10.1). Although varices and gastric carcinoma are each responsible for only 3% of bleeds (Fig. 10.1) they carry mortalities in the region of 45% and 35% respectively (Fig. 10.2). Their combined mortality is greater than that from duodenal ulcer, which is the commonest cause of bleeding.

As gastrointestinal haemorrhage occurs with varying severity from a variety of causes, one problem in management is how extensive the diagnostic procedures should be in the early stages. Accurate diagnosis leads to the identification of the patient who is at great risk. As treatment cannot be separated from diagnosis in this situation, both will be discussed below.

Urgent treatment may sometimes have to precede establishment of a firm diagnosis. In up to 10% of patients, a precise diagnosis may never be made. This somewhat unsatisfactory state of affairs can be tolerated in younger patients since this group carries a good prognosis. Now that early gastroscopy is performed, it is found that many of the previous undiagnosed group have acute ulcers, erosions or so-called Mallory–Weiss (M–W) tears at the gastro-oesophageal junction caused by the trauma of repeated vomiting. These lesions will usually only be seen in the first 48 hours.

ESTABLISHING THAT GASTROINTESTINAL BLEEDING HAS OCCURRED

This is rarely in doubt, although patients can sometimes be remarkably uncertain as to whether blood has been coughed or vomited. Occasionally blood from the upper respiratory tract, for example from a nose bleed, may trickle into the pharynx. If the material produced is acid on testing, it strongly suggests a gastric origin, although in carcinoma of the stomach or acute erosion, there may be associated achlorhydria. Haematemeses are almost always associated with some degree of blood in the stools, from a frank tarry melaena to dark stools which give a positive reaction on testing for occult blood. A source of confusion here is the black stool associated with oral iron therapy or with bismuth-containing antacid tablets. As in all other fields of medicine there are malingerers who say they have vomited blood, or may go to some lengths to simulate it. Passage of fresh blood per rectum without haematemesis usually suggests a source in the colon or rectum.

CONSEQUENCES OF HAEMORRHAGE

The important factors are the amount of blood lost and the rate at which it is lost. The effectiveness of the patient's compensatory mechanisms will depend on age, and the extent of any associated cardiorespiratory and cerebrovascular disease. Acute blood loss may be superimposed on chronic.

Initially the problem is more one of reduction in circulating volume, i.e. shock, rather than impaired oxygen-carrying ability, i.e. anaemia. The more rapid the bleeding the more likely the patient is to present as haematemesis and, conversely, slower haemorrhage presents as melaena. In one series, patients presenting with haematemesis had twice the fatality rate of those presenting with melaena alone (12.0% versus 5.4%). By the time the adaptive mechanisms break down, with rapid pulse and fall in blood pressure, a young patient can have lost up to 50% of the circulating volume. After such a severe bleed, haemodilution occurs over the next 24 hours. This means that the initial haemoglobin concentration may be normal and will only be a true estimate of blood loss 24 hours after the event. By then, in the more severe cases, replacement by transfusion will have been initiated. In the absence of routine rapid and accurate blood volume estimation, the decision regarding transfusion is based on the age and condition of the patient (sweating, vasoconstricted), pulse rate (>100/minute), blood pressure (<100 mm Hg systolic or a postural drop >20 mm Hg). In addition an initial haemoglobin concentration below 10 g/dl is regarded as an indication for transfusion. There is a risk of overtransfusion and the precipitation of left heart failure and pulmonary oedema.

This is particularly so in the elderly, especially if previous anaemia has resulted in a high output state. In these patients it may be valuable not only to examine regularly the lung bases and jugular venous pressure, but to monitor the central venous pressure (CVP) during transfusion, adjusting the transfusion rate accordingly. Where rapid transfusion is required and the patient is bordering on heart failure, a short-acting diuretic such as frusemide should be given. Digoxin may also be needed, especially if atrial fibrillation is present. Transfusion will treat shock and prevent ischaemic damage to other organs. Cerebral infarction and myocardial infarction may, however, occur, and the characteristic pain of the latter may be obscured. A moderate rise in blood urea disproportionate to the creatinine is a common finding attributed to the 'protein meal' effect of blood in the gut. However, in addition, renal blood flow is reduced and, rarely, acute renal failure may occur. In a cirrhotic patient, bleeding from varices, there will be a reduction in hepatic blood flow. This together with the 'protein meal' may precipitate liver failure and portosystemic encephalopathy. Retinal ischaemia can cause acute changes resembling malignant hypertension, and may result in optic

Table 10.1 The prevalence and mortality of gastric and duodenal ulcer haemorrhage related to age

	Under 60 years		Over 60 years	
	No. of cases	deaths	No. of cases	deaths
Gastric ulcer	57	1 (1.8%)	98	25 (26%)
Duodenal ulcer	122	1 (0.8%)	88	9 (10.2%)

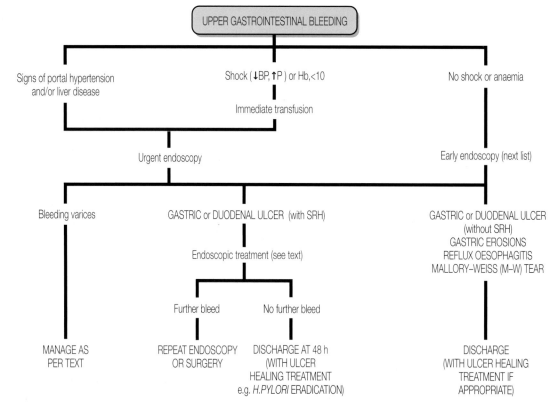

Fig. 10.1 A guide to the management of upper gastrointestinal bleeding.

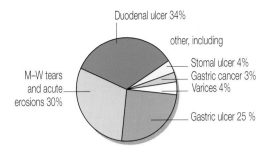

Fig. 10.2 Causes of gastrointestinal bleeding (excluding 10% undiagnosed).

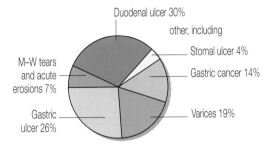

Fig. 10.3 Causes of fatal gastrointestinal bleeding.

atrophy. A further important reason for replacing blood loss, is that 15% to 20% of patients either continue to bleed or rebleed after admission, producing a dangerous deterioration in patients who have previously managed to compensate for the initial blood loss.

The other hazards of blood transfusion are well known. When large volumes of blood are transfused there is the additional risk of inducing a bleeding tendency. There are many related causes for this, such as reduction in clotting factors in stored blood and the binding of calcium by the citrate used as an anticoagulant. To prevent this, fresh frozen plasma may be necessary after large and rapid transfusions, especially in patients with cirrhosis with already impaired clotting factors and low platelets.

DIFFERENTIAL DIAGNOSIS

After establishing that gastrointestinal haemorrhage has occurred, blood should be taken for grouping, cross-matching (4 units), haemoglobin estimation and examination of the blood film. An intravenous infusion is set up at this stage using either saline to maintain access or colloid (gelatin) if the patient is shocked and awaiting blood transfusion. Before proceeding further a full history should be taken from patient and relatives and a complete examination must be performed to try

and establish the cause of bleeding as well as its effects. Although acute and chronic peptic ulcers (including the 25% presumed to be acute erosions) are responsible for 90% of admissions the less common causes comprising about 10% must always be considered, since specific treatment may be indicated.

Patients may give a history of preceding gastrointestinal symptoms, and some will have had a previous bleed, which will probably have been investigated resulting in a diagnosis of the underlying cause. However, a worrying trend in recent years with the increasing use of non-steroidal anti-inflammatory drugs (NSAIDs) in elderly arthritic patients is that the first manifestation of the presence of a peptic ulcer may be when it bleeds or perforates.

Duodenal ulcer

Some patients will give a history of epigastric pain occurring before meals, waking them at night, and relieved by food, milk, alkalis and belching. Ulcer pain often disappears when haemorrhage occurs; in fact if the patient continues to have severe or worsening pain after bleeding it should alert one to the relatively rare combination of events – haemorrhage and perforation. Other pointers to the diagnosis of duodenal ulcer are a positive past history, and a family history of the disorder. The patient's personality is often conscientious and ambitious, and there is frequently a history of recent stress.

Gastric ulcer

This is a much less common form of peptic ulcer than duodenal ulcer. However, gastric ulcers have a greater likelihood of bleeding, and constitute 25% of all cases of gastrointestinal bleeding, compared with duodenal ulcer which contributes 35% of all cases. Gastric ulcer occurs with greater frequency in the aged and this is a high risk group who might benefit from early surgery. Pain occurs usually after food, often making the patient afraid to eat and resulting in a loss of weight. Vomiting may relieve pain. When a gastric or duodenal ulcer is seen at early gastroscopy it may also reveal stigmata of recent haemorrhage (SRH), such as a visible vessel in the ulcer base, thrombus adherent to the ulcer or red spot within it. These indicate an increased risk of continuing or recurrent bleeding and would postpone the otherwise early discharge from hospital of low risk (of recurrence) patients.

Acute ulcers and erosions

A positive diagnosis can only be made by direct visualization by gastroscopy in the acute stage of the illness. The findings vary from a generalized haemorrhagic gastritis (diffuse gastrostaxis) to multiple or single acute superficial ulcers involving the gastric, duodenal or oesophageal mucosa. Only exceptionally is there a bleeding artery of significant size in the base of the ulcer, and there is unlikely to be further bleeding. Drugs and alcohol play an important part in causing acute erosions. Many patients will have taken one of the 40 prescribable aspirin preparations or, more likely, one of the many 'over the counter' remedies. While it may be argued that they would not have taken aspirin if they were not already feeling unwell, nonetheless the drug may be sufficient to convert simple indigestion into a haematemesis. NSAIDs, including aspirin, exert their beneficial anti-inflammatory analgesic effect by inhibiting prostaglandin synthetase. Unfortunately they simultaneously inhibit the synthesis of other prostanoids which have a cytoprotective effect on the gastric mucosa. Although a history of dyspepsia is a contraindication to anticoagulant therapy, this may be a cause of bleeding, either due to the prothrombin time getting out of control, or because of an associated gastric disturbance. In these patients vitamin K should be given in spite of a slight risk of rebound thrombosis from rapid reversal of anticoagulation.

In acute erosion there will usually be a history of a short period of preceding dyspepsia. The patient may have with him tablets or a steroid or anticoagulant clinic card. Examination will be noncontributory.

Oesophagitis

Reflux oesophagitis, often associated with a sliding hiatus hernia, is a recognized cause of iron deficiency anaemia due to chronic blood loss in obese elderly women. They frequently give little or no history of flatulent dyspepsia or acid regurgitation ('heartburn'). The problem of whether reflux oesophagitis causes acute bleeding can only be resolved by early gastroscopy, but it is probably unusual. Occasionally an ulcer may occur in the oesophagus of a patient with a sliding hiatus hernia, at the junction of secretory columnar epithelium and the normal squamous epithelium ('Barrett ulcer'). A rolling hiatus hernia with a fixed loculus above the diaphragm occurs less commonly but is more likely to bleed.

Mallory–Weiss syndrome

A tear occurs at the lower end of the oesophageal mucosa as a result of prolonged or severe vomiting. The point in the history which should arouse suspicion is that the patient has had a bout of vomiting, often after a drinking binge, or in the first trimester of pregnancy, but only at the end of the bout did the vomit contain fresh blood. A definite diagnosis can only be made by oesophagoscopy.

Stomal ulcer

Following both partial gastrectomy or vagotomy and pyloroplasty for bleeding from a peptic ulcer there is a risk of later bleeding in up to 5% of cases. This will usually be due to a stomal ulcer or recurrence of the original ulcer if left behind. A history of ulcer dyspepsia will generally be obtained, though surgery may have modified the location of the pain. The decline of elective and emergency gastric surgery makes this an increasingly uncommon cause.

Carcinoma of the stomach

This was formerly thought to be a cause of chronic rather than acute blood loss. However it is presenting more frequently as a cause of acute haemorrhage, particularly in the over 60s. The history will resemble that of gastric ulcer, with anorexia and weight loss, though pain may be less prominent. Examination may reveal an epigastric mass and sometimes an enlarged left supraclavicular node of Virchow. Diagnosis is by gastroscopy and biopsy. Biopsy should be undertaken in every gastric ulcer, however benign in appearance. If the ulcer is actively bleeding or shows SRH, biopsy may have to be deferred until the danger of rebleeding is receding after 48 hours, or until the mandatory follow-up endoscopy is carried out after a 4-week course of ulcer-healing treatment.

Gastro-oesophageal varices

The underlying portal hypertension is, in the majority of cases, due to cirrhosis of the liver with alcoholic cirrhosis a more common cause than postviral cirrhosis in the western world. There is a raised incidence of peptic ulcer in cirrhotics, especially in alcoholic and biliary cirrhosis. One must not therefore automatically attribute haematemesis to bleeding varices in a patient with cirrhosis but, nonetheless, assume it is the cause until proved otherwise!

Extrahepatic portal hypertension occurs rarely and is due to portal vein obstruction. This may date from infancy, following thrombosis of the portal vein due to umbilical sepsis, or be acquired as a result of malignant involvement from hepatoma or pancreatic carcinoma. Other causes are polycythaemia, cirrhosis itself, or portal pyaemia, for example due to an appendix abscess. Hepatic fibrosis due to schistosomiasis carries a better prognosis when bleeding occurs, because there is generally much better liver function. This is a major determinant in the outcome of variceal bleeding and is reflected in the different prognoses in the Child–Pugh grading (Table 10.2).

Haematemesis may be the first symptom in a cirrhotic patient, or there may be a history of chronic

Table 10.2 Child–Pugh grading of severity of cirrhosis at time of admission with variceal haemorrhage related to prognosis

	Score 1 pt	Score 2 pts	Score 3 pts
Bilirubin (µmol/l)	17–34	35–50	>51
Prolongation prothrombin time (sec)	1–4	5–6	7+
Albumin (g/l)	>35	28–34	<28
Ascites	None	Mild	Moderate/ severe
Portosystemic encephalopathy (grade)	0	1–2	3–4

Grade A (5–6 points) carries a 5% mortality during an admission for acute variceal bleeding compared with 20% mortality in grade B (7–9 points) and over 40% mortality in grade C (10–15 points)

ill health, oedema, and ascites. Whatever the cause of the portal hypertension, the spleen will nearly always be enlarged and usually be palpable, and collateral vessels may be seen in the abdominal wall. The liver need not be enlarged and, indeed, is often small and fibrosed. Other signs of hepatocellular damage such as palmar erythema, leuconychia, spider naevi, gynaecomastia, testicular atrophy, parotid enlargement and Dupuytren's contractures may be present. Ascites and jaundice indicate a bad prognosis. Careful and repeated neuropsychiatric assessment must be made for signs of portosystemic encephalopathy. Hepatic fetor is frequently masked by the equally unpleasant smell of altered blood. Mechanisms initiating haemorrhage are not clearly understood but may be related to intravariceal pressure. Immediate gastroscopy is essential to confirm this high-risk condition and initiate appropriate specific treatment (see below).

Rare causes of haemorrhage

Blood disorders such as thrombocytopenia, haemophilia and Von Willebrand's disease may cause upper gastrointestinal bleeding. One should look for purpura. Leukaemia can cause thrombocytopenia or portal vein thrombosis but may also cause gastric bleeding by infiltration and ulceration of the stomach. Inherited disorders include pseudoxanthoma elasticum, where the elastic tissue defect not only weakens vessel walls but is also responsible for the 'plucked chicken' appearance of the skin of the neck and angioid streaks in the retina. In the related Ehlers–Danlos syndrome there is a defect of supporting tissue which also pre-

disposes to haemorrhage; there may be characteristic hyperextensibility of the skin with delayed recoil. Hereditary haemorrhagic telangiectasia and multiple angiomas usually give rise to chronic blood loss. Similarly acute haemorrhage, except in children, is unusual in the Peutz–Jegher syndrome (intestinal polyposis associated with pigmentation of the lips). Diverticula of the gut rarely bleed massively with the exception of a Meckel's diverticulum, which may contain ectopic gastric mucosa which has ulcerated. Severe haemorrhage can occur in this condition and will present as melaena only.

FURTHER MANAGEMENT IN ACUTE AND CHRONIC ULCERS

Further management requires close collaboration with surgical colleagues who, in all but trivial bleeds, should see the patient jointly with the physician early on in the admission. Even though only a minority of patients will come to surgery (less than 20%) the surgeon will be able to make a baseline assessment before the patient has been resuscitated and sedated. Where the patient is over 60 and gives a clear past history of gastric or duodenal ulcer, with, perhaps, previous haemorrhage, SRH are present and transfusion exceeds 6 units, the case for surgery will be strong. It is preferable to operate electively after the bleeding has stopped, but the surgeon will also be prepared to go ahead if bleeding persists or recurs, especially if the patient's blood group makes further supplies of blood uncertain. In these circumstances when emergency surgery is indicated, delay and continuing massive transfusion increases the mortality. When similar situations arise in younger patients there is more reluctance to undertake surgery. However, though the vessels in the ulcer bed may not be as arteriosclerotic as in the elderly, scarring rather than healing is the best that is likely to occur, and there remains the likelihood that the patient may bleed again in the future.

The patient in whom there is not a clear-cut indication of the underlying pathology presents a problem should bleeding continue or recur. It is now common practice to gastroscope most patients with acute bleeding to try and make an early diagnosis. Gastroscopy is superior to radiology in that it is more accurate and the site of bleeding can be positively identified. It is particularly valuable when there is more than one possible source of blood loss and in detecting the sizeable number of bleeders who have gastric erosions in whom, in the past, radiology would have been negative. The need for surgery and risk of rebleeding is reduced by therapeutic endoscopy with laser, thermal or electrocoagulation of the bleeding point or its injection with adrenaline, to vasoconstrict, plus a sclerosant.

FURTHER MANAGEMENT IN BLEEDING VARICES

Apart from the basic problem of blood replacement there are two further objectives: stopping the bleeding and preventing hepatic coma.

The prothrombin time may be prolonged in cirrhosis and, although this is usually due to hepatocellular damage rather than to shortage of vitamin K, the latter should none the less be given parenterally. Glypressin and nitrates or octreotide (a somatostatin analogue) or balloon tamponade for not more than 24 hours, may temporarily arrest bleeding and 'buy time' to prepare for more definitive treatment of the varices by sclerotherapy or banding if this is not used as a first measure.

Treatment and prevention of hepatic coma requires emptying of the bowel of blood by means of lactulose and perhaps suppression of colonic bacteria by oral neomycin, with maintenance of both circulation and nutrition by transfusion and infusion of concentrated dextrose into a large vein.

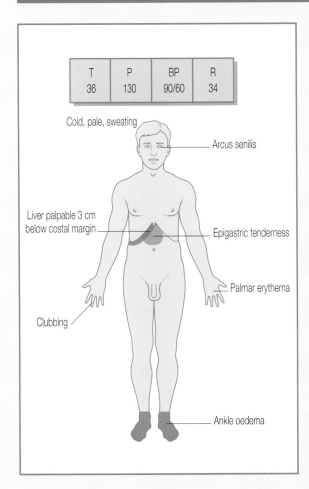

T	P	BP	R
36	130	90/60	34

Cold, pale, sweating

Arcus senilis

Liver palpable 3 cm
below costal margin

Epigastric tenderness

Palmar erythema

Clubbing

Ankle oedema

drinking although he agreed he was sociable! He smoked 30 cigarettes daily. He weighed 90 kg.

He had had winter bronchitis for the past 6 years. Four years previously he had been admitted to hospital with jaundice for 2 weeks and had been advised to reduce his alcohol consumption.

On examination, he was shocked, restless and pale; his blood pressure was 105/70, and pulse 115/minute regular. There was a marked arcus senilis but no jaundice. The JVP was not raised, although he had moderate pitting oedema of both ankles. In the chest there were scattered rhonchi but no crepitations. He had early clubbing of the fingers and palmar erythema. The abdomen was markedly obese and the spleen could not be felt. The liver edge was palpable 3 cm below the costal margin, seemed smooth and regular in outline and was not tender. There was diffuse tenderness in the epigastrium but no rebound tenderness. Ascites could not be detected. Melaena stool was present on rectal examination.

Haemoglobin was 9.6 g/dl and the film showed hypochromia and anisocytosis. He was transfused 3 units of blood over the next 6 hours. His pulse fell to 85/minute and his BP rose to 140/80.

One hour later the house physician was recalled to the ward because the patient had suddenly begun to complain of severe pain in the upper abdomen and lower chest. He now looked very ill, the skin being cold and pale. He was sweating profusely. The pulse was 130/minute, regular but thready. The BP was 90/60 and there was rapid shallow breathing. In the abdomen there was marked epigastric tenderness but bowel sounds were present.

An obese 55-year-old publican was admitted at 2 a.m. on a Saturday morning, having vomited a large quantity of fresh and altered blood 4 hours previously. He gave a history of increasingly severe epigastric pain over the previous 3 days. This occurred immediately after meals and on two occasions he had vomited his recent meal with relief of his pain.

For the previous 6 months he had had mild upper abdominal discomfort; his appetite had deteriorated and he had lost about 7 kg in weight. He denied excessive

Questions

1. What is the likely cause for his initial admission to hospital?
2. What might be the reason for his deterioration in hospital?
3. What other underlying diseases may be present?
4. How would you now manage the patient?

Discussion

The gastrointestinal haemorrhage is most likely to have arisen from a simple gastric ulcer. The symptoms of anorexia, weight loss and post-prandial pain could also occur with gastric carcinoma but this is less likely to cause massive bleeding. The pattern of symptoms is not typical of a duodenal ulcer. An acute gastric erosion, as may occur after alcohol, could bleed in this way but is less likely in view of the 6-month history of symptoms. The low haemoglobin on admission might be due to recent massive blood loss but the presence of hypochromia and anisocytosis on the blood film suggests that there has also been chronic bleeding. His occupation, past history, hepatomegaly, clubbing and palmar erythema all suggest that he may have alcoholic cirrhosis. However, there are no signs of portal hypertension such as splenomegaly to suggest bleeding from oesophageal varices. The presence of cirrhosis would also increase the likelihood of a peptic ulcer.

His further deterioration might be due to recurrence of bleeding. However, there has been no further haematemesis and the development of severe pain after haemorrhage would be most unusual. Indeed it should alert one to the possibility of perforation of an ulcer. Acute pancreatitis, perhaps precipitated by alcohol, can closely mimic ulcer perforation, but the pain frequently radiates to the back and is accompanied by vomiting. In either case, bowel sounds may continue to be heard or even be exaggerated until they disappear several hours later.

Myocardial infarction could also explain his later sudden collapse, and is a recognized complication of massive haemorrhage. Underlying coronary artery disease may be present but may have been previously asymptomatic. Although the pain of myocardial infarction may be poorly localized, the presence of epigastric tenderness is against this diagnosis. The clinical picture is compatible with massive pulmonary embolism but this is an unlikely complication at this stage, and there is no evidence of an underlying deep vein thrombosis.

The most likely diagnosis is a perforated and bleeding gastric ulcer which will require urgent surgical treatment. Investigation must therefore be immediately relevant and rapid. A straight X-ray of the abdomen is likely to be diagnostic by showing gas under the diaphragm. An ECG would probably be done even though it cannot exclude a myocardial infarction. The patient will require further intravenous fluid to resuscitate him sufficiently to allow surgery. In view of the pain which he has now developed, once the decision to undertake laparotomy had been made he would be given an analgesic such as diamorphine.

At laparotomy he was found to have bled from a lesser curve chronic benign gastric ulcer which had perforated into the lesser sac. He also had micronodular cirrhosis without evidence of portal hypertension. The ulcer was sutured but despite vigorous resuscitation he died 12 hours post-operatively.

11

Acute abdominal pain

The 'acute abdomen' does not always find its way to the surgical ward. Even when it does, it may be for a reason not requiring surgery. None the less the problem of making an early diagnosis is sharpened by the knowledge that undue delay in removing a gangrenous appendix, suturing a perforated ulcer or relieving an obstructed bowel may seriously endanger the patient's life. Although delay in operating may be dangerous it can be equally harmful, for example in pancreatitis, to perform an unnecessary laparotomy.

The temptation to relieve what is often very distressing pain with opiates or other potent analgesics must also be resisted, until a diagnosis or the decision to perform a laparotomy has been made. Premature treatment in response to the patient's urgent appeals for relief of pain may irretrievably cloud the symptoms and signs on which a diagnosis can be made. Another treatment which may also modify the clinical picture is long-term steroid therapy.

Previous surgery may lead to unusual presentations of abdominal disease. Thus the pain of recurrent or stomal ulcer may have quite a different site and characteristics from that of the original peptic ulcer which was treated surgically. Other complications of previous surgery include intestinal obstruction from adhesions or the symptoms of dumping or afferent loop obstruction following partial gastrectomy.

A multiplicity of scars and a history of repeated emergency admissions, often in someone who is without job or family, should alert one to the Munchausen syndrome of malingering. Unless such a person can be positively identified, medicolegal considerations require giving the benefit of the doubt.

The more common categories of abdominal pain, and their causes, are discussed below.

COLIC

Colic is a true visceral pain arising from the affected viscus and created by tension or spasm of the smooth muscle in its wall. Because it is often an exaggeration of the inherent peristaltic activity of the organ it is often taught that colic frequently builds up to a peak, fades and then recurs in cycles. This is by no means always the case, especially when it is renal or biliary in origin. Pressure over the painful area sometimes gives a little relief and may be the basis for the patient's restlessness. He may draw his legs up, twist or even walk about. In all cases of colic – renal, biliary or intestinal – there is obstruction to pelvis or ureter, cystic or common bile duct, or the gut.

Renal colic

The commonest cause is a stone lodged either at the pelviureteric junction or, more usually, in the course of the ureter, especially near the vesicoureteric junction. If there is gross bleeding from a kidney into the pelvicalyceal system, blood clots may cause colic. It is said that obstruction of the pelviureteric junction can be caused by pressure from an aberrant renal artery, but it is usually due to an ill-understood neuromuscular abnormality resulting in spasm at this point. In this latter condition episodes of colic may occur during the diuresis that follows a large and rapidly ingested water load.

The characteristics of renal colic are distinctive. The pain begins in the loin and, if ureteric colic follows renal colic as it usually does, radiates round the flank into the groin, testicle or labia, and thigh. The patient is prostrated by the pain and may vomit, while there is often associated pallor, sweating and tachycardia. Depending on the cause there may be a residual dull ache in the loin between acute attacks, which can last several hours. The urine will usually show some abnormal constituents such as red cells, or sometimes pus cells or protein. In most cases of renal stone there is no underlying disease detectable, but hyperparathyroidism or hypercalcaemia from some other cause should always be searched for. Some have idiopathic hypercalciuria. An emergency IVP is the most useful investigation, particularly to demonstrate pelviureteric obstruction, as this is usually intermittent. An acute attack of pyelonephritis often causes renal pain, but this is more constant and is associated with frequency, dysuria and pyuria, together with considerable constitutional disturbances such as high fever and rigors. Other conditions that may cause pain resembling renal colic are retrocaecal appendicitis, pancreatitis and gallbladder disease.

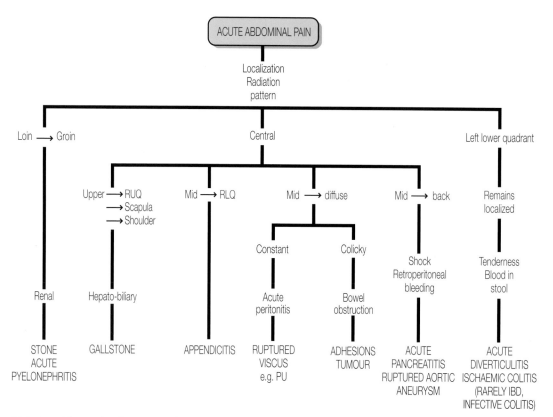

Fig. 11.1 A guide to the diagnosis of acute abdominal pain.

Biliary colic

This may be the first manifestation of the presence of gallstones. In an uncomplicated case a severe pain of sudden onset is felt in the epigastrium or under the right costal margin. It may follow a large meal but frequently there is no obvious cause. Nausea, vomiting and restlessness accompany it as it builds up over 10–40 minutes and there may be radiation of the pain to the right scapula. If the stone is not passed or does not drop back into the gallbladder from Hartmann's pouch, where it is frequently lodged, infection of the retained bile may occur and acute cholecystitis supervenes (Fig. 11.2). There will then be fever, marked tenderness over the gallbladder, especially on inspiration, and possibly pain in the shoulder tip. This pain is referred to this site because the inflamed overlying parietal peritoneum is innervated by the phrenic nerve derived mainly from C4. A mild degree of obstructive jaundice may occur in half the patients where the stone reaches the common bile duct. The obstruction is not usually complete but if the stone is not passed, ascending cholangitis may supervene with a hectic fever and rigors. Back pressure of bile will then cause

the liver to enlarge. Jaundice may also occur in acute cholecystitis. The cause is not clear but it is possible that the inflammatory mass may directly affect the adjacent liver or exert pressure on the hepatic or common bile ducts (Mirizzi's syndrome). Previous cholecystectomy by no means guarantees future freedom from further gallstones, colic, or jaundice, since stones may form in the stump of the divided cystic duct or in the hepatic ducts. When colic is accompanied by jaundice this is a valuable clue to its cause. In the absence of bilirubinuria or elevation of the serum bilirubin, other diagnoses must be considered – renal colic, pancreatitis, perforated peptic ulcer, myocardial infarction, appendicitis and upper intestinal colic for example. Plain X-ray of the abdomen is of little value because only 10–15% of gallstones are opaque; it has been superseded by abdominal ultrasound scanning as the initial investigation (Fig. 11.3).

Intestinal colic

Intestinal colic is the cardinal symptom of intestinal obstruction. It is the pain that is most likely to be truly colicky in nature, with freedom from pain between bouts. When due to small bowel obstruction in a thin person, visible peristalsis may be seen to coincide with the colic and loud borborygmi are heard simultaneously. The pain is usually situated in the centre of the abdomen, or slightly lower in the case of large bowel obstruction. Although colicky at the outset it may become more constant, particularly if strangulation or infarction of the bowel supervenes. Vomiting is an early feature of small intestinal obstruction and it may later become faeculent. Although absolute constipation must ultimately occur it may be preceded by diarrhoea. Circulatory effects such as tachycardia, hypotension, dehydration and peripheral circulatory failure result from hypovolaemia, due to large volumes of fluid sequestered in the lumen of the obstructed bowel, and to absorbed toxins.

The many possible causes of mechanical obstruction must be considered when examining the usually distended abdomen. Any previous abdominal operation could be a source of adhesions. External hernial orifices must be carefully checked and particular attention paid to the femoral triangle. A femoral hernia occurs particularly in thin elderly women, and the tender lump below the inguinal ligament may either not be seen, due to shyness on the part of the patient matched by reticence in the doctor, or it may be misdiagnosed as a tender lymph node. Other internal mechanical causes may be confined to particular age groups. The commonest cause of intestinal obstruction in children is intussusception, the pathognomonic features being the sudden onset of pain with screaming, flexing of the thighs and vomiting, and the presence of a sausage-shaped tumour. Blood may be passed in the stool, or found on rectal examination. In the elderly intestinal obstruction may be caused by volvulus due to twisting of a long redundant pelvic colon on its mesentery. Initially the swelling may be localized to the left side of the abdomen. Strangulation of the

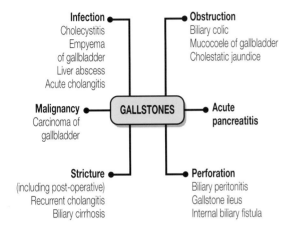

Fig. 11.2 The complications of gallstones.

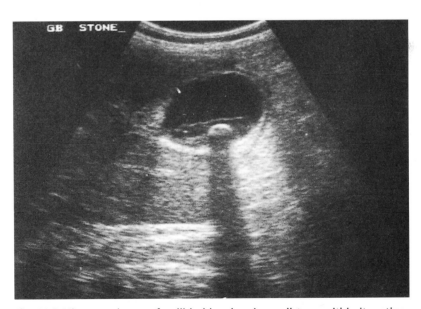

Fig. 11.3 Ultrasound scan of gallbladder showing gallstone within it casting a characteristic acoustic shadow. The gallbladder also contains 'sludge' and its wall is thickened, suggesting that episodes of cholecystitis have occurred. (Courtesy of Dr Hakhamaneshi.)

obstructed loop progressing to gangrene is a dangerous complication.

Carcinoma of the distal colon may present acutely as large bowel obstruction without much previous history. Other causes of stricture such as Crohn's disease, tuberculosis or lymphoma, particularly when affecting the ileum, usually cause subacute obstruction over a period and are associated with other signs of the underlying disease. Obstruction from within the lumen is an unlikely event. Gallstone ileus appears in every list of differential diagnosis but rarely in reality. Following a gastrojejunostomy the possibility of bolus obstruction arises, for example by a segment of an orange.

Patients with underlying cardiovascular disease, such as rheumatic mitral stenosis with recent onset of atrial fibrillation, recent myocardial infarction with mural thrombus, or widespread atherosclerosis, are candidates for mesenteric artery occlusion by embolism or thrombus. Infarction of the bowel with signs of obstruction will occur. The pain is continuous rather than colicky, the patient is shocked and blood is passed per rectum. The most common site of occlusion is the superior mesenteric artery affecting the small bowel.

The most valuable investigation in making a diagnosis of intestinal obstruction is a straight X-ray of the abdomen. Taken in the erect position it should show fluid levels in the small intestine as well as gas. The gas shadow pattern may help to localize the site of the obstruction. The gas shadow caused by the most distal loop of obstructed bowel cannot always be identified with confidence (Fig. 11.4).

Intestinal colic may be caused by a functional disturbance, such as spastic colon. The pain may be of sufficient severity to mimic other causes of acute abdominal pain.

Ischaemic colitis

Ischaemic colitis, affecting the region of the splenic flexure, which is the watershed area between the superior and inferior mesenteric artery, is a condition which is becoming more frequently recognized. In its most severe form there is large bowel obstruction due to infarction of the full thickness of the bowel with rapid deterioration and circulatory collapse due to toxaemia and septicaemia. Blood will be present in the stool. Plain abdominal X-ray may show evidence of obstruction together with a thumb-print or cobblestone appearance within the colonic lumen due to oedema of the mucosa. In less severe episodes, where the bowel muscle is preserved, shedding of the oedematous devitalized mucosa gives rise to acute bloody diarrhoea and pain, mimicking inflammatory or infective bowel disease; during healing the partly ischaemic

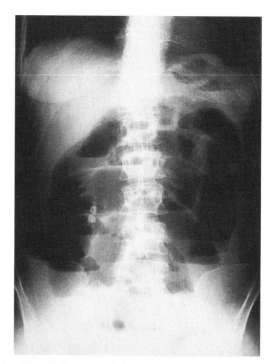

Fig. 11.4 Plain erect abdominal X-ray of a middle-aged woman presenting with acute central abdominal pain, distension and vomiting. Numerous fluid levels are seen in dilated loops of small intestine which was obstructed due to old adhesions. The dense opacities to the right of L4–5 are calcified lymph nodes. (Courtesy of Dr Hakhamaneshi.)

muscle may be replaced by lengthy fibrous strictures, typically in the region of the splenic flexure (Fig. 12.2A, p. 88).

Appendicitis

This is the commonest cause of acute abdominal pain. The classical textbook description is of central abdominal pain, often with colicky features, shifting after a few hours to the right iliac fossa. There is associated nausea, vomiting and slight rise in temperature. Initially there is localized tenderness with guarding in the right lower quadrant. When the overlying parietal peritoneum becomes inflamed, guarding and rebound tenderness can be elicited. Unfortunately less than half the patients present in such a characteristic fashion. Frequently the pain is right-sided from the outset. Depending on the position of the appendix, the signs may be most marked on rectal examination (pelvic appendix) or in the loin (retrocaecal appendix). Delay in diagnosis may result, and in a case of obstructive appendicitis where the lumen is blocked by a faecolith, perforation may occur as the rising intraluminal pres-

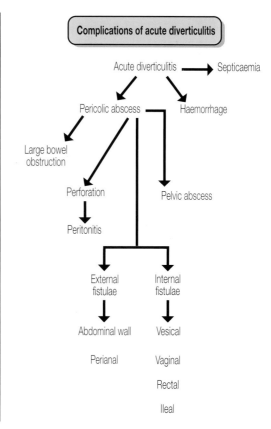

Fig. 11.5 The complications of appendicitis and acute diverticulitis.

sure leads to gangrene of the wall of the appendix. This will cause either local abscess formation, when a tender mass becomes palpable, or generalized peritonitis with abdominal pain, rigidity and distension, and loss of bowel sounds (Fig. 11.5).

The differential diagnosis includes right-sided pyelonephritis, renal colic, cholecystitis, or, in a woman, right-sided salpingitis, ruptured ectopic pregnancy or a twisted ovarian cyst. These additional gynaecological causes help to explain the higher proportion of incorrect diagnoses in women than men undergoing laparotomy for suspected acute appendicitis. Some young children in whom laparotomy is performed have a normal appendix removed. There may be some enlargement of neighbouring lymph nodes and a diagnosis, in retrospect, of mesenteric adenitis is made. There is no sure way of making the diagnosis prospectively and avoiding operation.

There are no specific investigations which confirm the diagnosis of appendicitis, though a leucocytosis and a sterile pyuria may be present. Atypical presentations are particularly dangerous in the aged and young. The condition is less common at the extremes of age but when it does occur is more likely to be misdiagnosed and thus have a worse prognosis.

Diverticulitis

Colonic diverticula, particularly in the sigmoid colon, are found with increasing frequency after the age of 40. In the majority of patients they are asymptomatic, the condition being termed diverticulosis. Some patients may have alternating diarrhoea and constipation with grumbling left-sided abdominal pain, this stage being designated diverticular disease. Other patients, either after a history of diverticular disease or having been symptom-free, develop acute diverticulitis. This has been likened to left-sided appendicitis with severe left iliac fossa pain, nausea, vomiting, fever and constipation. Local pericolic abscess formation may occur and blood and pus may be passed per rectum. Such an abscess, if it ruptures, rarely causes generalized peritonitis as the local inflammatory reaction and neighbouring organs wall it off. This may result in fistulae to the bladder or vagina. Ischiorectal abscess may form and result in a fistula to the surface (Fig. 11.5).

Acute peritonitis

This may be a complication of acute infection such as acute appendicitis, diverticulitis or septic abortion. It will rarely be the first symptom in any of these situations. An important and common cause is perforation of a peptic ulcer. Often there will be a history of epigastric pain following food, sometimes making the patient afraid to eat, suggesting a gastric ulcer. Alternatively there may be hunger pain, pain between meals, and pain waking the patient in the early hours, suggesting a duodenal ulcer. However, with the increased use of non-steroidal anti-inflammatory drugs (NSAIDs) for arthritis, a patient may present with bleeding or perforation of an ulcer without any preceding symptoms to indicate its presence. The sudden onset of severe upper abdominal pain is accompanied by intense, 'board-like' rigidity of the abdominal wall and great reluctance by the patient to make any movement. Vomiting may occur and result in the patient being referred to hospital as a haematemesis. Although pain may precede bleeding it is most unusual for it to persist and if it does so, should raise the possibility of the dangerous, but fortunately rare, combination of bleeding and perforation (see Clinical Problem, Ch. 10). Following the initial pain and shock some patients may appear to improve over the next few hours, though signs of abdominal rigidity, tachypnoea and tachycardia persist. Generalized peritonitis will usually develop after about 5 hours. Even though there may be little vomiting the patient will be dehydrated and haemoconcentrated due to the large outpouring of fluid into the peritoneal cavity. The resulting shock and hypotension may lead to the patient being nursed with the foot of the bed raised, which in turn will cause irritation of the diaphragm by the inflammatory exudate draining upwards. Signs of this will be shoulder-tip pain and often hiccups. A plain X-ray of the abdomen in the erect position (to show gas beneath the diaphragm) is the crucial investigation.

Various non-surgical conditions, like myocardial infarction, basal pneumonia, sickling crisis in HbS disease, diabetic ketoacidosis, diabetic crisis or acute porphyria, may enter the differential diagnosis in a less typical case, apart from many other of the causes of acute abdominal pain already discussed. One further condition that requires urgent surgery is a ruptured ectopic gestation. Shock may be great as rapid exsanguination can occur. There is often a tender mass in the pouch of Douglas on rectal examination and a blood-stained vaginal discharge. A history of a missed period may not always be forthcoming. A rare sign is of bluish discoloration around the umbilicus due to retroperitoneal tracking of blood from the retroperitoneal space (Cullen's sign).

Acute pancreatitis

This condition is characterized by severe upper abdominal pain which may radiate to the back. Although some fluid loss may occur due to vomiting, large internal losses from the acutely inflamed, and sometimes haemorrhagic, pancreas may occur. In addition there is release of vasoactive peptides into the circulation. A profound state of shock results.

On examination the abdomen is not as rigid and tender as in the peritonitis of a perforated ulcer – which is the main differential diagnosis. The bluish discoloration around the umbilicus or in the flanks due to retroperitoneal bleeding is rarely seen. Most identified cases in Britain are due to gallstones with alcohol the next most common cause; 20% of cases remain idiopathic.

An elevated serum amylase is the best diagnostic test available but has the limitation that it is also raised in many of the other causes of acute abdominal pain discussed above. The elevation may be transient but values above 1000 units are strongly suggestive of acute pancreatitis when the normal upper limit is 280 units.

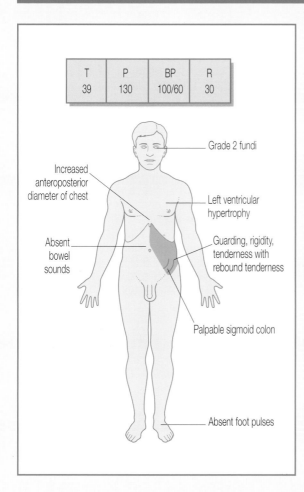

T	P	BP	R
39	130	100/60	30

Grade 2 fundi

Increased anteroposterior diameter of chest

Left ventricular hypertrophy

Absent bowel sounds

Guarding, rigidity, tenderness with rebound tenderness

Palpable sigmoid colon

Absent foot pulses

vomited and the fluid contained bile, but no blood. He had passed a liquid stool containing fresh and altered blood.

He had had increasingly severe chronic bronchitis for some years, which now limited his exercise tolerance to one flight of stairs or 200 yards on the flat. With this amount of effort he would also develop constricting central chest pain. This followed a myocardial infarction 6 years previously. At the age of 28 he had had an appendicectomy.

He had been constipated for many years and had haemorrhoids which sometimes bled. During the last two years he had lost 4 kg in weight.

On examination he was febrile, sweating, and appeared dehydrated. T 39°C. In the cardiovascular system he had a BP of 100/60 and a tachycardia of 130/min regular with a poor volume pulse. The foot pulses and left popliteal pulse were not palpable. The fundi showed AV nipping with narrowing and tortuosity of the arteries. There was left ventricular hypertrophy but no signs of heart failure. Examination of the chest showed evidence of emphysema, but there were no signs of acute infection. The abdomen was not distended but there was marked tenderness and rebound tenderness on the left side. Palpation was difficult because of localized guarding and rigidity. The sigmoid colon could be felt in the left iliac fossa but was only slightly tender. Bowel sounds were absent, and no bruits could be heard. The hernial orifices were clear. There was a midline lower abdominal scar. On rectal examination there were no masses or tenderness but there was both fresh and altered blood present without pus or mucus.

A 73-year-old retired printer had lived alone for 2 years since the death of his wife. He was admitted to hospital complaining of left-sided abdominal pain, bloody diarrhoea and vomiting which had begun abruptly 6 hours previously. At first the pain had fluctuated but became constant later. The pain was not relieved when he

Questions

1. What is the probable cause of his presenting symptoms?
2. What immediate investigations would help in diagnosis and management?

Discussion

The most likely causes of his abdominal symptoms are ischaemic colitis, acute diverticulitis or carcinoma of the colon, each causing large bowel obstruction. Ischaemic colitis is especially common in this age group and to support this diagnosis he has evidence of both peripheral vascular disease and coronary artery disease. In addition, although his present blood pressure is low, the presence of left ventricular hypertrophy and Grade II retinopathy indicate that he was previously hypertensive. The signs of fever, tenderness and bloody diarrhoea are all compatible with infarction of the bowel, and suggest that this is present in addition to obstruction. It is very likely that a constipated old man will have some degree of diverticular disease but the onset of his symptoms and the rapid deterioration argue against the diagnosis of acute diverticulitis. Carcinoma of the colon may present with large bowel obstruction, but the abrupt onset and marked tenderness with rebound are against this diagnosis. A sigmoid volvulus is common in old people, and strangulation may be present from the start, but rectal bleeding is not a feature. Furthermore, in this patient there is no abdominal distension such as would usually be present.

Other causes of bloody diarrhoea, such as ulcerative colitis or Crohn's disease, would not present for the first time with signs of peritonitis. Bacillary dysentery would not explain the peritonitis and there is no pus in the stool. Other causes of acute peritonitis such as a perforated peptic ulcer or diverticulum would not cause bloody diarrhoea.

A straight abdominal X-ray is likely to confirm the diagnosis of large bowel obstruction and may also show evidence of the mucosal oedema sometimes seen in ischaemic colitis, even on the plain film. Blood culture should be taken. An ECG is important as it may show a recent silent myocardial infarction which could be a source of systemic embolism. However, none of these measures should delay the immediate preparation of the patient for emergency laparotomy. This will include taking blood for grouping and cross-matching of at least 4 pints of blood. The haematocrit, urea and electrolytes would also be estimated. An intravenous infusion line would be set up and his dehydration treated with normal saline while the blood was awaited. In an elderly man with ischaemic heart disease it would be especially valuable to set up a central venous pressure line to control the rate of intravenous infusion and so prevent pulmonary oedema. Blood cultures should be taken before starting broad spectrum antibiotics (a combination of gentamycin, cloxacillin and metronidazole is widely used) and intravenous hydrocortisone could also be given (see Ch. 5 for treatment of septic shock).

At laparotomy there was an extensive infarction of the transverse and descending colon with widespread thrombotic occlusions of the branches of the inferior mesenteric artery. Despite resection of the infarcted bowel he died 24 hours later.

12

Change in bowel habit

Many serious or unpleasant diseases vie for the title of the English Disease, but perhaps national pride prevents its application to constipation. There is no doubt that a morbid preoccupation with the bowels leading to injudicious and sometimes ferocious purgation can promote and perpetuate symptoms, thereby causing considerable anxiety or actual harm. As with most hobbies there is a large market to cater for the public's needs and indeed to encourage them with appeals for the need to achieve 'inner cleanliness'. Fact, as opposed to folklore, is hard to come by in establishing the norms of bowel habit. Surveys have shown that in 99% of normal people defaecation occurs between thrice daily and once every 3 days.

As with all presenting symptoms the patient's self-diagnosis of constipation or diarrhoea must not be accepted without a full description of the complaint being obtained. Much more significance should be attached to a recent change in bowel habit than to a very long history of diarrhoea or constipation. As always, the associated symptoms are vital in distinguishing between the various causes. Physical examination, including inspection of the stool, rectal examination, proctoscopy and sigmoidoscopy must always be undertaken before embarking on more detailed investigation. A malpractice which is still very common is to order a barium enema without prior sigmoidoscopy. A normal radiological appearance in no way excludes a carcinoma of the rectum, as the region proximal to the rectosigmoid junction cannot be confidently visualized radiographically. Rectal examination and sigmoidoscopy are therefore the means of establishing this diagnosis.

It is the functional nature of many bowel disorders that makes this particular symptom complex such a treacherous field. Unfortunately much teaching ignores this, so that the diagnosis of irritable bowel syndrome (IBS) is made by exclusion only. This can result in many unnecessary radiological examinations and other investigations which tend to reinforce the patient's view that there is some serious underlying cause. It may culminate in the rather negative reassurance that the clinician 'can find nothing wrong'. It is therefore important to make a positive diagnosis of a functional disorder, and to follow this by an explanation to the patient of the mechanism of the production of his symptoms. The patient can then be advised of the necessary modifications to everyday life, and supportive drug therapy given if needed.

Since diarrhoea and constipation frequently coexist both in functional disorders, like the irritable bowel syndrome, and organic lesions, such as carcinoma of the sigmoid, the two symptoms will be dealt with together rather than separately. Furthermore, acute causes of diarrhoea, such as dysentery, gastroenteritis, food poisoning and cholera, and acute constipation due to obstruction or dehydration, will not be specifically discussed here.

PATHOPHYSIOLOGY OF THE COLON

Steatorrhoea due to the various causes of malabsorption syndrome is dealt with in detail in Ch. 13. This group of disorders can usually be distinguished from other forms of diarrhoea by inspection of the stools. These are typically pale grey or putty-coloured, soft, bulky and greasy, or when associated with pancreatic disease, may contain oil droplets. They are offensive and tend to float in the lavatory pan, requiring repeated flushings. The patient invariably loses weight and has evidence of various nutritional deficiencies of which anaemia, which may be megaloblastic, is the commonest. Some of the mechanisms responsible for steatorrhoea give insight into the functioning of the colon.

The prime activity of the colon is the absorption of water from the liquid contents entering the caecum, thereby creating the semisolid stool evacuated from the rectum. Absorption of water and electrolytes is not as effective or as rapid as in the small intestine. If the small intestine fails to reabsorb fully the daily 7 litres of gut secretions, and the products of digestion entering it, this will present an excessive load for the colon. The large bowel normally reabsorbs 500 ml and has a reserve capacity to reabsorb about 3 litres of water. The nature of the material entering the colon will also influence its function. Bile salts that have not been reabsorbed in the terminal ileum act as irritants, and indeed have been used therapeutically as purgatives. Unabsorbed sugars undergo fermentation to lactic acid by colonic bacteria. The lowered pH increases the frequency of defaecation and may promote a change in the bacterial flora to lactobacilli; this forms the rationale for the use of the non-absorbable sugar lactulose, as a laxative. Likewise the unabsorbed products of fat digestion have an irritant action on the bowel.

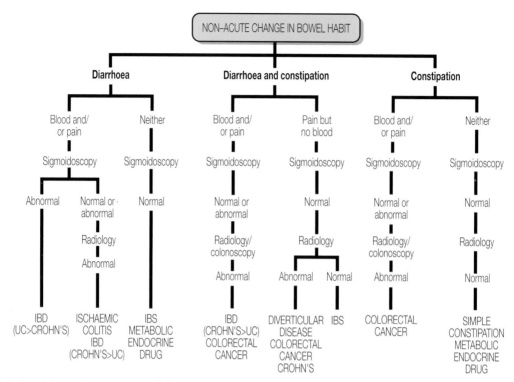

Fig. 12.1 A guide to the diagnosis of change in bowel habit.

Mechanisms of transit through the colon are not clearly understood. The orderly onward peristalsis preceded by a wave of relaxation that occurs in the oesophagus (see Ch. 9) does not happen in the colon. Instead various non-progressive segmental contraction waves occur. The main propulsive act is called the mass movement: this occurs infrequently and an important initiating stimulus is eating. In humans there is some doubt whether this is the same neural gastrocolic reflex shown in animal experiments. It seems more likely that it is humorally mediated by cholecystokinin (CCK) or a related peptide. There are many excitatory and inhibitory neural and chemical stimuli which exert their effect on the motility of the colon.

Defaecation occurs when the rectum has filled to a critical level so that stretch receptors in its wall are stimulated, giving rise to the desire to defaecate. At the same time reflex relaxation of the internal anal sphincter occurs, allowing rectal contents to stimulate the sensitive area of anal mucosa. This region alone can distinguish whether the contents of the rectum are solid, liquid or gas. Thus the final control of defaecation is voluntary and is brought about by relaxation of the external sphincter, fixation of the diaphragm and contraction of the abdominal and pelvic floor muscles. The acquisition of this voluntary control in childhood results in the change from the infant state of defaeca-

tion following most meals to the socially acceptable adult habit. However, if the urge to defaecate is repeatedly ignored, the rectum, like the bladder, relaxes to accommodate larger volumes without increase in pressure. Ultimately this results in infrequent defaecation from diminished rectal sensation. This illustrates how important an effect childhood toilet training can have on adult habits.

IRRITABLE BOWEL SYNDROME

This common condition is a cause of considerable misery to many young adults and presents a frequent diagnostic problem. The patients are usually tense and anxious, and concern about their symptoms creates further anxiety. They are often in situations at home or work which in other patients give rise to other psychosomatic syndromes such as palpitations or dyspepsia. There are probably inherited or acquired factors which determine which organ bears the brunt of the stress. Some patients give a history of previous migraine or bilious attacks. They may also have experienced the same bowel symptoms acutely before examinations or athletic events.

Two patterns are commonly seen. In the first, the minority, the complaint is of persistent painless diarrhoea, sometimes with mucus but never blood. There is no weight loss and general health is good. Interestingly the symptoms may date from a holiday abroad in which other members of the same party had the same attack of 'tourists' diarrhoea' but all except the patient made a full recovery. Bacteriological and virological studies are invariably negative at this stage, although it is particularly important to exclude amoebic, giardia and salmonella infections. In the second group, which constitutes the majority, the patient experiences flatulence with diarrhoea, in which several loose motions are passed each morning or after meals. This alternates with constipation, which is associated with the passage of either small dry hard pellets or thin ribbon-like stools. Preceding defaecation there may be considerable abdominal pain. When this is located in the left iliac fossa and associated with a palpable and tender sigmoid colon there is little diagnostic difficulty.

Sigmoidoscopy shows a normal mucosa but can also be helpful in making a positive diagnosis. The bowel clamps down tight on the sigmoidoscope, and its passage, together with air insufflation, may accurately reproduce the pain. Pressure recordings from the colon have shown that there is an exaggerated response to various stimuli, including stressful interviews arousing hostility, entry of food into the stomach and cholinergic drugs such as prostigmine. Indeed the patient may experience pain during such a recorded contraction; this is in contrast to the diminished activity seen in the painless diarrhoea subgroup.

If the clinical picture is not sufficiently clear one may, despite normal blood count, ESR and negative stool occult bloods, feel it necessary to perform a barium enema to exclude organic disease of the colon. In such an unphysiological procedure one is hardly likely to detect what is essentially a physiological disturbance. There may be some evidence of spasm if the bowel has not been too vigorously prepared.

Diagnostic difficulty occurs if the pain arises from spasm of the splenic or hepatic flexure. This may mimic peptic ulcer or gallbladder disease (see Ch. 11).

In a small minority of patients a careful history supported by an elimination diet may incriminate certain dietary factors in the causation of diarrhoea. A relevant and perhaps overpublicized factor is intolerance to milk and milk products. This may be associated with a deficiency of lactase in the small intestinal epithelium. Lactose from milk therefore passes unsplit into the colon where lactobacilli convert it to lactic acid with consequent diarrhoea. Although lactase deficiency may occur secondary to other gut disorders such as gluten enteropathy, it is also present in many otherwise normal people. Certain ethnic groups such as Blacks and Cypriots show a high incidence of lactase deficiency but they are usually asymptomatic.

DIVERTICULAR DISEASE

This in some ways provides a bridge between the irritable colon syndrome and organic disorders since both a functional and structural abnormality are present. As in irritable colon it can be shown that there is a heightened response of colonic muscle to the same psychological, physiological and pharmacological stimuli. This occurs particularly in the sigmoid colon, the commonest site of diverticula, where pathological and radiological studies show thickening of the circular muscle. The point of interest is whether the irritable colon syndrome of the younger adults goes on to become the diverticular disease found in the over-40 age group. Certainly in the uncomplicated form the symptomatology is very similar, but diverticulosis without any symptoms is probably even more common and seems almost part of the ageing process.

The differential diagnosis from carcinoma of the colon is important in this age group, and a barium enema is an essential investigation. The symptoms of pain, tenderness in the left iliac fossa, and alternating diarrhoea and constipation are due to over activity of the circular muscle of the colon.

The diverticula may become inflamed causing acute diverticulitis, which has been called 'left-sided appendicitis'. It is usually associated with guarding, fever and leucocytosis. This may subside, but complications can occur of pericolitis and pericolic abscess formation may go on to a local peritonitis. There may be rupture to cause a generalized peritonitis. Perforation into the neighbouring organ such as bladder, vagina or another part of gut will cause fistula formation. Obstruction of the bowel and haemorrhage can also result, and clear differentiation from a sigmoid carcinoma may not be possible until after surgical resection (see Fig. 11.5, p. 81). The previous demonstration of colonic diverticulosis in such a patient must not induce temporizing optimism in the surgeon as there may be coexisting carcinoma (see Ch. 11).

CARCINOMA OF THE COLON AND RECTUM

Because of the fluid nature of the ileal contents which enter the caecum and the greater diameter of the ascending colon, disturbance of bowel habit is less likely to occur with right-sided tumours but is a feature of left sided lesions. Passage of fresh or altered blood, and sometimes mucus, occurs with sigmoid and rectal lesions in contrast to the occult bleeding presenting as an iron deficiency anaemia that occurs from the right side.

With lesions of the ascending colon pain, often related to meals, may occur, and a mass may be palpable. In left-sided lesions pain due to partial obstruction is common and acute large bowel obstruction is a frequent presentation. Pain, however, is uncommon in rectal carcinoma although there may be a vague discomfort associated with a sensation of inadequate defaecation. Passage of mucus is particularly associated with carcinoma of the rectum. Early diagnosis by sigmoidoscopy followed by colonoscopy or barium enema is particularly important in this group of cancers since radical surgery may carry a relatively good prognosis depending on the Duke's staging of the operative specimen.

ULCERATIVE COLITIS AND CROHN'S DISEASE

All age groups can be affected by either of these inflammatory disorders. In ulcerative colitis bloody diarrhoea is nearly always present, and the diagnosis is strongly supported by the presence of a granular proctitis on sigmoidoscopy. Although ulceration and pseudo polyps are not usually seen in the rectum, the appearance of the mucosa and the ease with which it bleeds on contact are characteristic. The disease spreads proximally in continuity and, if extensive, there may be systemic disturbances with fever, malaise, weight loss and anaemia. Rarer manifestations such as clubbing, erythema nodosum, pyoderma gangrenosum, and sacroiliitis may be of diagnostic value. Barium enema or colonoscopy should confirm the diagnosis and indicate the extent of the disease (Fig. 12.2E).

In recent years a condition has been delineated from ulcerative colitis in which the colon around the splenic flexure is mainly involved. Formerly called segmental colitis, it presents initially with pain as well as bloody diarrhoea and later barium enema may show a char-

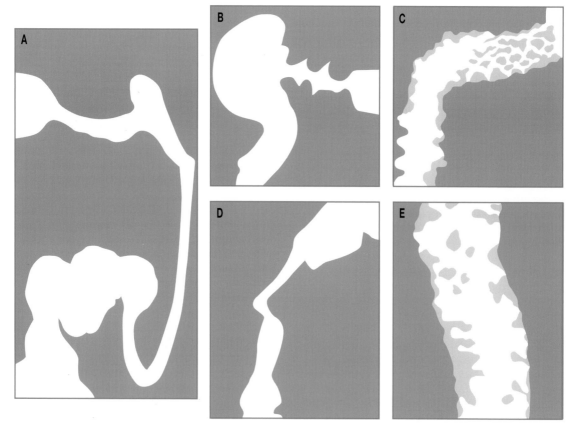

Fig. 12.2 Barium enemas in colonic disease.

A) Ischaemic stricture of splenic flexure and descending colon.

B) Crohn's disease of transverse colon.

C) Crohn's disease of colon showing 'cobble-stone' appearance.

D) Recurrent Crohn's disease causing a stricture at an ileocolic anastomosis.

E) Ulcerative colitis of descending colon showing pseudopolyposis.

acteristic long length of stricture (Fig. 12.2A). It is now known to be of ischaemic aetiology, occurring in the watershed region of bowel between superior and inferior mesenteric artery territories. It occurs in elderly patients, often with other evidence of cardiovascular disease, and is due to occlusion or low flow in the inferior mesenteric artery (see Ch. 11).

Crohn's disease may not only involve the terminal ileum but the colon as well. In retrospect, cases had been misdiagnosed as atypical ulcerative colitis. Apart from the pathological differences of colitis being a superficial mucosal disorder, and Crohn's involving the full thickness of bowel wall with granuloma formation, there are important clinical differences (Table 12.1). Only half the patients with colonic Crohn's have rectal lesions seen on sigmoidoscopy. When present, these are patchy rather than uniform, with areas of oedema but not much bleeding. Deep fissuring ulcers may be seen and give a characteristic 'rose thorn' appearance on barium enema (Fig. 12.2, B and C). The lesions are discontinuous. Perianal lesions are seen in over three-quarters of patients and include one or more painless anal fissures, associated with oedema, anal tags and discoloration of the adjacent skin. Perianal abscesses and fistulae are also common. Biopsy of these lesions may be of diagnostic value. Abdominal pain and the absence of blood from the diarrhoea are further differentiating points. Nonetheless when Crohn's disease is confined to the colon real difficulty may be encountered in differentiating it from ulcerative colitis. This results in up to 15% of cases of colitis being designated 'indeterminate colitis', the final diagnosis being resolved by the pathohistological findings after surgical resection or the subsequent behaviour of the illness. Of course the more classical disease of the terminal ileum alone, or with colonic involvement, will cause diarrhoea; there may be colicky pain if a stricture is causing subacute obstruction and a mass may be palpable in the right iliac fossa (Fig. 12.2D). Small-bowel enema, barium follow-through or colonoscopy will confirm the diagnosis. Scanning with the patient's leucocytes labelled with various radioactive isotopes can be used to detect and demonstrate the extent of inflammatory bowel disease and any complicating abscess.

SIMPLE CONSTIPATION

Two main categories occur and it is of importance to distinguish them since the approach to the treatment

Table 12.1 Differential diagnoses of ulcerative colitis, colonic Crohn's disease and ischaemic colitis

	Ulcerative colitis	Crohn's disease	Ischaemic colitis
Age at diagnosis	20–40 years	0–50 years	Over 50 years
Symptoms			
Bleeding	Very common	Unusual	Very common
Abdominal pain	None	Common	Very common
Signs			
Abdominal tenderness	None	Sometimes	Very common
Abdominal mass	None	Sometimes	May develop over a few weeks
Anal lesions	Rarely, secondary to infection	Common, often painless May precede bowel disturbance	None
Sigmoidoscopy			
Rectal involvement	95–100%	50%	? 1%
Appearances	Uniform hyperaemia, granularity and contact bleeding	Discontinuous, oedematous and occasional ulceration	Very rarely engorgement of mucosa, oedema and bluish-purple discoloration
Radiology			
Distribution	Continuous with rectum	Often discontinuous with normal intervening colon	Left colon especially around splenic flexure
Internal fistulae	None	Sometimes	None
Strictures	Carcinomatous only	Common	May be lengthy and develop some weeks after onset
Mucosal lesions	Shallow granular ulceration and pseudo polyps	Fissuring deep ('rose-thorn') ulcers with oedema in between ('cobble-stones')	Mucosal oedema ('thumb-printing') and irregularity in early acute stage

of each will be different. The condition called rectal dyschezia has been alluded to in the discussion of defaecation. These patients have normal colonic transit with delay occurring in rectal emptying. Large volumes of stool may be felt on rectal examination. In geriatric patients, actual faecal impaction with a spurious overflow diarrhoea may occur. Infirmity, confusion and similar disorders may render them immobile and unable to answer the call to stool, and are common contributory factors. In this condition the diet is often low in roughage and fluid content, while painful anal lesions such as haemorrhoids or fissures may further inhibit defaecation.

The second group of patients seem, by transit studies, to take an abnormally long time for caecal contents to reach the rectum, with the result that stools are hard and dry and may be painful to pass. The condition merges with the spastic variety of irritable colon. A variant of this type of constipation is the idiopathic megacolon. This differs from Hirschsprung's disease of children and Chagas' disease (infection with *Trypanosoma cruzei*) in that there is no evidence of destruction of ganglion cells.

Constipation is an important symptom of depression; a change in sleep pattern as well as bowel habit, often with early waking and inability to get back to sleep, may alert one to this diagnosis.

METABOLIC, ENDOCRINE AND DRUG CAUSES

Hypercalcaemia from any cause causes constipation, and is usually associated with nocturia, due to failure of renal concentration, lethargy, abdominal pain, nausea, vomiting, and mental disturbance even amounting to psychosis.

Thyrotoxicosis may be accompanied by diarrhoea whereas constipation is a common symptom of myxoedema.

The carcinoid syndrome, due to liver metastases from the 5-hydroxy tryptamine secreting tumour, is characterized by diarrhoea, flushing attacks, asthma and tricuspid and pulmonary valve disease.

A rare endocrine tumour causing diarrhoea is the gastrin secreting non-beta islet cell pancreatic tumour giving rise to the Zollinger–Ellison syndrome. In most cases gross gastric hypersecretion of acid causes recurrent and multiple peptic ulceration with diarrhoea, attributable to inactivation of pancreatic and intestinal enzymes and conjugated bile salts by acid and the large volume of gastric fluid. Another pancreatic islet tumour causing profuse watery diarrhoea associated with hypokalaemia and achlorhydria is the VIPoma. The severity of the diarrhoea has led to the term pancreatic cholera and the diagnosis can be confirmed by measuring VIP (vasoactive intestinal polypeptide). In the rare medullary carcinoma of the thyroid there is diarrhoea in half of the patients.

A record of drugs is an essential part of history-taking. Opiates, codeine, aluminium hydroxide and anti-muscarinic drugs (atropine, phenothiazines and tricyclic anti-depressants) are amongst constipating drugs whereas magnesium trisilicate, aminosalicylates, non-steroidal anti-inflammatory drugs (NSAIDs), beta adrenergic blockers, and digoxin may cause diarrhoea. A wide range of antibiotics can cause diarrhoea by a variety of mechanisms including alteration of the colonic bacterial flora. This may allow *Clostridium difficile* to flourish causing pseudo-membranous colitis – a potentially dangerous disease in debilitated hospital patients.

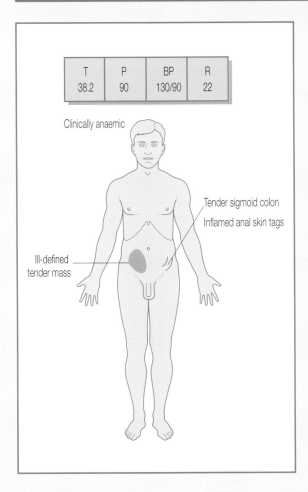

T	P	BP	R
38.2	90	130/90	22

Clinically anaemic

Tender sigmoid colon

Inflamed anal skin tags

Ill-defined
tender mass

A 54-year-old market gardener was admitted to hospital for investigation. He complained that for 4 months he had had left-sided abdominal pain. At times the pain was colicky and was sometimes relieved by defaecation.

During this period he had had alternating episodes of diarrhoea and constipation. He had also noticed streaks of blood in the stool which he had attributed to 'piles'. He had felt unwell with poor appetite and had lost 5 kg in weight.

For the previous 15 years he had had recurrent episodes of central and right-sided abdominal pain associated with diarrhoea but never constipation. The pain occurred about an hour after meals. His symptoms might persist for several months and his weight would fluctuate.

He had had two barium-meal examinations 10 and 5 years previously, which were normal, except that on the second occasion a sliding hiatus hernia had been demonstrated. Two years previously he had had a sigmoidoscopy which was normal and a barium enema which showed a few sigmoid diverticula only.

On examination he was thin, clinically anaemic and appeared unwell. He was mildly febrile (temperature 38.2°C). The only abnormal findings were in the abdomen. He was tender in both lower quadrants. In the right iliac fossa there was an ill-defined tender rounded swelling in the region of the caecum. On the left side the sigmoid colon was palpable, tender and could be rolled under the fingers. On rectal examination no masses could be felt. Proctoscopy showed first degree internal haemorrhoids and there were also prominent and inflamed skin tags around the anus. Sigmoidoscopy to 20 cm was normal.

Questions

1. How would you account for his present symptoms?
2. What are the likely causes of his past symptoms?
3. What further investigations would you perform?

The illness leading to this patient's admission to hospital suggests a stenosing lesion of the left side of the colon. In this age group such a stenosis is very likely to be due to carcinoma, especially if it presents in a patient who was previously well. There are two situations however where previous illness might be associated with the development of cancer.

The risk of cancer in ulcerative colitis is related to the extent and duration of the colitis. It is probably only significant in patients with total colitis which has been present for 10 years. This patient's 15-year history is unlikely to be due to colitis for several reasons: the diarrhoea was never associated with blood loss until recently; sigmoidoscopy in the past, and on admission, showed no evidence of proctocolitis which is invariably present and may extend any distance back towards the ileocaecal valve. Finally, a barium enema 5 years earlier showed no evidence of colitis.

Single and multiple colonic polyps are associated with carcinoma of the colon. When multiple the condition is usually inherited as a dominant characteristic and carries a particularly high risk of malignancy. The condition may be asymptomatic or cause diarrhoea and bleeding. In this patient the intermittency of the past symptoms, with pain as one of its features, and the absence of polyps on barium enema make their presence unlikely.

Diverticulosis of the colon, which has been radiologically demonstrated in this patient, can give rise to large bowel obstruction if a pericolic abscess develops. The illness is more acute than in this patient. Diverticula in the absence of inflammation may give rise to symptoms indistinguishable from the irritable colon syndrome of either the spastic or simple diarrhoea variety. This patient's previous history does not fit easily into any of these categories as he has had recurrent episodes of diarrhoea and pain without constipation and they have been associated with loss of weight.

Stricture of the left side of the colon may follow some weeks after an episode of subacute ischaemic colitis. There is no such antecedent history in this patient and this diagnosis does not explain his past history.

Crohn's disease can affect the gut anywhere from mouth to anus, although the terminal ileum is the commonest site. Colonic lesions, in isolation or associated with those elsewhere, are well recognized. The clinical presentation in this patient shows many of the features of Crohn's disease. Recurrent episodes of diarrhoea, right-sided abdominal pain with a vague mass and weight loss and malaise over many years are a feature of involvement of the terminal ileum. Attention has been drawn to the long interval between the first symptoms and the establishment of the correct diagnosis in the past. If this patient's disease had been confined to the terminal ileum a barium meal without a follow-through examination of that area would have been negative. Likewise a barium enema can be negative though often the terminal ileum, and disease within it, is demonstrated. Unlike ulcerative colitis the rectum is frequently spared in colonic Crohn's disease but anal and perianal lesions are common. Considerable significance should be attached to the inflamed skin tags seen in this patient.

Further radiological studies must be undertaken, with a barium enema first. This will show the site of the presumed stenosis and may also provide a clue to the underlying disease. If Crohn's disease is present the lesion will be segmental with adjacent normal bowel. The mucosa may show a coarse cobble-stone appearance and there may be deep ulcerating fissures, giving a spiky 'rose-thorn' appearance. A stricture will probably be seen. A small-bowel enema of the small intestine, especially ileum, will be necessary. The detection and delineation of disease elsewhere in the gut is of importance in deciding the vexed question of the best treatment. Biopsy of the skin tags is of great help in establishing a histological diagnosis, as is colonoscopy, or, for left-sided lesions, flexible sigmoidoscopy.

> Barium studies confirmed the presence of strictures of the descending colon and terminal ileum. Biopsy of the skin tag showed non-caseating granulomata with giant cells. The diagnosis was Crohn's disease.

13

Steatorrhoea and malabsorption syndrome

The importance of steatorrhoea as a symptom is that it invariably indicates malabsorption not only of fat but also of other essential nutrients. The reverse may not always be true in that some patients with malabsorption may have seemingly normal bowel actions, though stool fat content is usually raised on analysis. Further, if digestion of fat is impaired for whatever reason, then, inevitably, it cannot be absorbed. Steatorrhoea has, therefore, been promoted from being synonymous with malabsorption to being the most important symptom and sign of malabsorption. Sometimes symptoms or signs associated with malabsorption of nutrients other than fat dominate the clinical picture, and may bring the patient to the haematologist, neurologist or dermatologist. For all these reasons the more comprehensive term of malabsorption is preferred.

PRESENTATION

Gastrointestinal symptoms

The patient with steatorrhoea usually complains of frequent passage of semiformed stools. In place of a normal daily stool volume of 200 ml he may pass up to 2500 ml. In appearance, the stools are pale yellow or grey and are abnormally offensive. Sometimes they may appear greasy and, in the case of pancreatic steatorrhoea, oil droplets may be seen. In the absence of pancreatic lipase, fat digestion cannot even begin and the grossest steatorrhoea is often pancreatic in origin. When steatorrhoea is due to impairment of intestinal absorption of fat, oil droplets are not usually seen in the stool as some degree of fat digestion will have taken place. The stools are often lighter than water and float, and may contain undigested food; characteristically, the patient will say that he has to flush the toilet repeatedly. Frequent inspection and weighing or measurement of stool volume is a good guide to response to treatment.

Abdominal distension is a common finding which may be accentuated by loss of muscle and fat in the rest of the body. It is particularly prominent in children with gluten enteropathy but can occur in all forms of malabsorption syndrome. It may be associated with discomfort and flatulence. Various factors contribute, including muscular weakness due to muscle wasting and hypokalaemia, and gas, due to fermentation of the bulky stools in transit.

Abdominal pain is an uncommon feature confined to patients with pancreatitis and those with strictures causing subacute intestinal obstruction, of which the commonest cause is Crohn's disease. However, some patients with coeliac disease remark on the disappearance of abdominal discomfort when a gluten-free diet is instituted.

Vomiting is unusual, occurring chiefly in children with coeliac disease.

Change in appetite is an important symptom which may be overlooked. In a minority of patients, for example with a 'mechanical' cause such as resection of the ileum for mesenteric infarction, there may be an increased or ravenous appetite associated with weight loss resembling uncontrolled diabetes or thyrotoxicosis. In many other intestinal causes such as gluten enteropathy, however, there is marked anorexia. The resultant diminution in calorie intake contributes significantly to the weight loss in addition to the calorie wastage in the stools due to the malabsorption.

Nutritional symptoms

Weight loss is a prominent symptom which can only in part be attributed to the increased faecal loss of long-chain fatty acids, lactic acid and nitrogen due to malabsorption of fat, carbohydrate and protein respectively. The accumulation of oedema as a result of hypoproteinaemia in severe cases may mask the loss of weight. In some cases the calorie loss is compensated for by an increase in appetite. In other patients, with less severe malabsorption, weight may be maintained although other deficiencies may still be present.

Anaemia is frequent, and is sometimes the only presenting symptom. Iron deficiency occurs commonly but is often associated with a macrocytic megaloblastic anaemia, giving rise to a dimorphic blood film. It is therefore important to measure the serum iron in patients with malabsorption even though red cell indices do not suggest iron deficiency. Malabsorption of folic acid is the commonest cause of megaloblastic anaemia. When vitamin B_{12} deficiency is present it suggests that the cause of the malabsorption is either disease of the terminal ileum, which is the site of its absorption, or the contaminated bowel syndrome where the dietary vitamin B_{12} is utilized by bacteria in the small intestine.

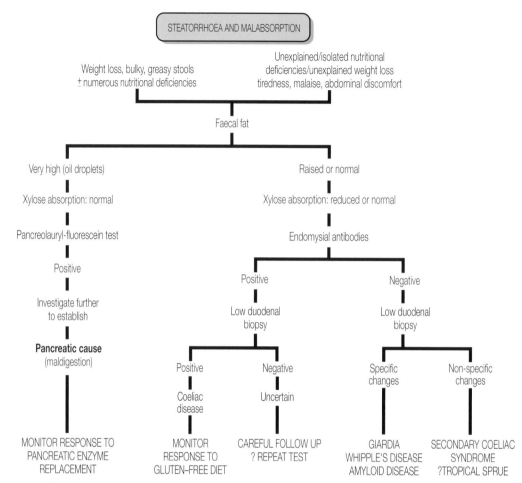

Fig. 13.1 A guide to the diagnosis of malabsorption.

Failure to grow will only be apparent in childhood. The limbs are affected more than the trunk and in an adult with presumed adult coeliac disease comparison of the crown–pubis with pubis–heel, or half-the-span, dimensions, may show the trunk measurements to be more than one inch (2.5 cm) greater in addition to an overall reduction in height. Additional evidence from the greater heights of siblings or parents and a vague history of abdominal symptoms dating back to childhood often suggest that adult coeliac disease has been present for longer than suspected.

Metabolic bone disease may cause changes in height due to vertebral collapse, or, in children, bowing of the legs due to rickets. Malabsorption of vitamin D and calcium causes rickets in children and osteomalacia in adults, whereas protein deficiency predisposes to osteoporosis. When these develop acutely, bone pain can be a distressing symptom. Apart from obvious radi-

ological changes, pseudo fractures are characteristic (Looser zones). These may be painless. They involve only the cortex of the bone, particularly in the scapulae and pelvis. Long-standing untreated osteomalacia may induce a compensatory or secondary hyperparathyroidism which may further complicate both the clinical and radiological picture. Bone biopsy may be necessary to disentangle the situation.

Tetany may develop acutely due to the great loss of calcium, which combines with fat in the stools. Calcium loss can very easily exceed the average daily intake of 1000 mg when it is remembered that normally 400 mg is secreted in saliva, bile, pancreatic juice and succus entericus, and may fail to be reabsorbed. Obvious bone disease may not be present. The role of coexistent magnesium deficiency contributing to tetany has become apparent in recent years with the interesting observation that correction of magnesium deficiency alone may raise the serum calcium and relieve tetany in some cases. Trousseau's and Chvostek's signs should be looked for to detect latent tetany.

Peripheral neuropathy occurs rarely and is usually due to vitamin B_{12} deficiency when a myelopathy may also be present, giving subacute combined degeneration of the cord. In contaminated bowel syndrome these changes may be marked, for not only is there vitamin B_{12} deficiency but the responsible intestinal bacteria may also synthesize folic acid, giving rise to supranormal blood levels. Nature thus commits the cardinal therapeutic error of treating vitamin B_{12} deficiency with folic acid! Thiamine deficiency may be responsible for a pellagra-like peripheral neuropathy in rare cases. Mental changes such as depression and irritability are relatively frequent but often tend to be overlooked or underestimated and only appreciated in retrospect by patient and physician.

Oedema is due to hypoalbuminaemia which has several causes. Not only is there failure of absorption of ingested protein but there is often an increased loss of protein into the gut lumen and failure of hepatic synthesis.

Keratitis and impaired dark adaptation or night blindness may be caused by vitamin A deficiency.

A wide variety of skin changes which seem secondary to malabsorption in that they improve when the malabsorption is corrected, are recognized. The commonest skin lesion is a nondescript eczema of patchy distribution which may be associated with itching. Sometimes a more characteristic psoriasiform eczema accompanied by pigmentation is seen. A gluten enteropathy is the usual cause of the underlying malabsorption and both gut and skin respond to gluten withdrawal from the diet. Protein depletion may cause fissuring of the keratin layer, giving rise to a crackled skin appearance. Oral lesions including glossitis, angular stomatitis, cheilosis and buccal ulcers may occur due to deficiencies of riboflavin, nicotinic acid, folic acid and other unidentified deficiencies. Bleeding gums, due to scurvy from ascorbic acid deficiency, and skin purpura from vitamin K deficiency may also be seen.

In dermatitis herpetiformis, where bullous lesions occur symmetrically over the extensor aspect of the limbs, buttocks and shoulders, over three quarters of patients have some degree of villous atrophy of the small bowel. This is rarely associated with clinical malabsorption, and usually there is only a mild anaemia due to deficiency of iron or folate. These deficiencies respond to gluten withdrawal; in over 70% of patients the skin will also improve, so that after about 6–24 months, dapsone, a specific remedy for the skin lesions, can be withdrawn.

CONFIRMATION OF MALABSORPTION

Normally about 93% of the dietary intake of fat is absorbed. Demonstration of increased faecal fat excretion remains the 'gold standard' test in demonstrating the presence of malabsorption, despite inaccuracies in adequate stool collection and the unpleasantness of the laboratory procedure. Attempts have been made to circumvent it by measuring absorption of radioactive fatty acids (palmitic or oleic acid). The passive absorption of the non-metabolized carbohydrate D-xylose, measured by its subsequent urinary excretion and sometimes blood levels, is usually abnormal in mucosal disease (and normal in maldigestion). It is relatively easy to perform but subject to error if there is delayed gastric emptying or renal impairment, but may be used to monitor response to treatment, for example in children with gluten enteropathy.

ASSESSMENT OF EXTENT OF DEFICIENCIES

The further battery of tests usually undertaken serves several purposes. First, treatment of the patient can be planned to replace the deficient substances. Second, demonstration of these deficiencies lends further support to the diagnosis of malabsorption syndrome. Third, the pattern or profile of these deficiencies may give strong clues as to the underlying cause of malabsorption in a particular patient; for example, steatorrhoea with impaired vitamin B_{12} absorption and high, rather than low, folate levels would suggest terminal ileal disease or contaminated bowel syndrome. It will already be obvious from the many ways in which the syndrome presents that a wide range of tests will be necessary.

DIAGNOSIS OF THE UNDERLYING CAUSE

Intestinal biopsy is invariably required and is now much more easily undertaken by multiple low duodenal sampling at gastroscopy, which is replacing the more cumbersome jejunal biopsy by Crosby capsule. However, the abnormalities seen may be relatively non-specific, because any disease process affecting the division and migration from the crypts to the tips of the villi of the intestinal mucosal cells will produce much the same effect. In place of the normal finger-like villi there may be leaves, ridges or convolutions. This is called partial villous atrophy. This is accompanied by an increased cellular infiltrate of the lamina propria. These findings occur in gluten enteropathy, tropical sprue and other mucosal disorders. A balder appearance of flat cobble-stones is called subtotal villous atrophy and is virtually pathognomonic of gluten enteropathy. Only in such rare disorders as Whipple's disease, intestinal lymphangiectasia, amyloidosis, and some cases of intestinal lymphoma may there be characteristic diagnostic findings. Intestinal biopsy may often therefore confirm the presence of malabsorption rather than clearly indicate its cause. However, when repeated after a period of specific treatment such as a gluten-free diet in coeliac disease, broad-spectrum antibiotics and folic acid in tropical sprue, or broad-spectrum antibiotics in Whipple's disease, improvement may be seen which, in conjunction with clinical and biochemical improvement, helps to clinch the diagnosis.

Where a structural abnormality such as diverticula, fistulae or previous surgery is the suspected cause, small bowel contrast radiography will be indicated. A small-bowel enema by intubation is replacing the older barium follow-through in most instances. A plain abdominal radiograph is generally unhelpful unless looking for the calcification sometimes found in chronic pancreatitis.

CAUSES OF MALABSORPTION SYNDROME

Other diagnostic procedures will be mentioned below in the discussion of individual causes. Although one particular disease may exert its effect by several mechanisms (e.g. Crohn's disease) a simple classification based on the disorders of intestinal function is instructive.

Inadequate digestion

- Pancreatic insufficiency   mucoviscidosis, chronic pancreatitis
- Inactivation of pancreatic enzymes   gastric acid hypersecretion (Zollinger–Ellison syndrome)
- Inadequate mixing of chyle, bile and pancreatic enzymes   Polya gastrectomy
- Bile salt deficiency   biliary obstruction, ileal resection, bacterial deconjugation in contaminated bowel syndrome.

Mucosal cell disorders

- Coeliac disease (gluten enteropathy)
- tropical sprue
- Whipple's disease

- amyloidosis.
- intestinal ischaemia
- intestinal lymphoma.

Inadequate digestion

Pancreatic disease. The confirmation of pancreatic insufficiency used to involve intubation tests stimulating pancreatic function such as the secretin–pancreozymin or Lundh test. 'Tubeless' tests have replaced them such as the pancreolauryl–fluorescein test relying on pancreatic enzymes to split the compound and allow the fluorescein to be absorbed and subsequently estimated in the urine. Pancreatitis of sufficient severity to cause steatorrhoea will always be associated with abnormal ducts visualized by ERCP (endoscopic retrograde cholangiopancreatography).

Gastric disease. Hypersecretion of hydrochloric acid of sufficient degree to inactivate pancreatic enzymes in the lumen of the intestine occurs in the rare Zollinger–Ellison syndrome due to a pancreatic tumour secreting gastrin.

One of the several mechanisms whereby partial gastrectomy combined with gastrojejunostomy gives rise to malabsorption is the mechanically obvious one where chyle rapidly enters the jejunum 'missing' the bile and pancreatic juices secreted into the afferent loop.

Disorders of bile salt metabolism. (See Fig. 13.2). Conjugated bile salts are essential to the emulsification of fat, which is a prerequisite of its digestion by lipases. They also facilitate the absorption of the products of fat digestion in the jejunum by forming micelles with them. After fulfilling this function in the jejunum 95% of bile salts are reabsorbed and return to the liver. The site of reabsorption is largely by a specific transport mechanism confined to the ileum, i.e. distal to the site of fat absorption. The liver is therefore required to supplement this enterohepatic circulation by producing about 5% of the body's bile salt pool daily. The maximum bile salt production of which it is capable is probably 20% of the total body bile salt pool. Steatorrhoea due to conjugated bile salt deficiency may therefore be due to failure of hepatic synthesis, due to chronic liver disease; obstruction to flow of bile, as in biliary cirrhosis; failure of ileal reabsorption, usually due to ileal resection; increased deconjugation of bile salts as in contaminated bowel syndrome.

Contaminated bowel syndrome. Primary bile salts (cholic and chenodeoxycholic acid) are conjugated in the liver with glycine and taurine. In this form they are highly dissociated at the normal intestinal pH giving them their detergent properties of being both water-

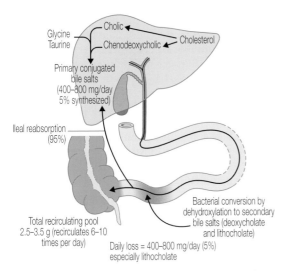

Fig. 13.2 The pathways of metabolism of bile salts.

and fat-soluble. Deconjugation can be brought about by bacteria and the deconjugated salts are very much less dissociated and therefore less effective. Furthermore, the specific ileal reabsorption mechanism is for the conjugated form. These factors are important in producing contaminated bowel syndrome which occurs in conditions associated with stasis in the small intestine. This may be due to strictures (congenital, tuberculous, Crohn's disease or following radiotherapy); diverticula of jejunum or duodenum; blind loops, such as the afferent loop of a Polya gastrectomy; or disturbances of motility, such as muscle degeneration in systemic sclerosis or autonomic neuropathy in diabetes mellitus. Bacteria, normally confined to the colon, will then multiply in the small intestine producing significant counts greater than 1 million/ml. Another means whereby infection may be introduced is through a fistula (jejunocolic due to a stomal ulcer, colonic diverticulitis or Crohn's disease), or by resection of the ileocaecal valve. Reduced gastric secretion and impaired humoral or cellular immunity may also sometimes be contributory factors.

E. coli and anaerobes including *Bacteroides* are the most commonly found organisms. The latter seem more important since they will cause deconjugation of the bile salts and hence steatorrhoea. In addition these bacteria utilize vitamin B_{12} and may synthesize folic acid as mentioned above. The resultant vitamin B_{12} malabsorption can be confirmed by the Schilling test and will not be corrected by intrinsic factor as in pernicious anaemia. Urinary indican excretion may be raised due to excess bacterial activity, but intestinal aspiration and culture is the definitive test. The ^{14}C glycocholate breath test depends on bacterial deconjugation of the radioactive glycine, allowing its absorption

and metabolism to $^{14}CO_2$ as shown by the estimation of exhaled radioactive carbon dioxide. In a normal subject the conjugated glycine remains attached to cholic acid in its enterohepatic circulation, with no ensuing radioactivity in the breath. Furthermore, whatever the cause of the contaminated bowel syndrome, nearly all cases will show at least a temporary improvement when given broad spectrum antibiotics.

Mucosal disorders

Coeliac disease and coeliac syndrome. Coeliac disease in children, responding rapidly to withdrawal of gluten from the diet, does not usually present any diagnostic difficulties. Its presumed autoimmune aetiology is supported by the finding of IgA antibodies to endomysium, the antigen being tissue transglutaminase. This has become a sensitive and specific screening test for coeliac disease as well as using falling levels to monitor response to gluten free diet. There was semantic confusion regarding its presentation in the adult before it was appreciated that one could often trace symptoms back to childhood, however mild they might have been. The adult disease was formerly called idiopathic steatorrhoea. Since 70% of cases may show a complete mucosal response to gluten withdrawal (albeit more slowly than in children), some prefer to call it primary coeliac syndrome, rather than adult coeliac disease as this would imply that it is always due to gluten sensitivity. Another reason for the introduction of the term coeliac syndrome was to embrace the large number of conditions in which a secondary, and often transient, malabsorption syndrome was demonstrable. Secondary coeliac syndrome may occur in a wide variety of conditions in which damage to the rapidly dividing intestinal mucosal cells occurs. Such a situation can arise during the use of cytotoxic drugs such as methotrexate and colchicine. Other drugs have also been incriminated, such as neomycin and biguanides. Severe protein malnutrition (Kwashiorkor) and extensive skin disease such as psoriasis and eczema affecting more than 60% of the body surface, may also be responsible (dermatogenic enteropathy). Several debilitating diseases such as infectious hepatitis, ulcerative colitis or disseminated malignancy, may give rise to secondary coeliac syndrome. Although impaired xylose absorption, partial villous atrophy, and sometimes steatorrhoea occurs, thereby resembling coeliac disease, there is not usually a response to gluten withdrawal, but the condition resolves with successful treatment of the underlying cause. In most instances malabsorption is not clinically significant.

The relationship of malignancy and malabsorption is of great interest. Lymphoma, usually affecting the distal jejunum and ileum, should always be considered when malabsorption presents for the first time in middle or late life. Of greater interest still is the finding of localized areas of lymphoma in the jejunum (an unusual site) or small bowel carcinomas (even more unusual) in association with long-standing coeliac disease, particularly when it has not been treated by gluten withdrawal. This possibility should always be considered if there is a sudden unexplained deterioration in a previously well-controlled patient with long-standing coeliac disease. It also suggests that all such patients should be treated with a gluten-free diet however mild their symptoms may be. Infections superimposed on underlying mucosal disease like latent gluten enteropathy may bring it to clinical notice or may in their own right cause diarrhoea with malabsorption. Giardiasis is well recognized as such an agent. The increasing number of immunocompromised patients as a result of HIV infection or cytotoxic treatment may allow other pathogens to flourish, such as the protozoa *Cryptosporidium* or *Isospora belli* and *Mycobacterium avium intracellulare*. Despite a high index of suspicion it is frequently impossible to identify the presumed pathogen in AIDS patients and treatment is accordingly very difficult; the HIV virus itself may damage enterocytes.

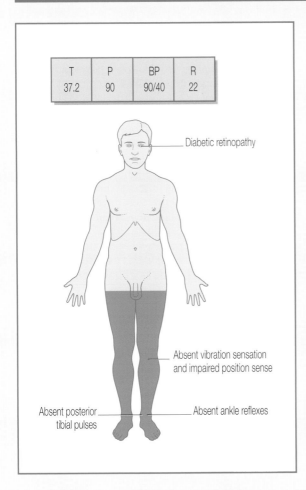

T	P	BP	R
37.2	90	90/40	22

Diabetic retinopathy

Absent vibration sensation and impaired position sense

Absent posterior tibial pulses

Absent ankle reflexes

A 42-year-old accountant was admitted from the diabetic clinic for investigation. In the previous 3 months he had become impotent and had also noticed dizziness on getting out of bed. He had been very happily married for 15 years. There had been no previous sexual problems and he had had intercourse once or twice weekly over the previous 10 years. He had also recently experienced episodes of diarrhoea, which began suddenly, often at night, and lasted for 3 to 4 days.

For the past year he had complained of epigastric discomfort, distension and nausea after food, which had responded to an alkali mixture from his GP. During this time he had also had episodes of angina, which usually occurred when he was hurrying for his morning train. Although he had not altered his diet he had recently lost 4 kg in weight. He had found his diabetes more difficult to control, having experienced hypoglycaemic episodes in the early morning, while he had noticed occasional heavy glycosuria after meals.

He had developed diabetes 14 years previously at the age of 28. For most of this time he had taken 16 units soluble and 32 units protamine zinc insulin each morning. There was no family history of diabetes. He had healthy twin sons aged 12.

His only other past illness had been an attack of mumps parotitis at the age of 26. This had been an unpleasant attack associated with right-sided orchitis, and severe epigastric pain. There had later been atrophy of the affected testis.

His job was a secure one, and he enjoyed his work. He was financially very successful and he had had no recent domestic worries.

On examination he had a pulse of 90/min, regular. The posterior tibial pulses were absent in both legs, the skin of the legs being cool and dry to the touch. The blood pressure was 110/60 lying and 90/40 standing. The fundi showed bilateral blot haemorrhages, while hard exudates were seen at the periphery. In the nervous system the ankle reflexes were absent, and the plantar responses were flexor. There was loss of vibration sense below the hips, with some impairment of position sense in the feet.

Urinanalysis showed 2% glucose and 200 mg/l albumin. The stools were unformed, clay-coloured and greasy. Laboratory analysis of a 3-day collection taken shortly after a recent episode of diarrhoea showed a faecal fat loss of 10.5 g/day.

Questions

1. What is the likely cause for his symptoms over the past 3 months?
2. What is the relevance of his past history of mumps to his present illness?
3. What further investigations would you undertake?
4. What treatment would you recommend?

Discussion

Not all of this man's symptoms can be attributed to malabsorption, some being due to the underlying diabetes. There are several clues as to the cause of the steatorrhoea.

If a patient has diabetes this suggests he may have disease of the pancreas. If steatorrhoea is also present then the exocrine as well as the endocrine function may well be affected. The usual sequence of events is nearly always that malabsorption develops some time before the diabetes. Furthermore, a history of chronic pancreatitis, often presenting with acute recurrent attacks, is usually obtained, though cases of painless chronic pancreatitis are described. In this patient diabetes antedated steatorrhoea by nearly 14 years.

This patient's history strongly suggests that during an attack of mumps 16 years ago he suffered from acute pancreatitis. Although pancreatitis due to mumps may be associated with transient glycosuria it is very doubtful whether it is ever a cause of chronic pancreatitis, with the development of permanent exocrine and endocrine deficiencies. Sterility, which should not be confused with impotence, may occur with bilateral orchitis but this was not the case here. His past history of mumps is therefore not relevant to his present illness.

This patient, like many diabetics, has evidence of accelerated vascular disease in his symptom of angina and the finding of absent foot pulses. It is becoming increasingly recognized that mesenteric ischaemia may occur in such a setting. This is an important condition to detect as in a proportion of patients the state of chronic insufficiency is a prelude to the more catastrophic and lethal small bowel infarction. Post-prandial discomfort with repeatedly negative barium meal examinations of the stomach and duodenum often occurs in this syndrome. The patient learns by experience that smaller meals cause less pain, and as a result may consequently lose weight. Sometimes the mesenteric ischaemia causes malabsorption, but this is usually not gross. It would not, however, explain the episodic and nocturnal nature of this patient's diarrhoea.

The known association between Type 1 diabetes and coeliac disease is unlikely here and could be excluded by a negative endomysial antibody test.

With evidence of retinopathy and nephropathy it is very likely that neuropathy, the remaining member of the triad of diabetic complications, is present. Peripheral nerve involvement would explain his absent ankle reflexes and loss of vibration and position sense, while autonomic neuropathy would explain his impotence, his postural hypotension (the cause of his dizziness), and his cold dry legs.

There is a well-recognized association between autonomic neuropathy and diarrhoea. The diarrhoea frequently occurs episodically and, for ill-understood reasons, nocturnally. It has been shown that gut motility is impaired by the autonomic neuropathy, giving rise to stagnation in the small intestine and its colonization by bacteria. This in turn gives rise to the contaminated bowel syndrome described above. Gastric atony with delay in emptying and vomiting may also occur. In the presence of a diabetic peripheral neuropathy it would be unnecessary to invoke vitamin B_{12} deficiency as a cause for this patient's signs in the legs but it should, none the less, be excluded.

Despite further investigations it may not be possible to make the diagnosis of contaminated bowel with absolute certainty. The autonomic neuropathy could be confirmed by the lack of response of pulse and blood pressure to Valsalva's manoeuvre. Barium meal and follow-through might show evidence of stasis and dilatation of loops of small intestine and possibly of the stomach. Aspiration and culture of small intestinal contents is a difficult procedure and the screening test of urinary indican estimation is frequently within normal limits. A vitamin B_{12} absorption test and a serum folic acid should be done.

The response to therapy would also be of diagnostic value. Improvement in the symptoms and steatorrhoea after a 5-day course of a broad-spectrum antibiotic such as tetracycline would be expected.

> The presence of an autonomic neuropathy was confirmed. He was able to curtail subsequent episodes of diarrhoea by courses of antibiotics.

14

Jaundice

The differential diagnosis of jaundice embraces the whole of liver disease. The majority of patients who present with jaundice can usually be placed into the categories of obstructive, hepatocellular or haemolytic jaundice on the basis of history, examination and bedside tests of urine and stools. More sophisticated tests may be necessary to diagnose the precise cause within these categories, but the greatest problem is the minority of jaundiced patients whose illness obstinately refuses to follow textbook descriptions. In the production of jaundice more than one mechanism may be responsible. The 'pharmaceutical explosion' of recent years has produced its own considerable problems, since drugs can produce nearly all the different patterns of jaundice, and probably account for at least 10% of patients presenting to hospital with jaundice.

BILIRUBIN METABOLISM

The correct clinical approach to jaundice must be based on an understanding of bilirubin metabolism (see Figs. 14.2 and 14.3).

The first step in the production of bilirubin is the breakdown of red blood cells by the reticuloendothelial system to release haem and produce unconjugated (prehepatic) bilirubin. This is relatively water insoluble and when estimated in the serum requires the addition of alcohol as a solvent before it will react with the diazo dye used in the van den Bergh reaction. This addition of alcohol is the basis of the indirect van den Bergh reaction. The normal amounts of bilirubin found in the blood are almost all in this form. Any cause of increased haemolysis may cause jaundice but because of its water insolubility, unconjugated bilirubin will not appear in the urine and haemolytic jaundice is therefore termed acholuric. Conjugated bilirubin on the other hand is water soluble and therefore will react directly with the dye in the van

den Bergh test and will appear in the urine. Conjugated hyperbilirubinaemia occurs in all forms of obstructive jaundice.

The unconjugated bilirubin is transported in the blood bound to the plasma proteins, especially albumin. If it is displaced from its protein binding sites it has an affinity for lipids and may be taken up by the brain in neonates but in adults does not cross the blood–brain barrier. Certain drugs such as sulfonamides and salicylates may interfere with protein binding. In the newborn, where a 'physiological' jaundice may occur due to immaturity of the conjugating enzymes of the liver, administration of these drugs may sometimes precipitate or exacerbate such jaundice and cause kernicterus.

The next steps are uptake of bilirubin by the liver cells and transportation to the endoplasmic reticulum, which is the site of the enzyme glucuronyl transferase. Here bilirubin is conjugated with glucuronide to form conjugated, water-soluble (post-hepatic) bilirubin. Defects in these steps occur in the congenital hyperbilirubinaemias, of which the commonest is Gilbert's disease. Inheritance of this condition is by an autosomal dominant character. The defect is chiefly one of uptake of unconjugated bilirubin by the liver cell but occasionally conjugation itself is impaired. When this is the case, production of the enzyme glucuronyl transferase can be induced by phenobarbitone. Male fern, once used in the treatment of tapeworm infestation, may interfere with transport of bilirubin to the endoplasmic reticulum, and novobiocin with its conjugation, and cause jaundice.

The conjugated bilirubin is then concentrated in the liver cell and excreted into the canaliculus and thence into the larger branches of the biliary tree. The hereditary defect associated with failure of excretion is the Dubin–Johnson type of hyperbilirubinaemia characterized by brownish-black pigmentation of the liver, probably due to melanin. Cholecystographic media compete with conjugated bilirubin and therefore will not be concentrated in the presence of excess bilirubin or, conversely, may precipitate jaundice. Methyl testosterone jaundice (and that due to other oral C 17 alkyl-substituted testosterone compounds) is due to impaired canalicular excretion of bilirubin. This is a dose-related phenomenon unlike the hypersensitivity type of intrahepatic cholestasis seen in susceptible patients taking phenothiazines.

Virtually all the conjugated bilirubin is excreted into the gut, where it is converted to stercobilinogen and then to stercobilin. Some of the former is reabsorbed from the gut and mostly re-excreted into the bile, while a small amount is excreted into the urine as urinary urobilinogen. The inability of the liver cell to re-excrete stercobilinogen, with its appearance as excess urinary urobilinogen, is a simple but sensitive

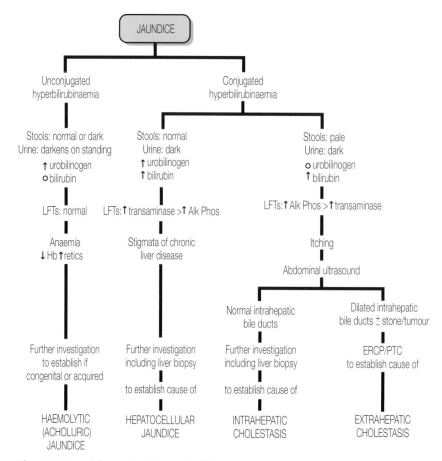

Fig. 14.1 A guide to the diagnosis of jaundice.

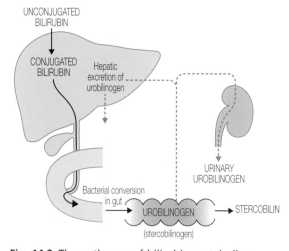

Fig. 14.2 The pathways of bilirubin metabolism.

test of liver function. It is also of considerable diagnostic value in jaundice. In the presence of total obstruction from whatever cause, urobilinogen must disappear from the urine since no bile is passing into the gut. In viral hepatitis there may be excess urinary urobilinogen in the early stage, due to liver cell damage. If, in viral hepatitis, a phase of intrahepatic cholestasis supervenes, urobilinogen will disappear from the urine and reappear when the cholestasis subsides. In obstructive jaundice pale stools are due to the absence of bile pigments, whereas they may be darker than usual with the excess production of stercobilinogen in haemolytic jaundice. Continuing complete obstruction with prolonged absence of urinary urobilinogen suggests a carcinoma of the head of the pancreas, since a stone impacted in the common bile duct will usually allow some bile to escape into the gut. Daily examination and recording of the stool appearance and urine urobilinogen are therefore simple but important measures in both the diagnosis and prognosis of jaundice.

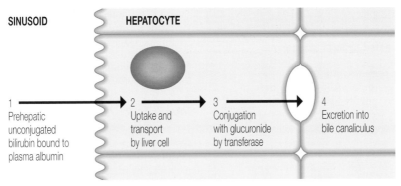

Fig. 14.3 The metabolism of bilirubin in the liver cell.

TYPES OF JAUNDICE

Cholestatic jaundice

The differential diagnosis between extra- and intra-hepatic causes of cholestasis is greatly facilitated by early upper abdominal ultrasound imaging looking for evidence of dilatation of intra- and extrahepatic bile ducts (remembering that it takes a few days after the appearance of jaundice for this to occur).

Extrahepatic. Not every patient with gallstones will be 'fat, female, fair, fertile and forty'. A family history of cholelithiasis may be obtained. A preceding history of flatulent dyspepsia may culminate in an attack of central abdominal pain, not always colicky, or right upper quadrant pain radiating to the scapula. Vomiting is a common feature. Fever is not invariable and, if pronounced, may indicate cholangitis. With the jaundice there is often pruritus due to retention of bile salts (see Fig. 13.2, p. 97). Examination usually reveals tenderness in the epigastrium and over the gallbladder. Dark urine and pale stools are the hallmark of obstructive jaundice. A neutrophil leucocytosis and raised sedimentation rate are due to the associated cholangitis. Apart from the raised direct-reacting bilirubin, the serum alkaline phosphatase will be disproportionately raised with respect to the transaminase which may indeed be normal.

If the obstruction were not relieved, biliary cirrhosis might eventually develop. An earlier complication is acute cholangitis due to ascending infection of the bile ducts. This renders the mucosa oedematous, making the obstruction complete. Bouts of fever with rigors ensue and septicaemia, usually due to *E. coli*, may occur. This syndrome of Charcot's intermittent biliary fever is more likely to occur after previous biliary tract surgery, when it may be due either to stricture formation or to residual calculi.

Carcinoma of the head of the pancreas is a rather loose term embracing carcinoma of the ampulla of Vater, the lower end of the bile duct, or of the acini of the pancreas. In its diagnosis and differentiation from gallstone obstruction there are several helpful pointers and investigations:

- Patients are more often male and over 50 years old.
- Onset is insidious, often with weight loss and malaise preceding the onset of jaundice. The jaundice progresses steadily, compared with the more acute and intermittent pattern seen with gallstones.
- Contrary to older textbook description, pain is a common feature and is often felt in the back; it may result in the patient adopting a hunched position or sitting bent over the bed. The pain is not colicky. Pruritus may occur.
- Examination may reveal an enlarged gallbladder, palpable in half the patients, although present at laparotomy in three-quarters.
- An associated thrombophlebitis may occur in the adjacent splenic vein, resulting in congestive splenomegaly. A remote effect is the occurrence of thrombophlebitis elsewhere in the body.
- There may be evidence of metastases such as an enlarged left supraclavicular gland of Virchow.
- Stools may contain occult blood, in addition to showing pallor due to obstruction. Their fat content may be raised although clinical steatorrhoea is uncommon and most of the patient's weight loss is attributable to the cancer.
- In addition to the persistent absence of urinary urobilinogen, glycosuria may be present.

Box 14.1 Causes of jaundice

Prehepatic unconjugated hyperbilirubinaemia
Haemolysis
Congenital defects: Gilbert's syndrome
                (uptake/conjugation defect)
                Crigler-Najjar (conjugation defect)

Hepatocellular jaundice
Acute
Viral hepatitis A, B, C, D
Other viruses: glandular fever, cytomegalovirus
Drugs – dose-dependent, e.g. paracetamol
      – idiosyncratic: numerous, e.g. halothane
Toxins
Autoimmune hepatitis
Alcoholic 'hepatitis'

Chronic
Chronic viral hepatitis (B, C)
Chronic autoimmune hepatitis
End-stage liver disease: cirrhosis of any cause
          alcoholic
          hepatitis B/C
          autoimmune
          haemochromatosis
          Wilson's disease

Cholestatic jaundice
Extrahepatic obstruction of biliary tree
Gallstones
Carcinoma of head of pancreas
Benign (usually post-operative) stricture
Carcinoma of ampulla of Vater or bile ducts
Sclerosing cholangitis

Intrahepatic
Drugs: numerous, e.g. chlorpromazine
Primary biliary cirrhosis
Cholestatic phase of viral hepatitis
Alcohol: acute fatty infiltration
Primary and secondary cancer
Lymphoma
Pregnancy

Percutaneous transhepatic cholangiography is more hazardous but is more likely to visualize the biliary tract.

With these diagnostic advances it is unusual to have to perform a laparotomy to make a diagnosis.

Intrahepatic. As the causes of intrahepatic cholestasis are often initially obscure even after history, examination and simple tests, it is sometimes desirable to perform liver biopsy. Provided duct dilatation has been excluded by ultrasound, clotting is normal, or has been corrected by parenteral vitamin K, the platelet count is greater than 50000 and the patient can cooperate in breath-holding, the procedure should be safe. A typical biopsy appearance of intrahepatic cholestasis with an eosinophilic and mononuclear portal zone reaction and some liver cell degeneration may be due to drug hypersensitivity, and could prevent an unnecessary laparotomy.

Hypersensitivity to phenothiazine, chlorpropamide, thiouracil, or phenylbutazone is the commonest cause of intrahepatic cholestatis. It can occur several weeks after stopping the drug and even after a single dose. There may be a rash, fever and eosinophilia accompanying the obstructive jaundice. Though usually self-limiting, obstructive features may persist for months or even years, closely resembling primary biliary cirrhosis. Hypercholesterolaemia, xanthoma formation and secondary malabsorption from bile salt deficiency could then develop, and histological differentiation may be impossible. The mitochondrial immunofluorescence test (where the antibody is directed against pyruvate dehydrogenase in the mitochondrial membrane) could then be positive in most patients with primary biliary cirrhosis and will differentiate it from prolonged drug cholestasis. Apart from the cholestatic phase of viral hepatitis and acute alcoholic hepatitis mentioned below, the other rare causes of intrahepatic cholestasis are cholangiocarcinoma and sclerosing cholangitis when confined to the intrahepatic bile ducts.

Hepatocellular jaundice

Viral hepatitis is the commonest cause. The clinical presentation of types A and B is very similar. Glandular fever and cytomegalovirus (CMV) may also cause hepatitis. A history of recent contacts of injections of any type must always be sought as well as sexual contacts and transfusion of blood or blood products. In all forms of hepatitis, the presenting symptoms are similar with a flu-like illness, fever, sore throat, malaise, depression, loss of libido and of taste for alcohol and tobacco. The disappearance of fever heralds the arrival of jaundice which rapidly deepens. Bilirubinuria,

- Pancreatic scanning by ultrasound or CT scan may show a mass in the head of the pancreas rather than gallbladder, as well as confirming the presence of dilated bile ducts. It may also reveal liver metastases.
- Contrast radiology includes ERCP (endoscopic retrograde cholangiopancreatography) in which the pancreatic ducts may be visualized as distorted by tumour, and the dilated common bile duct, if visualized, may enable a distinction to be made between tumour and gallstones. The endoscopic examination may show a carcinoma of the ampulla of Vater.

which may have preceded overt jaundice, increases, but urobilinogen may disappear from the urine if cholestasis develops. The stools initially are not pale. Liver tenderness and slight enlargement is a common finding but spontaneous pain does not occur. The spleen may be moderately enlarged.

If, instead of the usual pattern of recovery beginning in the second week of the illness, jaundice, pyrexia, and malaise persist, the illness may be entering the phase of chronic hepatitis. This carries a bad prognosis, for as liver cell failure progresses, splenomegaly appears and either cirrhosis develops, sometimes with portal hypertension, or death occurs from liver failure. All these complicated forms of hepatitis are more commonly seen with type B hepatitis and in middle-aged women, in whom the prognosis must therefore always be guarded. Laboratory investigations usually give strong support to the diagnosis. There is no leucocytosis, but a relative lymphocytosis with atypical morphology (viral lymphocytes) is seen. Alkaline phosphatase is usually only slightly raised whereas the transaminase is markedly elevated. The gamma globulins rise and, if the illness is prolonged, the albumin falls.

Diagnostic difficulty also arises if the complication of cholestasis develops, with the stool and urine changes previously mentioned, together with equivocal biochemical tests. The possibility is that an atypical painless cause of 'surgical' extrahepatic obstruction responsible for the jaundice is being missed. Ultrasound examination would be the next step, preceding either liver biopsy or visualization of the biliary tract by contrast radiography as discussed above. Serological tests for hepatitis B and C are helpful, though hepatitis A never progresses to chronic hepatitis or cirrhosis.

The most dangerous dose-related drug cause of hepatocellular jaundice is paracetamol poisoning. When presentation is delayed, lessening the efficacy of acetylcysteine as antidote, the condition may progress to fulminant hepatic failure and death.

Drug hypersensitivity may cause a hepatitis indistinguishable from the viral type. The hydrazine derivatives such as the monoamine oxidase inhibitors used in the treatment of depression are notorious in this respect and have resulted in fatalities. The incidence is, fortunately, low. The anti-TB drugs isoniazid and pyrazinamide (which are also hydrazines), ethionamide and the anaesthetic halothane are other idiosyncratic causes.

Direct hepatotoxicity related to dose occurs with carbon tetrachloride, this having been extensively studied in experimental animals. Other causes include cytotoxic drugs, large doses of tetracycline, especially in pregnancy, and overdoses of metals such as iron.

Cirrhosis is only accompanied by jaundice as a late and serious manifestation of the disease. An exception is primary biliary cirrhosis where jaundice is present before advanced liver failure. Mitochondrial antibodies are detected in most cases. In cirrhosis the presence of jaundice indicates that there is little hepatic reserve and is therefore usually found in conjunction with other signs of liver failure: ascites and oedema, hepatic precoma or chronic encephalopathy, and portal hypertension. There may be an acute cause for the deterioration of liver function such as gastrointestinal haemorrhage from a peptic ulcer or varices, a drinking bout in an alcoholic, injudicious drug therapy, or infection.

Chronic active hepatitis occurs in young, often obese and hirsute women, and may progress imperceptibly to cirrhosis over months or several years. It is characterized by gross elevation of gamma globulin (above $40\,g/l$). The involvement of other systems such as skin, joints, pleura and, rarely, kidneys suggests an autoimmune mechanism. These features do not however warrant the misleading name of lupoid hepatitis. Smooth muscle antibodies and ANF are usually present.

Acute alcoholic hepatitis typically occurs in an alcoholic without previous symptoms of liver disease, who suddenly develops a large tender liver, jaundice and ascites. Although the liver shows fatty infiltration, the damage may be reversible and need not progress to cirrhosis. The jaundice, curiously, may have the features of obstructive rather than hepatocellular jaundice.

Haemolytic jaundice

The presenting symptom is rarely jaundice. Symptoms are due more often to the underlying cause, the rate of haemolysis, or the degree of anaemia. The degree of haemolysis may vary from the lemon yellow tinge of an elderly patient presenting with pernicious anaemia, to a severe haemolytic crisis precipitated by drugs or broad beans (favism) in a patient with an inherited red cell deficiency of glucose-6-phosphate dehydrogenase (G6PD). In these more severe episodes there may be malaise, fever, headache, aching pains in the limbs, and sometimes, collapse. If the haemolytic process is chronic there may be splenomegaly and pigment stones in the gallbladder, which might give rise to the further complication of obstructive jaundice. The stools are dark, due to excess stercobilin, and the urine, containing excess urobilinogen, darkens on standing. Rarely, haemolysis is so great that haemoglobinuria occurs, darkening the urine (as in blackwater fever due to falciparum malaria). Apart from the raised indirect reacting bilirubin, other liver function tests may be normal. The blood picture shows a normocytic normochromic anaemia with reticulocytosis and immature red blood cells.

Important hereditary causes include hereditary spherocytosis, G6PD deficiency and haemoglobin disorders such as sickle cell disease and thalassaemia.

Acquired causes include the idiopathic autoimmune type of haemolytic anaemia and that associated with collagen diseases and chronic lymphatic leukaemia. Rhesus incompatibility in the newborn and mismatched transfusion at any age can produce severe jaundice. Drugs such as phenylhydrazine may have a direct lytic effect. Others such as methyl dopa may initiate an autoimmune reaction, while primaquine may expose an underlying G6PD deficiency, a condition particularly common in Afro-Caribbeans.

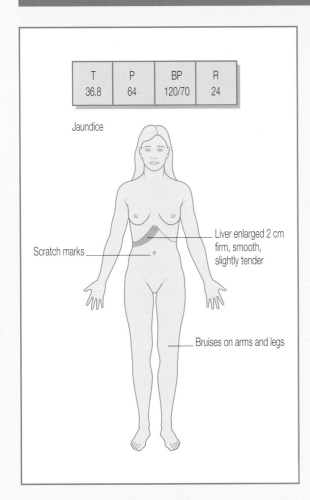

T	P	BP	R
36.8	64	120/70	24

Jaundice

Scratch marks

Liver enlarged 2 cm firm, smooth, slightly tender

Bruises on arms and legs

A 55-year-old divorced secretary was admitted to hospital with a history of increasing jaundice for 4 weeks. She had noticed that her urine had become darker and that her stools had become pale during this time. Over the past 3 months she had had a poor appetite and had lost 7 kg in weight. Apart from some flatulent dyspepsia, especially after fatty food, she had not had any abdominal pain. There had been no fever.

She had a long history of psychiatric problems since the age of 30. She had suffered from depression and anxiety with bouts of heavy drinking. She had had two admissions to psychiatric hospitals and also had been admitted to a general hospital after an overdose of barbiturates. She had been treated with a variety of psychotropic drugs in the past and for the last 4 months had been prescribed phenelzine and trifluoperazine for agitated depression. She smoked 30 cigarettes per day.

On examination she was jaundiced and had obviously lost weight. The skin showed scratch marks on the trunk and several bruises over the arms and legs for which she could not account. No lymph nodes were palpable and the respiratory, cardiovascular and central nervous systems were normal. In the abdomen the liver could be felt 2 cm below the right costal margin. It was firm and smooth with a regular edge and only slightly tender. The spleen and gallbladder were not palpable and ascites could not be detected. Pelvic examination was normal. The urine contained bilirubin but urobilinogen was absent.

Questions

1. What are the likely diagnoses?
2. What investigations would you undertake to establish the diagnosis?
3. What would be your further management?

Discussion

The patient has the features of obstructive jaundice with bilirubin but no urobilinogen in the urine, and pale stools. The presence of scratch marks, even though the patient has not complained of itching, is in keeping with cholestasis.

The insidious painless onset and steady progression together with the preceding ill-health is unlike the history of gallstone obstruction of the common bile duct. Various other causes of extrahepatic and intrahepatic cholestasis must be considered. Carcinoma of the head of the pancreas is a likely cause and would account for the preceding weight loss. Other forms of cancer may cause obstructive jaundice due to metastases in the lymph nodes of the porta hepatis pressing on the main hepatic ducts, or to secondary deposits within the liver. The latter would probably result in greater, more irregular, and possibly more painful enlargement of the liver than is present here. Primary sites to be considered would be stomach, bowel, bronchus or breast. In Western Europeans hepatomas invariably occur only after a lengthy history of cirrhosis. Although there is a history of alcoholism in this patient there are no stigmata of chronic liver disease (spider naevi, palmar erythema, parotid swelling or Dupuytren's contracture) to suggest cirrhosis. Furthermore, obstructive jaundice is not a common early feature in the development of a hepatoma. Carcinoma of the bile duct is rare but presents in much the same way as a carcinoma of the head of the pancreas.

The drug history of this patient could be relevant. Phenelzine is a monoamine oxidase inhibitor which may cause jaundice; this however is hepatocellular rather than obstructive. Trifluoperazine is a phenothiazine and may cause intrahepatic cholestasis. The illness preceding the jaundice makes drug cholestasis unlikely. The duration and progression of the jaundice seen here is not usual in phenothiazine jaundice but may occur and lead to difficulty in distinguishing it from primary biliary cirrhosis. This latter condition occurs particularly in middle-aged women and is characterized by intense pruritus, xanthomata of skin and tendons, and pigmentation of the skin in addition to jaundice.

Viral hepatitis may take a complicated course in middle-aged women and a cholestatic phase may develop. A prodromal illness of 2 months before the appearance of jaundice is rather lengthy.

The purpose of investigation is first to confirm that the jaundice is primarily obstructive rather than hepatocellular and then to establish the site of obstruction. When jaundice has been present for 4 weeks the biochemical pattern may not be clear-cut, as hepatocellular damage can supervene as a result of obstruction. However, if the liver alkaline phosphatase is proportionally more raised than the transaminase, the jaundice is more likely to be obstructive. The gamma glutamyl transpeptidase will also be raised in obstructive jaundice and more elevated than the alkaline phosphatase if the jaundice is due to alcoholic liver disease. The prothrombin time will also be prolonged but should be correctable with parenteral vitamin K if there is no significant hepatocellular damage. Hepatitis A and B should be excluded by looking for the anti-HA (IgM) antibody and surface antigen (HB$_s$Ag). Mitochondrial antibodies and other non-organ specific antibodies might be found in primary biliary cirrhosis or the less likely autoimmune chronic active hepatitis and a high titre of alpha-fetoprotein would suggest a hepatoma.

A chest X-ray should always be done to look for bronchial carcinoma and bone secondaries. The best investigation would be ultrasound scanning of the liver, pancreas and biliary tree; alternatively a CT scan would serve a similar purpose. These tests should determine whether the cholestasis is extrahepatic. If the biliary tree is not dilated the cause is likely to be intrahepatic and liver biopsy to determine its cause will be a relatively safe procedure. If the ultrasound shows dilated bile ducts it may also suggest the cause of extrahepatic cholestasis by revealing gallstones or an abnormal pancreas. Contrast radiology either by ERCP or transhepatic percutaneous cholangiography would be the next and, probably, final step before laparotomy. An alternative palliative treatment to be considered in a carcinoma of the head of pancreas would be the endoscopic placement of a stent through the obstructed lower common bile duct.

> The patient came to laparotomy and was found to have a carcinoma of the head of the pancreas. Adjacent lymph nodes were involved and a liver secondary was present. A choledochojejunostomy and gastrojejunostomy were performed.

15

Swelling of the abdomen

Many patients who present with the complaint of abdominal distension are describing a symptom rather than a visible or measurable physical sign. Such a feeling of bloatedness is a common feature in the acid–ulcer–dyspepsia syndrome and in irritable bowel syndrome (IBS). The patient has a great desire to belch which may give him a certain amount of relief. Sometimes he will swallow air repeatedly to provoke eructation in the hope of achieving this. However, there is little evidence that distension of the stomach by gas is the true cause of the discomfort experienced. Although it is rightly unfashionable to attribute too many symptoms to spasm, this would nonetheless seem to be the relevant factor. The patient's insistence that his abdomen visibly swells after meals, necessitating loosening of garments, is not usually confirmed by examination. The associated symptoms of pain, relieved by food or antacids, and perhaps heartburn, should help to eliminate this as a cause of the symptom of abdominal distension.

Paradoxically, many patients exhibiting the physical signs of abdominal swelling may have few symptoms directly caused by it. Unless the swelling is great or rapid they may not even be aware of it.

Whilst the old adage of swelling of the abdomen being due to fat, fluid, fetus, faeces or flatus provides a starting point in differential diagnosis, it will be necessary to consider the causes and their differentiation in greater detail. The need for careful examination of the abdomen under ideal conditions of relaxation in the fully flat position cannot be sufficiently emphasized. This must be combined with a full general examination which may reveal important clues to the underlying causes – for example anaemia, jaundice, lymphadenopathy or congestive cardiac failure. A well-known diagnostic trap is the patient with constrictive pericarditis. This is insidious in its onset and may present with abdominal swelling due to ascites. The jugular venous pressure may be so greatly elevated that its upper border is lost behind the angle of the jaw and it is therefore overlooked.

Gaseous distension

Having previously discussed the symptom of distension, one must consider it as a physical sign. Whatever the cause of gaseous distension there is usually swelling of the whole abdomen. In thin people loops of bowel may be discerned and percussion of the abdomen will give a resonant note.

In malabsorption syndrome, particularly coeliac disease (gluten enteropathy) in children, a pot-belly appearance is characteristic. This is pronounced when standing, probably because associated protein malnutrition and, perhaps, electrolyte deficiency, cause weakness and hypotonia of the abdominal wall musculature. The similar appearance in starvation and Kwashiorkor is an all too familiar appearance when famine strikes in an underdeveloped country. As discussed in Ch. 13 – steatorrhoea and malabsorption syndrome – there will be other important clues in a patient with malabsorption syndrome, such as a history of frequent, soft, bulky, pale, greasy, offensive stools and weight loss, together with such deficiency disorders as anaemia or metabolic bone disease.

Distension of the abdomen due to obstruction of large or small bowel is an acute surgical emergency and will be dominated by other symptoms of pain, vomiting and absence of stool or flatus. If diagnosis is delayed, signs of localized or generalized peritonitis develop. The various causes will be revealed by the ensuing laparotomy. Plain abdominal X-rays in erect and supine positions will confirm the presence of gas and fluid levels. Intestinal obstruction should always be considered in the elderly patient with gaseous abdominal distension, even if the other features are not prominent.

Fat

Excess adipose tissue both in the subcutaneous layers of the abdominal wall and in the mesentery does not require detailed description. The dependent Falstaffian paunch is an all-too-common feature of overfed western society. Sometimes fat is deposited selectively in the trunk and abdomen as in Cushing's syndrome or in patients receiving long-term steroid therapy. Such abdominal swelling associated with a moon face is in contrast with the spindly limbs caused by muscle wasting as a result of enhanced protein catabolism. Rapid fat deposition leads to stretching of the skin with the appearance of striae in flanks and thighs. When due to steroids the striae are livid or pigmented, whereas this is not the case in simple obesity. Additional physical signs of steroid excess such as acne, hirsutism, dorsal fat pad giving a buffalo hump, osteoporosis perhaps causing vertebral collapse, and kyphosis will support the diagnosis.

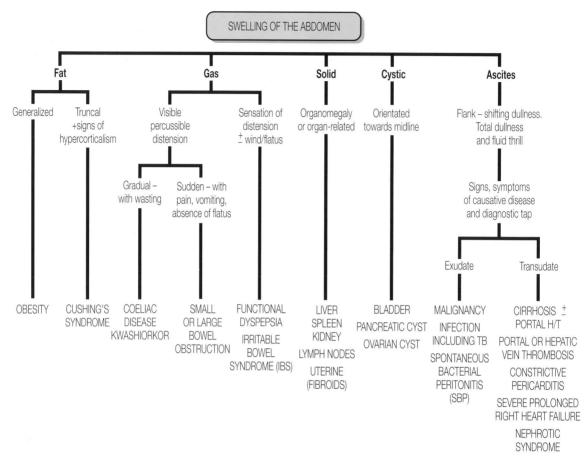

Fig. 15.1 A guide to the diagnosis of swelling of the abdomen.

The main problem presented by fat is that it may be confused with other causes of abdominal swelling. The sheer amount of fat present makes percussion of the abdomen unreliable and palpation uncertain.

SOLID SWELLINGS

Every pathological museum contains some tumours impressive for their size alone. In life these rarely present great diagnostic problems. Large solid swellings are usually due to enlargement of an organ which is normally present and will conform to the physical signs associated with that organ.

Gross splenomegaly may present as a dragging sensation in the left half of the abdomen with a superficial mass moving downwards and medially on inspiration. Palpation confirms the presence of a firm mass with sharp borders and a notch on the medial aspect. The upper border cannot be defined. It will be dull to percussion. Because of its size it may, unlike a

moderately enlarged spleen, be palpable bimanually, sharing this sign with an enlarged kidney. Gross splenomegaly in the UK is usually due to the myelo-proliferative disorders – myelosclerosis (myelofibrosis) and chronic myeloid leukemia. A blood count will be the next important step, showing a leucoerythroblastic anaemia in the case of myelosclerosis or an anaemia with neutrophil leucocytosis with some immature cells in chronic myeloid leukemia. Disorders of the reticuloendothelial system, particularly giant folli-cular lymphoma and less commonly Hodgkin's disease, may cause similar gross enlargement of the spleen. Here there will usually be associated lymph node enlargement and biopsy of one of these will be nec-essary to establish the diagnosis. In tropical countries additional causes such as kala-azar and chronic malaria would have to be considered. The latter is the cause of big spleen disease described in Africa, where there may be considerable difficulty in demon-strating the parasite in the peripheral blood. The splenomegaly represents an exaggerated immune response reflected in grossly elevated immunoglobulins (IgM).

Gross hepatomegaly will be confirmed by percussion and palpation. A malignant cause due to secondary or primary cancer is most likely. The latter, a hepatoma, is found increasingly as a terminal complication of cirrhosis of all aetiologies. The co-existent cirrhosis may, in turn, give rise to signs of hepatocellular dysfunction. These include palmar erythema, leuconychia, spider naevi, skin pigmentation, gynaecomastia and testicular atrophy, parotid swelling and Dupuytren's contractures. Hepatomas may rapidly reach a large size, giving rise to pain, tenderness and nodular enlargement of the liver. The same blood and reticuloendothelial disorders as cause gross splenomegaly may similarly affect the liver.

The commonest cause of uterine enlargement is, of course, pregnancy. The history of amenorrhoea may have been withheld, but the associated breast changes cannot be suppressed. The swelling will arise from the pelvis and should be confirmed by vaginal examination. Fibroids may assume huge proportions, and are then prone to develop complications of torsion or haemorrhage. Menorrhagia is a frequent accompaniment. Again bimanual pelvic examination should confirm the diagnosis.

The only likely cause of huge kidneys presenting as abdominal swelling is polycystic disease. Although both kidneys are involved they are frequently asymmetrical (Fig. 15.2). They are bimanually palpable, move downwards on inspiration and may be resonant to percussion because of overlying bowel.

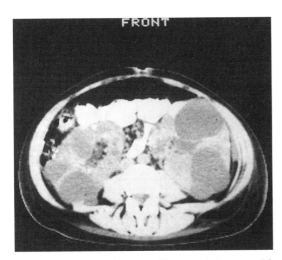

Fig. 15.2 Transverse CT scan of lower abdomen with oral contrast showing grossly enlarged kidneys with rounded areas of different attenuation. The diagnosis was polycystic disease. (Courtesy of Dr Hakhamaneshi.)

Rarely, large retroperitoneal tumours such as dermoids, sometimes undergoing sarcomatous change, cause swelling of the abdomen. Retroperitoneal lymph node enlargement due to lymphosarcoma may present similarly. It is particularly important to examine the testes for a primary site of a tumour giving rise to retroperitoneal metastases.

Fluid swellings

This category resolves itself into the differentiation of fluid-containing swellings, such as an enlarged bladder, ovarian or pancreatic cyst, from fluid in the peritoneal cavity. Having detected ascites, its cause must then be determined.

Cystic swellings, as they enlarge, will tend to adopt a central abdominal position irrespective of their site of origin. The two common sites are ovarian and pancreatic. Ovarian cysts can assume large sizes without causing symptoms and are first noticed by the patient because of increasing lower abdominal swelling. Frequently they are found accidentally on routine examination. They rise out of the pelvis, are rounded in outline and do not usually exhibit a fluid thrill or shifting dullness. They may be bimanually palpable on pelvic examination. Diagnostic confusion may be created by a distended bladder. Painless retention with overflow characteristically occurs in males with a longstanding obstruction due to prostatic enlargement. It may rarely occur in women with a neurogenic bladder caused by tabes dorsalis or spina bifida.

Cysts of the pancreas most commonly occur as a complication of pancreatitis. They are usually lesser sac pseudocysts, the walls of which are formed by adjacent structures as a reaction to the released pancreatic enzymes. The development of a palpable abdominal mass some days or weeks after an attack of acute pancreatitis, sometimes associated with a re-elevation of the serum amylase or a continuing elevation of the urinary amylase, suggests the diagnosis. Abscess formation can also occur in this situation, but the patient is usually more ill and has a persistent fever and neutrophil leucocytosis. True pancreatic cysts and mesenteric cysts are much rarer and do not follow any clear-cut illness. All these pancreatic swellings occur, of course, in the upper abdomen.

The physical signs leading to a diagnosis of ascites will depend on the amount of fluid present in the peritoneal cavity. Gross ascites will cause generalized abdominal distension with bulging of the flanks and eversion of the umbilicus. There will be generalized dullness to percussion, a fluid thrill can be elicited, and the liver and spleen, even if enlarged, may not be palpable, or, perhaps, only ballotable. Abdominal wall veins may be prominent, but are not necessarily diagnostic of the underlying cause. Thus, branches of the inferior epigastric system draining normally towards the groin are often prominent. If flow is in the opposite direction it suggests the development of a collateral circulation between branches of the inferior and superior venae cavae. This is usually due to the pressure of the ascitic fluid on the IVC rather than thrombosis, since venous flow returns to normal with disappearance of the ascites. When portal hypertension is present a collateral circulation between portal and systemic venous system may develop. The veins involved are in the ligamentum teres and appear as a caput medusa; that is veins radiating from the umbilicus, or as veins in the flanks. When less ascitic fluid is present the area of dullness may be horseshoe shaped, i.e. the centre of the abdomen is resonant and the dullness can be shown to shift on turning the patient from side to side.

The differential diagnosis of abdominal swellings has been greatly aided by modern imaging techniques, particularly ultrasound scanning, which is inexpensive and effective.

Causes of ascites

Ascitic fluid may be an exudate or a transudate and this is partly reflected in the protein content. Exudates may be due to malignancy, or infections due in turn to tuberculosis, *E. coli* or pneumococcus and have a raised protein concentration (>25 g/l). Transudates are usually due to a combination of raised portal venous pressure (portal hypertension) and lowered plasma colloid osmotic pressure due to hypoalbuminaemia and have a low protein concentration (<25 g/l). However vascular causes such as constrictive pericarditis and other causes of venous outflow block (hepatic vein thrombosis/Budd–Chiari syndrome) may have a high protein despite transudation being the mechanism of ascites formation. Portal hypertension will usually lead to splenomegaly, but whether the liver is enlarged will depend on the underlying cause. Other mechanisms involved in the formation of a transudate are an associated increased hepatic lymph flow and sodium and water retention by the kidneys due to secondary hyperaldosteronism, resulting from activation of the renin-angiotensin system, and increased anti-diuretic hormone (ADH) activity. Although large amounts of fluid may be present in the abdomen, the circulating plasma volume may be low due to hypoalbuminaemia, resulting in lowered colloid osmotic pressure allowing loss of salt and water from the intravascular compartment. This will reduce renal blood flow and glomerular filtration. This, together with stimulation of postulated volume receptors, resulting in aldosterone secretion, causes sodium and water retention and potassium loss (see Ch. 3). Furthermore if liver function is impaired, the hepatic

inactivation of aldosterone, ADH and other steroids such as oestrogens may be reduced.

The causes of transudates include:

Hepatic causes of portal hypertension. In the majority of cases this is due to cirrhosis of any aetiology, or fibrosis, as in schistosomiasis. An additional factor is that hepatic albumin synthesis is reduced. The liver may be shrunken (e.g. post-necrotic cirrhosis), enlarged (e.g. alcoholic portal cirrhosis) or normal sized.

Extrahepatic portal hypertension. This may be caused by thrombosis of the portal vein, possibly because of adjacent or remote malignancy, infection, such as an ascending pyelophlebitis from an appendix abscess, or a thrombotic tendency such as in polycythaemia. The liver need not be enlarged.

Thrombosis of the hepatic vein (Budd–Chiari syndrome) or of its intrahepatic branches. The cause in the majority will be a thrombophilic disorder such as myeloproliferative disorders (e.g. polycythaemia rubra vera) or the more recently discovered genetic deficiencies (protein S and C and Factor V Leiden). These are all more likely to manifest themselves clinically in association with use of the contraceptive pill or in the puerperium. Veno-occlusive disease associated with drinking bush teas, first described in the West Indies, and lupus anticoagulant are other causes. The liver will be enlarged and tender, and the patient usually jaundiced.

Raised systemic venous pressure transmitted back to the portal venous system. This may occur in severe congestive cardiac failure of long standing whatever the cause. The liver will be enlarged, tender and may be pulsatile if tricuspid regurgitation is present. Constrictive pericarditis is another cause.

Gross hypoalbuminaemia from other causes. This is usually due to excess urinary or gut loss of protein, of which nephrotic syndrome is the most frequent cause.

Ascites with the features of an **exudate** can result from bacterial infection of a pre-existing transudate. Spontaneous bacterial peritonitis is a common complication of ascites due to portal hypertension. The possibility of an infection is one reason for always performing a diagnostic paracentesis of 100 ml or more of fluid. The protein content of the fluid will be above 25 g/l in an exudate, and below this figure in a transudate. A transudate will usually appear clear whereas an exudate may be cloudy, turbid or bloodstained, depending on the cause. Culture for tuberculosis and pyogenic organisms should be undertaken, together with examination of the centrifuged deposit. Malignant cells may be difficult to distinguish from the normally shed peritoneal cells, but should none the less be sought. A raised white cell count of more than 250 neutrophils per mm^3 in the fluid suggests spontaneous bacterial peritonitis and is used as a criterion for initiating antibiotic treatment.

The ascitic protein content may be in the transudate range (<25 g/l) whereas in secondary bacterial peritonitis the neutrophil count is higher, greater than 1000 per mm^3 and the protein content in the exudate range (>25 g/l). Needle biopsy of the peritoneum may improve the accuracy of diagnosis of tuberculosis.

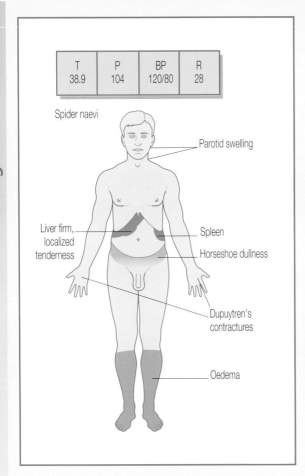

T	P	BP	R
38.9	104	120/80	28

Spider naevi

Parotid swelling

Liver firm, localized tenderness

Spleen

Horseshoe dullness

Dupuytren's contractures

Oedema

A 54-year-old freelance journalist was admitted from the outpatients clinic. He was complaining of swelling of the abdomen and pain in the right upper quadrant which had come on rapidly over the previous 10 days. For the past few months, he had felt unwell, with poor appetite and a lack of desire to smoke or drink. He had also lost nearly 12 kg in weight.

He had been attending hospital intermittently for the preceding 16 years, having initially presented with jaundice and a tender enlarged liver following a pro-longed alcoholic bout. He had only been partially successful in controlling his alcohol problem, and every few years would break loose with several weeks of continuous drinking. This had resulted in two further hospital admissions with jaundice, malaise and tender enlargement of the liver, which improved while in hospital. His wife had, despairingly, left him two and a half years previously. He had never before had oedema, ascites or splenomegaly. He had been gaining weight steadily over the years until at the time of his separation he weighed 89 kg. He smoked 40 cigarettes daily, and for the past 2 years some cough had been constantly present. His stools and urine appeared normal to him.

On examination, he looked ill and had a temperature of 38.9°C and a sinus tachycardia of 104 bpm. This fever persisted during his hospital admission. He was not visibly jaundiced. He had bilateral ankle oedema, and there were numerous spider naevi present on the arms and chest. He had bilateral Dupuytren's contractures and parotid swelling. In the abdomen, there was ascites, as shown by swelling of the flanks with a horseshoe area of dullness. There was generalized, firm, smooth, slightly tender enlargement of the liver, the left lobe was palpated with difficulty through the rectus sheath but contained an irregular hard tender area. The spleen was felt 2 cm below the left costal margin.

Initial investigations showed Hb 12.8 g/dl with normal indices and normal appearance of red cells on the film. WBC 7.4×10^9/l with normal differential. ESR 37 mm. Platelets: 330×10^9/l. Prothrombin time: 19 sec (control 12 sec). Serum bilirubin: 34 µmol/l. AST: 42 i.u./l (normal 2–20). Alkaline phosphatase: 300 i.u./l (normal 30–100). Serum albumin: 21 g/l. Serum globulin: 49 g/l. Electrophoretic strip showed decreased albumin and an increase in alpha-2 and gamma globulin.

Questions

1. What are the likely causes for the recent deterioration in this patient?
2. What are the possible causes of the ascites?
3. What further investigations should be performed?

Discussion

There is little doubt from the history, examination and investigations that this patient has cirrhosis. The strong history of alcoholism with earlier episodes suggestive of acute alcoholic hepatitis, makes alcohol the most likely cause and the presence of Dupuytren's contractures and parotid swelling supports this diagnosis.

When deterioration in health occurs in a cirrhotic patient, the first causes to be considered are whether the cirrhosis has progressed to the stage of decompensation and whether portal hypertension has developed. Weight loss, anorexia and malaise are common, though not very specific, symptoms of advanced cirrhosis. Likewise, low grade pyrexia may be associated with decompensation. Spider naevi indicate active liver disease. A falling serum albumin concentration with rising bilirubin and transaminase levels are signs of a poor prognosis.

Two features in this patient suggest that there is more than decompensation. Abdominal pain and liver tenderness do not occur in simple cirrhosis and suggest the complication of hepatoma. The disproportionate elevation of alkaline phosphatase, in the absence of obstructive jaundice, also suggests an expanding intrahepatic lesion. Hepatoma is an increasingly common terminal event in all forms of cirrhosis, though its incidence is greatest in the relatively rare form associated with haemochromatosis.

The development of splenomegaly and ascites in a patient with cirrhosis is generally due to portal hypertension. Portal hypertension more commonly occurs in the macronodular type of post-hepatitic (post-necrotic) cirrhosis than in the micronodular type associated with alcohol. The late development of the signs of portal hypertension in this patient, coinciding with the suspicion of a hepatoma, suggests that the block may be extrahepatic due to portal vein thrombosis, which can complicate hepatoma.

Ascites can result from a primary infective peritonitis due, for example, to tuberculosis which is more common in alcoholics. A more probable complication is secondary tuberculous infection of pre-existing ascites caused by portal hypertension. Similarly, secondary infection of ascitic fluid with Gram-negative bacteria can also occur and give rise to pyrexia. Secondary deposits in the peritoneum from either a hepatoma or a carcinoma of the bronchus, stomach or pancreas may cause malignant ascites and a tender nodular liver.

Other diseases occur more commonly in patients with cirrhosis. Pain suggests the possibility of peptic ulcer but would not explain the other features present. Gallstones are found more frequently in cirrhotics but this patient has not had biliary colic, does not have obstructive jaundice and is tender over the left lobe of the liver rather than the gallbladder. Pancreatitis is associated with alcoholism; however, this patient has not been drinking recently and although he is losing weight he does not have steatorrhoea.

Investigation is unlikely to provide much further evidence for cirrhosis since this diagnosis has already been reasonably well established. The hepatic origin of the elevated alkaline phosphatase could be confirmed by electrophoretic fractionation or by estimation of the gamma glutamyl transpeptidase (γGT) or 5-nucleotidase; the urine will contain excess urobilinogen. Guided liver biopsy is the only means of making a certain diagnosis of cirrhosis, but is precluded by the prolonged prothrombin time. If considered essential clotting factors could be given to temporarily correct this.

The main purpose of investigation in this patient is to establish the cause of his deterioration in the hope that it may be treatable. An ultrasound or CT scan would confirm a cirrhotic pattern with an area of different density corresponding to the suspected hepatoma. The presence of high levels of alpha fetoprotein in the blood is highly specific in suspected hepatoma. The ascitic fluid must be examined for its protein content, to distinguish transudate from exudate, and for malignant cells; it must also be cultured for tuberculosis and other bacteria. It would also be reasonable to perform blood cultures to exclude Gram-negative bacteraemia. At the time of diagnostic paracentesis, a peritoneal biopsy could be performed to look for TB or malignant deposits.

A chest X-ray might show either a bronchial carcinoma or tuberculosis. A gastroscopy or barium meal would probably be undertaken to look for oesophageal varices, gastric cancer or peptic ulcer.

Liver ultrasound scan confirmed the presence of a large uniform density in the left lobe of the liver; the rest of the scan was compatible with the diagnosis of cirrhosis. Alpha fetoprotein was present. The ascitic fluid contained 40 g/l protein and highly atypical cells suggestive of malignancy were seen. He rapidly deteriorated over the next 5 weeks, his ascites failing to respond to treatment. A hepatoma with peritoneal involvement arising from a micronodular cirrhotic liver was found at postmortem.

Loss of weight

Patients often present with vague and non-specific symptoms which provide the physician with no immediate indication as to the underlying cause whether organic or psychological. Among such symptoms is loss of weight. It is a routine in medical history-taking to ask what the weight is, to confirm this, and to assess its significance against the height and build of the patient. Even more important is to enquire whether there has been any recent change in weight. Any loss of more than 5% of the normal body weight should be considered significant and a reason sought for its occurrence. Sometimes a patient's account of weight loss seems at variance with their appearance. Regular weighings over a few weeks will be necessary to confirm that progressive weight loss is occurring.

CLINICAL ASSESSMENT

Apart from the amount of weight lost it is important to know how rapidly the loss has occurred. The more rapid the loss, the more likely it is to be due to organic disease. The weight of most people, whether it is normal or not, remains constant over long periods, although in women there is commonly some fluctuation in weight with the menstrual cycle. With middle age, both men and women tend to gain weight and this is often marked in women after the menopause. Loss of weight is widely recognized as a common symptom of disease, so that even if the patient regards loss of weight as beneficial, other members of the family may regard it more seriously. This latter situation may occur in young girls, who for cosmetic reasons want to lose weight, and who may be unwilling to recognize when the weight loss has passed acceptable bounds.

In the evaluation of weight loss the most important variable to consider is appetite. Loss of appetite is a common symptom of many illnesses. Loss of weight may often be adequately explained by a primary alteration in intake. Assessment of how much a patient is eating can be difficult without an independent witness such as a spouse or parent, and on occasions even this is not sufficient. If the appetite has declined one should always try to relate this temporally to the alteration in weight, the situation being obviously more straightforward where the loss of appetite comes first.

In a few patients the striking feature is the presence of an excellent or even increased appetite and intake of food, with weight loss. The diagnosis here is usually obvious: diabetes mellitus, thyrotoxicosis and steatorrhoea are the commonest diseases producing this pattern.

In many patients, weight loss will seem to be excessive in relation to an intake of food which is said to be normal or only slightly depressed. Here the range of possible diagnoses is widest. If there is another associated symptom this allows enquiry along appropriate lines. If no other complaint is made, more detailed questioning is needed, bearing in mind the more likely diagnoses. Two conditions commonly associated with serious causes of weight loss are anaemia and fever, and these must always be specifically excluded both clinically and by appropriate investigation. The diseases of most concern will be malignancy, endocrine disorders, malabsorption states and chronic infections. These organic diseases must be distinguished from psychological causes of weight loss which will often be the most difficult differential diagnosis. Disseminated malignancy arising from any site, or multifocally as in the lymphomas, may also be responsible. In most of these patients the diagnosis will already have been established. Weight loss is an almost invariable feature of advanced cancer especially when metastatic to the liver. It is often accompanied by anorexia and altered taste and sometimes by nausea. The cause of this cachexia syndrome is not well understood. The many abnormalities such as opportunistic infections, lymphoma and Kaposi's sarcoma complicating the immunosuppressed state created by HIV infection may present in non-specific ways such as weight loss and malaise.

Respiratory symptoms such as cough, sputum, haemoptysis, chest pain or shortness of breath may be indications of the underlying cause. Pulmonary tuberculosis is still common in many parts of the world. Weight loss in a young adult raises this possibility. The other symptoms are cough, haemoptysis and night sweats with fever. A middle-aged patient with weight loss and haemoptysis will be more likely to have carcinoma of the bronchus, particularly if a cigarette smoker. In this condition widespread dissemination can occur even though the primary remains occult. Some patients with bronchiectasis may produce very large quantities of sputum, and if this is associated with poor appetite, some degree of weight loss easily ensues. This diagnosis will be suggested by the large volume of sputum, the production of which is often related to the posture of the patient. It is often purulent and foul-smelling in character, and usually results in halitosis. In emphysema weight loss can be marked because extreme dyspnoea makes eating difficult. This diagnosis should be considered if severe breathlessness is the main complaint.

Polyuria occurs commonly with diabetes mellitus, and is often marked, the patient being also aware of the associated polydipsia. In uraemia there may be some degree of cachexia and there is a characteristic loss of the diurnal rhythm of urine secretion with resulting nocturia. In the treatment of uraemia a low protein diet may exacerbate the weight loss. Blood in the urine is always abnormal, whether macroscopic or microscopic, and may be the only indication of an underlying hypernephroma.

Weight loss may be due to heart disease – cardiac cachexia. It is uncommon and a reflection of severe heart disease, with a low cardiac output and congestive failure resulting in impaired perfusion and nutrition of the tissues. The other symptoms of heart disease will usually be present, and the diagnosis will not be in doubt.

IMPORTANT CAUSES OF WEIGHT LOSS

Gastrointestinal causes

Simple failure to eat enough food in mentally normal individuals is an uncommon cause of weight loss in developed countries. While many people have a poor diet, either because of ignorance or poverty, the total number of calories consumed is usually adequate, as the cheaper foods usually have a high fat content. In the elderly, lack of money may be combined with lack of drive and a loss of interest in food, together perhaps with ill-fitting and painful false teeth. Weight loss is an inevitable result. Vomiting or diarrhoea for any reason will rapidly lead to loss of weight, which in the more acute and severe cases will be mainly due to dehydration. Long-continued vomiting always suggests a mechanical obstruction of the upper bowel, such as pyloric stenosis following on a longstanding duodenal ulcer. **Gastric cancer** may also cause vomiting but here the anorexia will be more marked and the history shorter and of more rapid progression. Retching and vomiting, particularly in the mornings, are common in the chronic alcoholic, but weight loss occurs later, probably because of the high calorific value of the alcohol consumed. Very marked emaciation results from obstruction of the oesophagus, the cause usually being a carcinoma, when dysphagia rather than vomiting will be the major complaint.

Many patients who have in the past been treated for their peptic ulcer by partial gastrectomy will have found that they lost weight post-operatively and that regaining their pre-operative weight proved difficult. The causes of this are several and include reduced intake because of the small gastric remnant and some degree of malabsorption due to gastrointestinal hurry. The loss of weight does not usually require treatment even though more specific deficiencies of iron, folate, B_{12} and calcium may require attention.

Any inflammatory cause of **chronic diarrhoea**, particularly if it is caused by disease of the small bowel, will usually lead to weight loss – for example Crohn's disease and ulcerative colitis. Weight loss will also occur with the steatorrhoeas and here it may at times be difficult to arrive at the diagnosis. Diarrhoea is not always present nor may the stools show the classical steatorrhoeic appearance. This is particularly the case in some patients with coeliac disease. In those patients suffering primarily from pancreatic disease the steatorrhoea is usually more obvious. Tuberculous disease of the small bowel is now very rare. **Lymphoma** of the small intestine may present in this way. Tropical sprue will usually be suggested by the history of past residence in the tropics, and is an important diagnosis as the response to treatment is normally good. Previous surgery resulting in excessive reduction in absorptive area, blind loops or fistulae will again be suggested by the history (see Ch. 12).

Cancer of the large bowel may cause weight loss, but this is a less striking feature than with carcinoma of the stomach. The major associated symptoms will be of alteration in bowel habit, blood in the stool with left-sided lesions, whereas carcinoma of the caecum and ascending colon present with anaemia or a palpable mass.

Malignant disease

It has already been emphasized that weight loss is an important feature in most gastrointestinal malignancies, particularly carcinoma of the stomach. It also occurs in the majority of cancers when the tumour is extensive, and may also occasionally occur for reasons which are not clear at an early stage when the tumour is small. In some cases it may be because of infection and fever associated with the primary tumour, but if marked must always suggest dissemination of the cancer. In the lymphomas weight loss may also occur early on. Fever, lymph node enlargement, anaemia and bone pain may all be present.

Chronic infections

These are not now a common cause in Northern Europe with the exception of infections occurring in HIV and AIDS (see below). Tuberculosis must be considered, but is usually easily excluded by chest X-ray. **Miliary tuberculosis** can still be a difficult diagnosis, but the presentation is unlikely to be that of a simple loss of weight. Some cases of infective endocarditis may progress only very slowly, with general debility, weight loss and fever as major features. There will usually be some pointer to a cardiac lesion and ultimately of course embolic phenomena will develop. Blood cultures are the essential investigation in infective endocarditis, and microscopic haematuria is often present.

Diarrhoea and weight loss frequently occur in patients with **chronic HIV infection**. Usually a pathogen is found but there is an enteropathy associated with HIV itself. Cryptosporidium is a protozoal gut infection causing diarrhoea and weight loss, occasionally accompanied by electrolyte disturbance. Other opportunistic protozoal infections are those caused by microsporidium and *Isospora belli*. Atypical mycobacteria may infect the gut. Bowel ulceration with herpes viruses (CMV and herpes simplex) may also occur. (For further investigation of FUO see Ch. 20.)

Psychiatric causes

Anorexia nervosa is increasing in frequency, and occurs predominantly in teenage girls and young women. It consists of a gradual and progressive reduction in food intake so that finally gross emaciation occurs which can be fatal. In contrast to the physical state they characteristically remain very active and restless. Amenorrhoea is almost invariable and a number of other minor physical changes occur, such as lanugo. Some patients have a history of obesity, for which they have dieted vigorously, and anorexia nervosa has supervened, perhaps interspersed with, or preceded by, bulimia (binge eating and self-induced vomiting). There is almost invariably a deeper disturbance of personality, mood and family background. Despite the apparent wellbeing professed by the patients, they may be seriously ill and may need admission to hospital for treatment. Management is difficult and is made more so by the lengths to which the patient will go to hide food or to induce vomiting surreptitiously. Patients will also be unreliable in taking any prescribed medication. The main differential diagnosis is hypopituitarism. Anorexia nervosa can itself cause endocrine disturbances through the hypothalamic–pituitary axis. Unlike organic causes of hypopituitarism, hypothyroidism is a relatively early feature.

Weight loss is a common feature of both anxiety and depressive states and is usually proportional to the severity of the disturbance. In depression the loss of appetite may be almost complete and the loss of weight correspondingly severe. In some cases of depression the presence of other somatic symptoms such as loss of libido, early waking and constipation will aid in the diagnosis. The depression and accompanying weight loss will often respond to antidepressants.

Anxiety states may occasionally prove difficult to differentiate clinically from thyrotoxicosis but this is not a diagnostic problem with the ready availability of thyroid function tests.

Some schizophrenics may show disinterest in food and lose weight, and patients in a phase of manic excitement may also fail to eat adequately as a result of their restlessness and easy distractibility. In neither case is the diagnosis likely to prove difficult.

Endocrine disorders

The commonest endocrine conditions causing weight loss are **diabetes mellitus** and **thyrotoxicosis**. The diabetic who presents with weight loss will usually be young and prove to be insulin dependent. The other typical symptoms of polyuria and polydipsia will normally be present and indeed the presentation is sometimes with ketoacidosis. Even if these features are absent, the diagnosis will rarely be missed if the urine is always tested for sugar.

Hyperthyroidism is usually associated with weight loss, and although in a young woman the clinical picture will often be typical and the diagnosis straightforward, in an elderly male it is much more easily missed. Important confirmatory symptoms will be a good appetite despite the weight loss, heat intolerance, sweating, diarrhoea, shortness of breath on exertion, palpitations, undue fatiguability and a general motor overactivity and nervousness. In the elderly, the symptoms of cardiovascular disease often dominate and the patient may present with angina pectoris, or congestive heart failure which is usually high output in type. Atrial fibrillation is common and may be either paroxysmal or permanent. There can be difficulty in distinguishing between the thyrotoxicosis and anxiety states, where weight loss is also common. In general an increase in appetite with a marked loss of weight will suggest thyroid overactivity rather than a psychological cause.

Weight loss is sometimes a feature of adrenal insufficiency. The clinical severity and rate of progression may be variable and may be exacerbated by any form of stress. The symptoms are often very non-specific, and include tiredness, lassitude and vague gastrointestinal complaints such as nausea and vomiting. They are easily attributed to psychological causes. Depression and other psychoses may occur secondarily and will respond only to adequate steroid replacement therapy. Pigmentation is perhaps the single most helpful sign in leading to the diagnosis. Dizziness and faints can result from the postural hypotension which may occur in addition to the overall lowering of the blood pressure. Loss of body hair may be marked, especially in women, and be a source of complaint, but sexual functions are otherwise unaffected and amenorrhoea is unusual.

Patients with **hypopituitarism** are usually of normal weight. In some, however, loss of weight with reduction in subcutaneous fat does occur, but this is rarely extreme. Very marked emaciation is more likely to indicate a diagnosis of anorexia nervosa. Failure of anterior pituitary secretion leads to a fineness and wrinkling of the skin. Libido is reduced and body hair lost. The genitalia show atrophy, and there is usually oligo- or amenorrhoea. Any or all of the features of hypothyroidism can be present. Pigmentation of the skin is generally reduced, as is the pigmentary response to sunlight. So-called pituitary cachexia, however, only occurs if the pituitary destruction has been caused by a wasting disease such as tuberculosis or secondary carcinoma.

Loss of weight

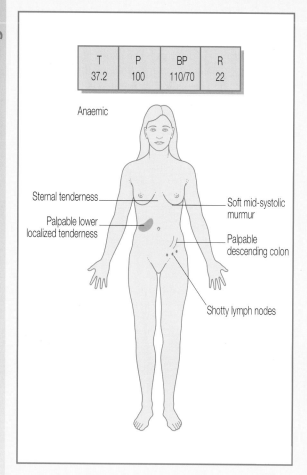

T	P	BP	R
37.2	100	110/70	22

Anaemic

Sternal tenderness

Palpable lower localized tenderness

Soft mid-systolic murmur

Palpable descending colon

Shotty lymph nodes

A 52-year-old woman was referred to the Outpatients clinic. She was Indian and spoke little English, although she had been in the UK for 5 years. The history given by her husband was that over the last 8 months she had lost a great deal of weight and had now become very thin. He denied that she had been attempting to diet and said that he had never objected to her previous weight. Her appetite had never been good, but had been worse recently. For the previous few months she had felt increasingly tired and had found difficulty in coping with her domestic responsibilities. She was very concerned about this, as she felt she was not caring adequately for her family. Over this time her sleep had been poor, but there had been no early waking. She also complained of occasional dyspepsia for some years, and of some generalized aching in her limbs more recently.

Previously she had been well except for malaria as a child and typhoid when she was 14. She did not smoke or drink alcohol. Her periods had been scanty for the last 8 months, but previously had been heavy and lasted about 8 days. Her parents were dead and she had seven siblings alive and well. She had four healthy children, two of whom were still at home.

On examination, she seemed quiet and withdrawn, and had obviously lost weight; her height was 158 cm, weight 45 kg. She was a little pale, but there was no abnormal bruising or bleeding. The pulse was 100/min regular and the blood pressure 110/70. No abnormality was present in the cardiovascular system except for a soft mid-systolic murmur, best heard just internal to the apex. No abnormal signs were present in the lungs, but pressure over the sternum elicited a little tenderness. The descending colon was palpable and slightly tender and the lower pole of the right kidney could be felt. Rectal examination was normal. A few shotty lymph nodes could be felt in both groins. Neurological examination revealed no abnormality. Urine examination was normal.

Questions

1. What are the most probable diagnoses?
2. What investigations would be of value?

Discussion

Although psychiatric causes of weight loss are common, organic disease must be first excluded and then, of the patients still undiagnosed, the majority will probably be found to be suffering from a depressive illness. Carcinomatosis could be responsible for this woman's loss of weight, but after 8 months it is a little surprising that no symptoms or signs have developed pointing towards the primary growth. A palpable right kidney is common in thin people and its significance uncertain since the urine is normal on routine examination. Sternal tenderness always suggests marrow infiltration with tumour or leukaemia. A depressive illness is a possibility, and may be occurring as a reaction to the disruption of old ties and the social isolation which many immigrant wives experience. Against this is the tachycardia and systolic murmur, which suggests anaemia, and also the body pains. Anaemia, however, is never a sufficient diagnosis in itself and one must always find the underlying cause. Lymphoma is not a common cause of this clinical picture, but could certainly explain this patient's illness. Tuberculosis must always be considered as a cause of loss of weight, especially in patients from India, who are prone to the extrapulmonary forms of the disease.

Management at this stage must be by further investigation and not by any therapeutic trial, whether of haematinics or of psychotropic drugs. A good history could not be obtained because of language difficulties and under such circumstances the physician is commonly forced to rely on a series of screening investigations. A blood picture is mandatory, not only for the haemoglobin but also for the white cell count and differential, and an examination of the stained film. The ESR and CRP are valuable screening investigations. Chest X-ray will always be part of the routine work-up of such a patient. It may show pulmonary tuberculosis, primary or secondary carcinoma and bony deposits. Sternal secondaries are not easily identified on routine chest films and spine views must be obtained. A bone scan will be more sensitive than radiology in the demonstration of bone lesions. A marrow examination, especially from the tender area, may give the diagnosis.

Investigation of this patient showed a normochromic normocytic anaemia of 8 g/dl. The ESR was very high at 95 mm. CXR revealed scattered osteolytic lesions in the ribs, and bone marrow examination established a diagnosis of secondary carcinoma. An IVP showed a left-sided hypernephroma.

17

Tiredness and fatigue

It is normal to feel tired at times, to suffer mental fatigue after sleepless nights and working long hours, and to be physically tired after unaccustomed exertion. It is normal, too, to feel tired during and after illness. *Persistent tiredness or physical fatigue*, with no obvious cause, is a common complaint and one that doctors often find difficult to manage to the satisfaction of the patient.

Fatigue is a common symptom of disease. When patients describe their symptoms, feelings of tiredness and exhaustion associated with diseases such as cancer, Crohn's disease and rheumatoid arthritis are often under-rated by doctors even though the symptoms may dominate the patient's life. Many patients on the other hand will have no discernible cause for the complaint. They are, nevertheless, concerned that it is diagnosed and treated. Fatigue as a symptom, rather than as a normal event, requires that the patient regards it as being of sufficient severity to prevent, or make difficult, normal activity. For the doctor the challenge is to exclude physical illness simply and reliably, and to offer guidance to management of the other causes.

THE CAUSES OF CHRONIC FATIGUE

Most chronic diseases are accompanied by varying degrees of fatigue. The main causes are shown in Box 17.1.

Cardiac

Fatigue is an invariable feature of 'forward' cardiac failure due to ischaemic or valvular heart disease. The reasons are not well understood. Resting skeletal muscle blood flow remains normal until heart failure is severe. However, in order to maintain blood pressure, there is a failure of vasodilatation in skeletal muscle on exercise. In addition there is wasting of skeletal muiscle in heart failure which is in part due to reduced exercise.

This reduction in muscle mass and deconditioning reduces muscle oxidative efficiency and causes fatigue, especially on exertion. Treatment of heart failure with ACE inhibitors and diuretics may give symptomatic improvement.

Anaemia

Chronic anaemia is often well tolerated, especially in the young. In the elderly, especially in those with a co-existing disorder such as ischaemic heart disease, even mild degrees of anaemia may cause fatigue. The diagnosis that anaemia is present is straightforward, but the diagnosis of the underlying cause may prove more difficult, especially of normochromic normocytic anaemia (see Ch. 18).

Infection

Infectious mononucleosis is usually accompanied by tiredness and fatigue typically lasting a few weeks. Occasionally the fatigue may persist, and the symptoms come to resemble that of the chronic fatigue syndrome (see below). Fatigue is a prominent feature of **AIDS** and, in an HIV-positive patient, may be an early symptom of the development of AIDS before the onset of other, opportunistic, infections.

Chronic infections such as **tuberculosis** and **brucellosis** also cause fatigue. The latter is now very uncommon in Europe and in North America. Tuberculosis may cause diagnostic difficulty when occult and disseminated. Nowadays this usually occurs in the context of HIV infection or in other situations where there is depressed immunity such as chronic immuno-suppressive therapy, malnourishment, or in frail elderly patients. **Lyme disease** causes fatigue in its chronic phase. The typical erythematous rash, occurring 3–20 days after the bite of the *Ixodes* tick, may have been overlooked. The spirochaete *Borrelia burgdorferi* goes on to cause arthritis, muscle and tendon pains, lymphocytic meningitis and radiculitis, and cardiomyopathy and arrythmias. These features lead to the diagnosis.

Malignancy

Fatigue and weight loss are important symptoms of cancer, especially when metastatic. The causes are not known, but may in part be due to cytokine release from tumour cells. Fatigue is a prominent component of the paraneoplastic syndrome of anorexia, altered taste and weight loss that is an almost invariable accompaniment of advanced cancer, especially when metastatic to the liver. Loss of muscle bulk leads to weakness and fatigue on exertion. Fatigue alone may be the present-

---

Box 17.1 Causes of chronic fatigue

Chronic fatigue syndrome
Post-viral syndrome
  Infectious mononucleosis, viral hepatitis
Depression
  Neurotic, psychotic
Anaemia
Malignancy
  Metastatic to liver or bone marrow
Chronic infection
  Tuberculosis, HIV, Lyme disease, brucellosis
Chronic inflammatory disease
  Crohn's disease, rheumatoid arthritis
Cardiac failure
Sleep disturbance
  Sleep apnoea, depression, sedatives, alcohol
Drug abuse
  Benzodiazepines, alcohol
Endocrine disease
  Myxoedema, Addison's disease

---

ing symptom of cancer although this is relatively uncommon. Other symptoms such as weight loss and those of the primary or metastatic tumour usually appear within a few weeks.

Sleep disturbance

Sleep disturbance causes sleepiness rather than fatigue. Nevertheless patients use the word 'tiredness' to describe both symptoms and a careful history of sleep patterns, and of daytime sleepiness, must be obtained to make the distinction.

Patients with obstructive sleep apnoea may have such disturbed sleep that daytime somnolence becomes a major disability and a great danger when driving. This may be accompanied by physical fatigue on moderate exertion but the complaint is more of sleepiness. Patients with sleep apnoea are usually considerably overweight and often have fat necks. The loss of muscle tone during sleep leads to narrowing of the upper airway and excessive snoring. Importantly this may be made more likely by alcohol and sedative drugs. Benzodiazepines and alcohol frequently lead to chaotic sleep patterns even in those who do not have obstructive sleep apnoea. Anxiety and depression also frequently disrupt sleep. Depression is especially important since it is easily overlooked and is often accompanied by physical fatigue.

Chronic fatigue syndrome

This syndrome is characterized by disabling physical fatigue often accompanied by difficulty in concentra-tion and aching muscles. Other terms used to descibe the condition are *post-viral fatigue* and *myalgic encephalomyelitis* (ME). Both are unsatisfactory since they ascribe an unproven infective or inflammatory cause to the syndrome. The condition, for which there are no generally accepted diagnostic criteria, presents a challenge in diagnosis and in management.

Typically the patient is a young adult. There is sometimes an antecedent history of ill-defined viral infection or of proven infectious mononucleosis. The patients describe physical tiredness of such a degree that they can only function for a few hours at a time. Exercise may be followed by hours or days of exhaustion. Mental fatigue is often present. As the weeks go by the symptoms interfere with work or study. Other symptoms add to the problem such as failure of concentration, sleep of poor quality, dizziness, muscle aches and depression. The symptoms fluctuate with periods of relative normality followed by disabling exhaustion.

A careful history is essential since treatable causes of organic or psychiatric illness must be recognized. The other organic causes of fatigue described in this chapter (Box 17.1) will usually be easily excluded by history, physical examination and simple investigations such as chest X-ray, full blood count, ESR, monospot and liver function tests. Drug and alcohol abuse may cause sleep disturbance and fatigue. Prescribed drugs such as benzodiazepines and beta-blocking agents may also cause excessive tiredness. Depression is the major differential diagnosis. The mental state should be assessed (see below). Often the topic must be approached carefully, since many patients with the chronic fatigue syndrome become resentful at the suggestion that their symptoms do not have an organic cause. Indeed patients, and their anxious relatives, may have specific diseases in mind, especially cancer, but sometimes infections such as HIV.

Management is often difficult because of the imprecision of the diagnosis, the chronicity of the symptoms and sometimes because of a belief by the patient and relatives that something is wrong that is not being diagnosed. The following guidelines are helpful:

- Patients should be told about chronic fatigue syndrome. They should be told that it is not due to a known viral infection; it is made worse by prolonged bed rest; it may be overlaid by understandable depression and anxiety; it will get better.
- The aim of management is to help the patient to get back to physical and mental activity by a programme of slow increase in physical activity. The advice and guidance of an experienced physiotherapist is invaluable.
- If there are symptoms suggestive of depression (whether primary or secondary to the symptoms) an anti-depressant may help preferably after spe-

cialist advice. However, patients may refuse formal psychiatric assessment or treatment.

For severely affected patients recovery may be slow although most are better in 2–3 years. Less severely affected patients will improve in a few months.

Endocrine disease

Patients with **myxoedema** commonly present with symptoms which include lethargy and tiredness. There may also be muscle cramps. These symptoms may be mistaken for chronic fatigue syndrome or depression. Mental depression, poor memory and concentration may occur in myxoedema concealing the diagnosis.

Patients with **Addison's disease** may present with ill-defined symptoms of fatigue, weakness malaise and muscle cramps. Other features of the disease may be present, such as hypotension, pigmentation, nausea and vomiting, but at the onset of the illness the symptoms may be vague and the diagnosis unsuspected.

Neuromuscular diseases

The characteristic presenting symptom of **myasthenia gravis** is muscle fatigue on exertion. In a mild case muscle weakness may only be demonstrable after exercise. Typically ptosis will also be present. The limb weakness is more proximal, but the small muscles of the hand are also usually affected. The reflexes are preserved and may be brisk. If they are absent, an alternative cause of muscle fatigue on exercise should be considered, such as the Eaton–Lambert syndrome which is a rare paraneoplastic complication of small cell lung cancer which may mimic myasthenia gravis.

Muscle fatigue and aching are prominent symptoms of polymyositis, polymyalgia rheumatica and **proximal myopathy** from any cause. The localized nature of the muscle weakness and fatigue usually leads to a diagnosis.

Depression

Depression often presents with somatic symptoms. Fatigue, loss of energy and tiredness may be prominent. There are associated features that make the diagnosis of depression more probable, although any prolonged illness may be associated with an associated depressive reaction. In depression there is depressed mood, sleep disturbance – either difficulty in falling asleep or early morning waking – loss of libido, low self-worth and other somatic features such as constipation. There may be suicidal thoughts and, in psychotic depression, there may be depressive delusions.

In a typical case there is little difficulty in distinguishing severe neurotic or psychotic depression from other causes of chronic fatigue. The differential diagnosis between depression and chronic fatigue syndrome may be much more difficult after a prolonged period of fatigue. The patient may have lost time from, or have had to give up, work or study, may see no sign of improvement in symptoms, and have lost confidence in the possibility of a return to normal health. In these circumstances anxiety and depression are understandable and add to the diagnostic difficulty.

AN APPROACH TO DIAGNOSIS

The history will be most important in diagnosis.

The patient

Chronic fatigue syndrome is most common in teenagers and young adults and especially in students. It is very uncommon after early middle age. Depression is more common in women aged 30 and over. In middle-aged and elderly people, the symptoms of chronic fatigue are more likely to be due to an underlying organic cause.

Onset

The history should enquire into an antecedent illness such as infectious mononucleosis or external events at work or in the family. Weight loss may suggest malignancy or depression, episodes of fever suggest a chronic infection such as tuberculosis. Cold intolerance will suggest myxoedema. Sleep disturbance will be present in sleep apnoea, and may be a prominent feature in depression, alcohol or sedative abuse.

Course

In chronic fatigue syndrome the illness may fluctuate from week to week and be temporarily relieved by rest, followed by further exacerbation on attempts to return to normal activity. In malignancy the symptoms are usually progressive and worsen inexorably. The same is true for endocrine deficiencies and infective illnesses. Neurotic depression may also fluctuate considerably with changing circumstances.

Physical examination

This must be meticulous, bearing in mind the diagnostic possibilities. In chronic fatigue syndrome and in depression there will be no abnormal signs. In malignancy, the liver may be palpable or there may be enlarged lymph nodes. Oral or vaginal *Candida* may raise the possibility of HIV infection. Proximal muscle weakness or tenderness will suggest a myopathy or

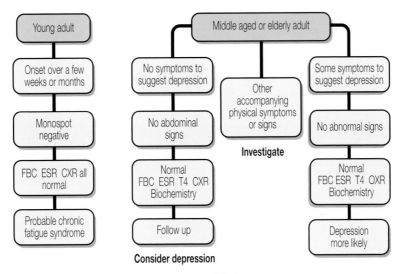

Fig. 17.1 An algorithm for diagnosis of fatigue.

myositis. Postural hypotension is usual in Addison's disease.

Preliminary investigation

A basic screening examination for organic disease should include the following:

- chest X ray: may show metastasis, lymph node enlargement or tuberculosis
- Full blood count and ESR: may show anaemia, leucocytosis, or suggest inflammatory or malignant disease
- Monospot test: if negative will exclude infectious mononucleosis
- Liver function tests will help to exclude hepatic metastases
- T4 and TSH will exclude hypothyroidism

- Blood urea, creatinine and electrolytes will exclude significant renal failure and hypercalcaemia.

Where possible a positive diagnosis of depression or chronic fatigue syndrome should be made *before* the investigations which, when negative, are presented to the patient as a previously agreed means of excluding illnesses that were anyway considered unlikely on clinical grounds. If, conversely, the investigations are presented as a means of trying to find out what accounts for a mysterious illness, the normality of the tests may not be reassuring. The doctor may then find that he or she engages in a process of multiple, and increasingly invasive, tests in order to find out 'what is wrong'. When each test is normal the position is not necessarily improved. Reassurance, and a planned approach to treatment of the chronic fatigue syndrome or depression, is then made more difficult.

CLINICAL PROBLEM

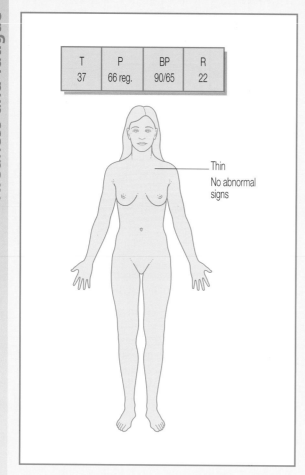

T	P	BP	R
37	66 reg.	90/65	22

Thin
No abnormal signs

A 26-year-old accounts clerk consulted her general practitioner with the complaint of increasing tiredness and fatigue over a 6-week period accompanied by a weight loss of about 8 kg. The symptoms had started after a particularly severe upper respiratory infection accompanied by an intensely sore throat, cough and muscle aches and pains. At first the symptoms were tolerable but, on return to work, she found that by mid-morning she was exhausted. Any form of physical exertion was difficult and followed by severe fatigue. She had taken two weeks off work and had rested but had found that the lack of energy and concentration did not improve.

Six months previously she had had a period of disturbed sleep characterized by waking at 2–3 a.m. This had followed the break-up of a four-year relationship, and had been associated with feelings of tiredness and loss of appetite. She had gradually recovered without treatment although she had consulted her GP and he had considered her to be mildly depressed.

Four years previously she had had an iron deficiency anaemia attributed to menorrhagia. This had responded to oral iron. She had been taking an oral contraceptive since that time.

On examination she was 5' 7" and weighed 50 kg. She looked tired. BP90/65. P66 regular She was not clinically anaemic. There was no lymph node enlargement. There were no abnormalities in the heart, lungs or abdomen. The optic fundi and CNS examination were normal.

Questions

1. What is your differential diagnosis?
2. What investigations would you perform in the first instance?

Discussion

In a person of this age the onset of severe fatigue, unaccompanied by other specific symptoms, suggests that she is suffering from the chronic fatigue syndrome. In this disorder there is sometimes a history that the symptoms followed an upper respiratory infection. However in this case the severity of the sore throat suggests that this might have been infectious mononucleosis, following which fatigue is often protracted. The worsening of symptoms during the day and following exertion are typical of chronic fatigue syndrome, but are non-specific since they can occur in many chronic diseases. The lack of physical signs on examination is typical of chronic fatigue syndrome and the fatigue that follows infectious mononucleosis.

However there are other diagnoses that must be considered. First among these is that she might be depressed. She has had a previous episode very suggestive of depression, associated with sleep disturbance and loss of appetite. This had a clear precipitating cause. These symptoms are not present now. Another feature of her illness that needs explanation is her weight loss. She is underweight for her height. This suggests a psychiatric explanation such as depression accompanied by anorexia, but could of course be caused by organic disease. She has previously had iron deficiency anaemia which, if present now, would cause fatigue and tiredness, but there are no clinical signs to suggest this.

The likelihood of chronic fatigue syndrome being the cause means that the patient should understand that investigation is not being undertaken in the expectation that this will lead to the disclosure of an underlying disorder that accounts for her symptoms, but to be certain that this possibility is excluded.

The appropriate first tests are a full blood count and monospot to exclude iron deficiency and infectious mononucleosis. In view of the weight loss the ESR and CRP should be measured and a chest X-ray obtained since if these are normal they will point away from an organic cause such as an underlying malignancy or chronic inflammatory disorder. Renal failure and myxoedema should be excluded by measurement of the blood urea and creatinine and the plasma T4 and TSH.

The history should be expanded to explore the possibility of depression further. One of the difficulties in the diagnosis of chronic fatigue syndrome is that the disruption to working and social life cause additional symptoms of anxiety and depression.

If these investigations are normal, the diagnosis of chronic fatigue is more likely and is suggested by the history. A gradual programme of rehabilitation, as described above, is then started.

> In this patient the investigations proved to be normal. A programme of graded return to activity was started, but it was many months before her symptoms improved.

18

Anaemia

Although many patients who are anaemic have become so from a cause which may easily be discovered and treated, the cause of anaemia can sometimes be difficult to determine. Certain symptoms and physical signs are common to all patients with anaemia regardless of its cause. Many patients complain of tiredness, fatigue and dyspnoea on exertion. The level of haemoglobin at which symptoms appear depends on age, the presence of associated medical conditions, occupation and the rapidity with which the anaemia has developed.

The symptoms are often due to a worsening of another, unrelated condition. Angina pectoris may be provoked, especially in the elderly population with ischaemic heart disease or left ventricular hypertrophy due to hypertension or aortic valve disease. If either heart disease or anaemia is severe, congestive cardiac failure may develop. Mental confusion may commonly be exacerbated in the elderly.

Specific features of history and physical examination relating to underlying causes are discussed later. Some signs are due to anaemia of any cause. Pallor of the nails and conjunctivae are the distinctive signs, but are often not noticeable even with quite severe anaemia. The physical signs of congestive cardiac failure may be present, and there is often a tachycardia with bounding peripheral pulses and a systolic ejection murmur.

The confirmation of the clinical suspicion of anaemia is by measurement of the haemoglobin. The automated cell counter measures haemoglobin concentration, the mean red cell volume (MCV) and number. The mean cell haemoglobin concentration (MCHC) and mean cell haemoglobin (MCH) are calculated automatically. The type of anaemia can then be divided into three broad categories according to the MCV: microcytic, normocytic and macrocytic.

Additional morphological information, often helpful in diagnosis, is then obtained by examination of the blood film.

MICROCYTIC ANAEMIA

The MCV (mean corpuscular volume) and the MCH (mean corpuscular haemoglobin) are the indices indicating microcytosis and hypochromia.

By far the commonest cause of hypochromic microcytic anaemia is iron deficiency. Absorption and loss of iron are normally in balance (see Fig. 18.1). Iron is taken up from the upper small bowel crossing the mucosal cells to be bound to plasma transferrin. It is transported to the marrow where it is incorporated into red cells, and to the reticuloendothelial (RE) system where it is stored as ferritin and haemosiderin. The body iron store is in haemoglobin and the RE system. Bleeding will cause a negative iron balance if absorption does not match loss. The plasma iron pool is very small, and is turning over rapidly as iron is supplied to the marrow from RE cellular stores. When the iron stores are exhausted, the plasma iron falls and insufficient iron is available to the marrow for haemoglobin synthesis, resulting in anaemia. Iron deficiency anaemia with a low plasma iron may also occur if the reticuloendothelial cells are unable to relinquish their iron into the plasma. This occurs in chronic infection and malignancy (the 'anaemia of chronic disease'). In sideroblastic anaemia, on the other hand, a hypochromic microcytic anaemia arises because the bone marrow cannot incorporate iron into red cells effectively. In this anaemia, however, the plasma iron level is not depressed. A hypochromic microcytic type of anaemia also occurs when synthesis of haemoglobin is impaired due to an inborn error of globin production, as in thalassaemia, when the storage, release and uptake of iron are all normal.

History and examination

The majority of patients with hypochromic microcytic anaemia have iron deficiency and most of these have blood loss as the cause. In pre-menopausal women iron deficiency is usually the result of loss in menstruation not matched by adequate iron intake. In all age groups, but especially in children and the elderly, dietary lack of iron may be an important contributory factor, and will only be discovered if a careful history is taken of what the patient actually eats.

If the symptoms of anaemia have developed over a few weeks then gastrointestinal haemorrhage is likely and symptoms of melaena or haematemesis may be obvious. Occult bleeding from the gastrointestinal tract is common. In elderly women oesophagitis due to gastro-oesophageal reflux is a common cause and is often asymptomatic. A history of anorexia, nausea, dysphagia or altered bowel habit may point to an underlying neoplasm. Malabsorption syndrome may

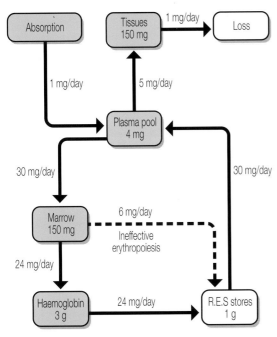

Fig. 18.1 Pathways of iron metabolism. Figures on the arrowed pathways indicate the amount of iron passing daily in this direction. Figures indicate the size of the various pools.

be suggested by the passage of bulky pale stools, but may be present even when the bowel habit is normal (see Ch. 13). Hookworm infestation usually presents with iron deficiency anaemia rather than with symptoms of the primary infestation.

Bruising and bleeding from sites such as the gums and urinary tract are serious symptoms suggestive of thrombocytopenia or bleeding from local malignancy as a reason for iron deficiency.

The anaemia of chronic infection may be hypochromic, and tuberculosis or localized collections of pus will be suspected by the characteristic fever and the local symptoms of the infection. Rheumatoid arthritis and other connective tissue disorders may all cause hypochromic anaemia but other signs of the disease will be present. Malignant neoplasms at any site can cause hypochromic anaemia, and weight loss, anorexia and other specific localizing symptoms such as haematuria may all be pointers to the diagnosis.

On examination the signs of iron deficiency may be present, with smooth tongue, cheilitis and koilonychia. An abdominal mass may indicate a gastrointestinal carcinoma or hypernephroma. The liver and spleen may be enlarged in a patient with hepatic cirrhosis and bleeding varices and also in patients with thalas-

saemia major. The latter condition should always be considered in patients who derive from Mediterranean regions, central Africa and parts of Asia. A moderate enlargement of the spleen may rarely occur in severe iron deficiency anaemia from any cause. Enlarged lymph nodes may indicate an unsuspected neoplasm, while more generalized lymphadenopathy occurs in lymphomas or tuberculosis. Rectal examination may reveal haemorrhoids, a melaena stool or a rectal carcinoma.

Investigation

Examination of the blood film and measurement of the serum iron and iron-binding capacity (TIBC) are the essential first steps. In iron deficiency the blood film will show anisocytosis, poikilocytosis and pencil cells. In thalassaemia there will be target cells and nucleated red cells. In sideroblastic anaemia the red cells may show a dimorphic picture of microcytosis and some normal cells. Thrombocytopenia may be present and the cause may be suggested by the white count (e.g. leukaemia). The serum iron may be low in iron deficiency anaemia with an increased iron-binding capacity (transferrin). In the anaemia of chronic disease (which may be mildly hypochromic) the serum iron is also low but there is no rise in the transferrin. In sideroblastic anaemias and in thalassaemia the serum iron will be normal or raised. The serum ferritin is a guide to the body iron stores and is low in iron deficiency.

A bone marrow examination will be helpful in difficult cases. In iron deficiency there will be erythroid hyperplasia and no stainable iron in the marrow. Iron will be present in the anaemia of infection and in sideroblastic anaemia. In the latter condition the iron is arranged in clumps around the cell nucleus of erythroid precursors – so-called 'ring sideroblasts'. A marrow aspirate may also show evidence of a primary blood disorder such as leukaemia, or secondary carcinoma.

In most patients with hypochromic microcytic anaemia the cause of iron deficiency will be discovered easily. This will usually turn out to be occult gastrointestinal blood loss, dietary deficiency or menstrual loss. If the serum iron is low and there is no stainable iron in the marrow, the problem is to find the cause of iron deficiency. Repeated examination of stools for occult blood, gastroscopy, colonoscopy, barium swallow and meal and barium enema examination may all be needed. In the elderly and in young children careful dietary assessment is necessary.

In some patients oral iron will have been given, without adequate response. The commonest reasons for a failure of response of anaemia to oral iron are that:

- iron deficiency is not present (in particular that the patient has the anaemia of chronic disease)
- occult bleeding is continuing
- the patient has not taken the tablets
- there is failure of absorption of iron such as occurs after gastrectomy and in malabsorption syndrome.

If the serum iron is normal the diagnosis may be sideroblastic anaemia or thalassaemia. Most cases of sideroblastic anaemia are acquired, and the disorder usually occurs in late middle age. Sideroblasts may be seen in the marrow in a variety of other conditions such as haemolytic anaemia, carcinoma, leukaemia and in nutritional and megaloblastic anaemias. Many acquired sideroblastic anaemias are idiopathic. The blood film usually shows anisocytosis and polychromasia, and some red cells are normochromic. The bone marrow appearance, with ring sideroblasts, is typical. Some of the idiopathic cases respond to large doses of pyridoxine, and in some an element of folate deficiency is present.

Thalassaemia major is a severe disease readily distinguished from iron deficiency anaemia because of the clinical and haematological characteristics. Patients with the less obvious condition of thalassaemia minor are often erroneously and harmfully treated with iron. The blood film usually shows target cells and basophilic red cells due to immature red cells. Diagnosis is by haemoglobin electrophoresis, which shows a moderate increase in HbA_2, and by finding affected relatives.

NORMOCYTIC ANAEMIA

It is in this group of anaemias that some of the most difficult problems in diagnosis arise. A classification of the causes is shown in Box 18.1.

History and examination

The diagnosis is usually suggested by the clinical details. Acute blood loss will be obvious, and occult bleeding has already been discussed. Malignancy is a common cause of normocytic anaemia in middle-aged and elderly patients. Although the history may be typical, and signs of a tumour may be present, it is not uncommon for the tumour to be occult. Malaise, fever, weight loss and anaemia may be the only indications of the underlying disease. An abdominal mass and enlargement of lymph nodes must be sought.

Chronic renal failure must be excluded in any patient with a normocytic anaemia. A history of polyuria and nocturia may be present, and the patient may show pigmentation and be hypertensive.

Box 18.1 Causes of normocytic anaemia

1. **Blood loss**
   Acute or subacute before iron deficiency occurs

2. **Inflammation**
   Pyogenic
   Infective endocarditis
   Tuberculous
   Connective tissue diseases (e.g. rheumatoid arthritis, polymyalgia rheumatica)

3. **Malignancy**
   Disseminated carcinoma
   Bone marrow replacement: myeloma, leukaemia, metastatic carcinoma, myelofibrosis (these often cause a leucoerythroblastic anaemia)

4. **Chronic renal failure**

5. **Aplastic anaemia**

6. **Endocrine disorders**
   Myxoedema
   Hypopituitarism
   Addison's disease

7. **Malnutrition**
   Protein calorie malnutrition
   Scurvy

8. **Haemolytic anaemias**
   Due to intrinsic red cell defects:

   - hereditary spherocytosis and elliptocytosis
   - abnormal haemoglobins; sickle-cell disease
   - enzyme defects (e.g. pyruvate kinase deficiency)

   Due to extrinsic factors:

   - autoimmune haemolytic anaemias due to drugs (usually in G6PD deficient individuals)
   - cold haemoglobinuria
   - hypersplenism
   - disseminated intravascular coagulation (e.g. due to septicaemia)

Myxoedema may be accompanied by mild normocytic anaemia, as may pituitary and adrenal insufficiency. There may be obvious features on history and examination to suggest these diagnoses, but the most important step is to consider these disorders in a patient with undiagnosed anaemia.

Conditions causing bone marrow infiltration, such as myeloma, will often be accompanied by bone pain and perhaps by pathological fractures. If there is thrombocytopenia there may be bruising and purpura. Myelofibrosis is almost always accompanied by splenomegaly.

Haemolysis may be suspected by a history of jaundice without dark urine. The spleen will usually be enlarged if the cause is hereditary spherocytosis or autoimmune haemolytic anaemia. Hereditary spherocytosis will be suspected if there is a family history of anaemia. Jaundice is often present, and recurrent haemolytic crises with deepening jaundice occur. Pigment gallstones frequently develop and may cause symptoms including obstructive jaundice.

In children, autoimmune haemolytic anaemia may follow viral infections, while in adults it may sometimes be associated with diseases such as SLE, lymphomas and chronic lymphatic leukaemia. If there is long-standing splenomegaly from any cause this may lead to anaemia as a result of hypersplenism.

If the haemolysis is acute and intravascular there will be haemoglobinuria. In paroxysmal nocturnal haemoglobinuria there is haemoglobinuria on waking which may be accompanied by abdominal or loin pain. In paroxysmal cold haemoglobinuria there is acute intravascular haemolysis after exposure to cold.

In glucose-6-phosphate dehydrogenase (G6PD) deficiency, the patient is usually Afro-Caribbean or Mediterranean. The disorder has a sex-linked inheritance of variable expression. The clinical picture is of acute haemolysis following exposure to a drug or broad beans (favism). There is jaundice and there may be haemoglobinuria. Occasionally acute infections may precipitate an attack. A wide variety of drugs can provoke haemolysis, such as antimalarials, sulfonamides, nitrofurantoin, analgesics and sulfones.

In aplastic anaemia the patient may present with anaemia or symptoms of infection due to neutropenia. A history of exposure to drugs such as chloramphenicol or chemicals such as benzene should be sought. Lead poisoning, although uncommon, is often accompanied by anaemia and may not be remembered as a possible cause of anaemia in young children. It may also occur in adults in the appropriate occupations.

Sickle-cell anaemia usually presents in early childhood. The symptoms of anaemia are present and sickling crises occur with bone and joint pain, abdominal pain, fever and cerebrovascular accidents. Although splenomegaly is common in children, in adults it is less so because of repeated splenic infarctions during sickling crises. There is commonly a mild degree of jaundice, which is more apparent during a crisis. Cardiomegaly is frequently present, and a systolic murmur is often heard. Leg ulcers are common.

A variety of inherited red cell enzyme defects are described which are often accompanied by a haemolytic anaemia. The commonest is pyruvate kinase deficiency which is inherited as an autosomal recessive character. The presentation is usually in childhood, and the degree of haemolysis varies from mild to severe. Slight jaundice is often present, splenomegaly is common and slight enlargement of the liver is not unusual. Inherited red cell enzyme defects should be thought of in any child or young adult with congenital haemolysis when spherocytosis is not present.

Investigation

Examination of the peripheral blood will often indicate the type of anaemia present. The red cells will show spherocytosis in hereditary spherocytosis, and some degree of spherocytosis is common in autoimmune haemolytic anaemias. Marked anisocytosis and poikilocytosis suggest bone marrow infiltration or disseminated carcinoma. In chronic renal failure there may be burr cells present, and target cells in liver disease. A reticulocytosis always suggests acute blood loss or haemolysis as a cause of the anaemia. Basophilic stippling is found in G6PD deficiency and in lead poisoning. Heinz bodies (haemoglobin precipitate) may be seen during haemolysis in G6PD deficiency and in some patients with inherited defects of haemoglobin which render the haemoglobin unstable (e.g. Hb Koln and Hb Zurich). Howell–Jolly bodies are found in hyposplenism, which is a feature of coeliac disease, where anaemia due to multiple deficiencies may be present. If there is bone marrow infiltration from myeloma, there is often marked rouleaux formation due to the paraprotein. Marrow replacement will also be suggested if a leucoerythroblastic blood picture is present with normoblasts, immature white cells and thrombocytopenia. A low white count may occur in aplastic anaemia or aleukaemic leukaemia, while a raised white count may occur in renal failure and disseminated malignancy as well as in infections.

The ESR may be helpful. It will not be raised in myxoedema or hypopituitarism or in blood loss from non-malignant causes. It will be raised in most other conditions, but very high values suggest myeloma or a connective tissue disease, especially polymyalgia rheumatica and polyarteritis.

Haemolysis will be suggested by spherocytosis, jaundice (indirect hyperbilirubinaemia), reticulocytosis, increased urinary urobilinogen and splenomegaly. Further investigation of the cause will be discussed later.

A chest X-ray is essential. It may show malignant deposits in the lungs, a primary bronchial carcinoma, and myeloma or secondary carcinoma in the ribs. Enlarged hilar or paratracheal nodes may be present, suggestive of lymphoma or tuberculosis. The lungs may also show tuberculosis, and a right-sided pleural effusion, perhaps with elevation of the hemidiaphragm, may point towards an underlying hepatic or subphrenic abscess although this will normally have been suspected on other grounds. Disseminated carcinoma and bone marrow infiltrations may be demonstrated by skeletal X-rays.

The urine may show red cells and white cells, suggesting renal infection or glomerulonephritis. Persistent microscopic haematuria is strongly suggestive of renal or bladder carcinoma. Proteinuria will usually be present in chronic renal disease. Culture of the urine is important, and a sterile urine with the presence of pus cells always suggests renal tuberculosis. Any of these findings will be an indication for further investigation, including blood urea and intravenous pyelography.

The gastrointestinal tract is a common site of hidden malignancy, and the stools may contain occult blood. Upper and lower GI endoscopy or barium meal and enema examinations will be necessary to exclude this possibility. The anaemia of blood loss is, however, much more likely to be hypochromic.

A bone marrow aspiration will usually demonstrate leukaemia or myeloma if present, but a bone marrow biopsy may be needed in some cases of aplastic anaemia and myeloma, and in many cases of secondary carcinoma of bone and myelofibrosis.

Liver function tests, tests for SLE, myxoedema and hypopituitarism will be carried out where appropriate.

If haemolysis is suspected on clinical grounds or because of jaundice and reticulocytosis, a variety of further investigations are needed. If haemolysis is suspected but not definitely present, then a raised urinary and faecal urobilinogen and decreased plasma haptoglobin may indicate its presence. Haemolysis can be confirmed by finding a decreased red cell half-life after injecting the patient's chromium-labelled erythrocytes intravenously. This test is only of value if there is no bleeding.

An osmotic fragility test will show a decreased resistance to hypotonic solutions in hereditary spherocytosis, and to a lesser extent in autoimmune haemolytic anaemias. The indirect antiglobulin test will be positive in the majority of cases of chronic autoimmune haemolytic anaemia during a relapse. In acute autoimmune haemolytic anaemias, only half of the cases have a positive antiglobulin test.

Further investigation of haemolytic anaemias will depend on the clinical picture. In autoimmune haemolytic anaemia, the presence of anti-DNA antibodies will support a diagnosis of SLE and biopsy of an enlarged lymph node may reveal an underlying lymphoma or chronic lymphatic leukaemia of which the anaemia is a manifestation. Sickle-cell anaemia will be demonstrated by the sickling test and by haemoglobin electrophoresis, and the latter test will show other abnormal haemoglobins. Estimation of G6PD activity can be made, and other red cell enzymes such as

pyruvate kinase can be estimated in cases of congenital non-spherocytic haemolytic anaemias. The Donath–Landsteiner antibody is detectable in paroxysmal cold haemoglobinuria, and the acid haemolysin and sucrose lysis tests are positive in paroxysmal nocturnal haemoglobinuria.

MACROCYTIC ANAEMIA

Macrocytes in the peripheral blood are usually the result of megaloblastic erythropoiesis in the bone marrow. Macrocytes are apparent on a blood film to the skilled observer, and increase in the MCV is a reliable guide to macrocytosis. However, it is not uncommon for a mixed iron deficiency and megaloblastic process to be present in the same patient and the automated red cell indices can then indicate normocytic cells, while examination of the blood film will show a dimorphic picture with microcytic hypochromic cells and macrocytic normochromic cells.

Although macrocytosis usually means that megaloblastic erythropoiesis is occurring, this is not always so, and normoblastic changes can be found under some circumstances. Some degree of macrocytosis is common in haemolytic anaemias and in post-haemorrhagic anaemia where larger, more immature erythrocytes are released into the circulation.

Many of the conditions where normocytic anaemia occurs may occasionally cause macrocytosis. These include myxoedema, hypopituitarism, bone marrow infiltration, acute leukaemia and aplastic anaemia. Macrocytosis is a frequent and sensitive accompaniment of alcohol excess, probably due to failure of folate utilization rather than folate deficiency. Liver disease from any cause may result in macrocytosis, part of which may be due to folate deficiency. The diagnosis of these conditions has been discussed. If there is any doubt as to the cause of a macrocytic blood picture, a bone marrow examination will be made. If normoblastic erythropoiesis is found then diagnosis will proceed along lines already discussed.

The main causes of megaloblastic erythropoiesis are summarized in Box 18.2.

History and examination

Pernicious anaemia occurs in the middle-aged and elderly, although a rare juvenile form occurs. The onset is insidious with symptoms of anaemia. Glossitis is common and may be present before anaemia. Central nervous system symptoms may also be the presenting feature, especially in men. The complaint is usually of paraesthesiae and numbness in the hands and feet due to neuropathy, and unsteadiness of gait with weakness of the legs. Mental disturbance is common, with

Box 18.2 The causes of megaloblastic erythropoiesis

1. Lack of vitamin B$_{12}$

Due to inadequate dietary intake:

- dietary deficiency in strict vegetarians
- fish tapeworm

Due to lack of intrinsic factor:

- pernicious anaemia
- total gastrectomy
- partial gastrectomy and gastric atrophy

Due to failure of intestinal absorption:

- disease or resection of terminal ileum
- stagnant loop syndrome contaminated bowel
- tropical sprue

2. Lack of folic acid

Due to inadequate intake:

- dietary deficiency (especially in the elderly and in alcoholics)
- pregnancy (increased demand)
- chronic haemolytic anaemia (increased demand)

Due to failure of intestinal absorption:

- coeliac disease
- tropical sprue
- anticonvulsant drugs

confusion and dementia. Loss of control of rectum and bladder occurs late, and external ocular palsy and retrobulbar neuritis are rare manifestations. Anorexia, weight loss and fever are common. Symptoms identical with those of pernicious anaemia may occur in any of the conditions which lead to lack of vitamin B$_{12}$ and a history of previous gastric or intestinal surgery may be present, or of terminal ileal disease such as Crohn's disease or tuberculosis (Ch. 13, p. 96). The fish tapeworm *Diphyllobothrium latum* does not usually cause symptoms other than those due to B$_{12}$ deficiency. It lives for many years and only a small proportion of those infested develop anaemia.

Folic acid deficiency also causes glossitis and loss of appetite, but neurological symptoms do not develop. There may be a history of underlying disease causing malabsorption syndrome, or the patient may be epileptic on anti-convulsant drugs when folate deficiency may occur possibly due to interference with folate absorption. Super-added folic acid deficiency may occur in chronic haemolytic states.

On examination, the physical signs will be those of anaemia, together with glossitis. In the case of per-nicious anaemia the patients are often prematurely grey, and a mild degree of jaundice is common. In the nervous system there may be mental confusion, peripheral neuropathy, upper motor neurone signs in the legs and also posterior column signs (SACD). In severe cases retinal haemorrhages occur.

In folate deficiency there may be other signs also related to an underlying cause such as gluten enteropathy, causing malabsorption (see Ch. 13).

Investigation

The blood film often shows hypersegmentation of neutrophils when there is megaloblastic erythropoiesis from any cause. There may be slight neutropenia and thrombocytopenia as well. Anisocytosis and poikilocytosis are marked in both B$_{12}$ and folate deficiency. Where the cause is nutritional, iron deficiency may co-exist and a dimorphic blood picture may be seen.

A marrow aspiration will establish whether there is megaloblastic erythropoiesis. Usually the cause will be clear, but serum B$_{12}$ and folate estimations will be diagnostic. Serum B$_{12}$ is especially helpful if the diagnosis of subacute combined degeneration (SACD) is suspected in a patient with little or no anaemia.

If the serum B$_{12}$ is low, a Schilling test (in which the absorption of radioactive B$_{12}$ is measured with and without intrinsic factor) will help to determine whether there is an intestinal defect of absorption or whether there is lack of intrinsic factor. Confirmatory evidence that pernicious anaemia is present will come from finding anti-intrinsic factor and anti-parietal cell antibodies in the serum. In juvenile pernicious anaemia, the antibody tests are negative. If intestinal malabsorption of B$_{12}$ is demonstrated by the Schilling test, radiological investigation of the small bowel will be required.

If folic acid deficiency is shown, investigation for steatorrhoea will be needed (see Ch. 13, p. 95), and an assessment of the patient's dietary intake will be necessary. The folic acid deficiency caused by anticonvulsants (phenytoin, primidone and phenobarbitone) responds rapidly to folic acid administration.

Finally, a possible cause of megaloblastic erythropoiesis, and an established cause of macrocytic anaemia is scurvy. The megaloblastic changes may be due to vitamin C lack itself or to a concomitant folic acid deficiency which is often present. The disease should be suspected in an anaemic patient with haemorrhagic manifestations and follicular hyperkeratosis in the skin. The white cell vitamin C content will be low.

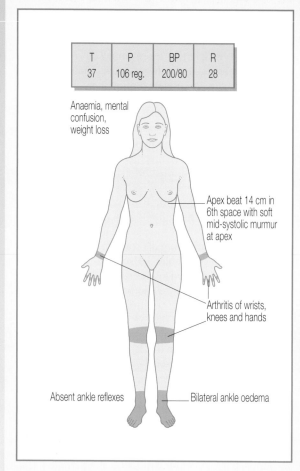

T	P	BP	R
37	106 reg.	200/80	28

Anaemia, mental confusion, weight loss

Apex beat 14 cm in 6th space with soft mid-systolic murmur at apex

Arthritis of wrists, knees and hands

Absent ankle reflexes

Bilateral ankle oedema

A woman of 82 was admitted to hospital having been found wandering in the street at night. She was confused and obstreperous and neighbours had called an ambulance when she refused to return to her own home. Her daughter said that following the death of the patient's husband 3 years earlier she had become depressed and withdrawn. She had not gone out of the house much and had refused all offers of assistance. Her daughter had tried to help by bringing in food and cleaning her flat. She had noticed that her mother had been losing weight over a 6-month period, and 3 months before admission the patient consulted her family doctor because of ankle swelling, and shortness of breath on exertion and at night-time in bed. These symptoms had responded to diuretic treatment. For 2 months she had been irritable and unco-operative, and her daughter had noticed that she had become untidy and forgetful.

She had had a hysterectomy 30 years previously for post-menopausal bleeding. For 20 years she had suffered from rheumatoid arthritis with deformity in the small joints of the hands and swelling and pain intermittently in the knees, wrists and hands. She had taken a variety of anti-inflammatory drugs for several years, and for the preceding 2 years her joints had not been troublesome and had not imposed any limitation on her activities.

On examination she was rather dirty and was clearly confused. Apart from absent ankle jerks there were no other abnormal signs in the nervous system. Temperature 37°C; pulse 106 regular; blood pressure 200/80; R 28/min. She was clinically anaemic, and her tongue was smooth and depapillated. The nails were cracked. The jugular venous pressure was not raised, but there was some ankle oedema bilaterally. The heart was enlarged with the apex beat 14 cm out in the 6th space in the anterior axillary line. A soft mid-systolic murmur was present at the apex. She had clearly lost some weight, but there were no other abnormal physical signs in the lungs and abdomen. Rectal examination was normal. She had rheumatoid arthritis involving the hands, knees and wrists, with some deformity but little pain on movement.

Investigations: Hb 8.2 g/dl; ESR 86 mm/h; MCH 29 pg; MCV 80 fl; WBC 4.2 × 10⁹/l with normal differential count. Platelets 259 × 10⁹/l. Chest X-ray showed cardiac enlargement with distension of upper lobe veins.

Questions

1. Which aspects of the history and physical signs might be related to the cause of her anaemia?
2. How would you interpret the red cell indices?
3. How would you investigate her further?

Discussion

Elderly people are prone to nutritional deficiencies and social isolation increases the likelihood of this occurring. The patient had been depressed and isolated since the death of her husband 3 years earlier. With respect to the anaemia, dietary deficiency of iron and folic acid are the likeliest causes, since dietary B$_{12}$ deficiency is very uncommon, unless very strict vegetarian diets are adhered to for a long time, as the liver stores are long lasting. Dietary iron deficiency will quickly cause anaemia if there is blood loss as well. The possible causes of blood loss in this patient are occult malignancy which is suggested by her weight loss over the preceding 6 months, and analgesic ingestion as treatment of her chronic rheumatoid arthritis although this had been inactive for some time.

The onset of congestive cardiac failure can be attributed to her anaemia. The physical signs of a wide pulse pressure, a large heart and a mid-systolic murmur support this, as does the radiographic finding of cardiomegaly and distension of upper lobe veins. A cardiac murmur in an anaemic patient with a raised ESR raises the possibility of subacute infective endorcarditis which must be excluded by blood cultures as other classical symptoms and signs may be absent.

The mental confusion may have several causes. Any severe anaemia in elderly people, who are likely to have some degree of cerebral arteriosclerosis, may provoke mental confusion and disorientation, especially in those who are socially isolated. The combination of mental confusion and anaemia raises the possibility of B$_{12}$ deficiency, and although there is nothing in the history to suggest a cause of B$_{12}$ deficiency in this patient, this must be excluded. Her confusional state may also be caused by cerebral secondaries from an occult malignancy, or by cerebrovascular disease alone.

Physical examination in this patient does not give much information as to the cause of the anaemia. The smooth depapillated tongue might be due to iron or B$_{12}$ deficiency. Absent ankle reflexes are common in old age and do not necessarily indicate peripheral neuropathy associated with B$_{12}$ deficiency or underlying carcinoma. There is no bruising or follicular hyperkeratosis suggestive of scurvy.

The red cell indices indicate a normochromic normocytic anaemia. This is unlike the findings in iron, folate or B$_{12}$ deficiency. Normochromic, normocytic anaemia suggests disseminated malignancy as a more likely diagnosis in this patient. Rheumatoid arthritis may also cause this type of anaemia and a raised sedimentation rate. The fact that the arthritis is quiescent at present is strongly against this as a cause.

The red cell indices may however be misleading if taken in isolation. Indices indicating normochromic normocytic anaemia may be found if there is microcytosis and macrocytosis present at the same time. Such a situation often arises if iron deficiency is combined with deficiency of folate or B$_{12}$. This combination of events is especially likely in the elderly. The meaning of these indices cannot be assessed unless a blood film is examined, when hypochromic cells may be seen, and macrocytes, with anisocytosis and poikilocytosis. There may be hypersegmentation of the nucleus of polymorphonuclear leucocytes in folate and B$_{12}$ deficiency. If the blood film suggests that a 'dimorphic' blood picture is present, then serum iron, folate and B$_{12}$ should be estimated. If these are normal then the likelihood of occult malignancy is strengthened. However chronic renal failure should also be excluded, especially in view of the history of analgesic treatment for years, which might have caused analgesic nephropathy. Thyroid function should be checked.

If investigations show that there is a deficiency of iron, folate or B$_{12}$ then most physicians would simply treat the anaemia appropriately, without a sternal marrow examination, in a patient of this age. Iron deficiency however should be investigated further in view of her weight loss, since a remediable condition may be found, such as giant gastric ulcer, or a slow-growing carcinoma of the colon, or chronic aspirin ingestion. Careful dietary assessment and endoscopy or barium studies will be needed.

If no deficiency is found, or if the result of treatment is only a small rise in haemoglobin, then GI studies may show the site of an underlying cancer. A CT brain scan and an ultrasound liver scan, both of which are non-distressing investigations, may be very suggestive of secondary deposits rendering further investigation and treatment inadvisable. Cerebral atrophy may be present.

> This patient had combined iron and folate deficiency. The latter was thought to be dietary in origin. The iron deficiency was attributed to gastrointestinal bleeding as a result of analgesic ingestion.

Bruising and bleeding

Many patients say that they bruise easily, but only a minority turn out to have an underlying blood disorder. The diagnosis of the cause of a bleeding tendency covers a wide range of medicine, but clinical evidence alone will often provide the answer without the necessity for complicated laboratory tests.

Purpura is due to bleeding into the skin. The appearance is of numerous small haemorrhages in the skin, clearly defined, not raised, and distinguished from telangiectases by the fact that they do not blanch on pressure. Ecchymoses are larger purpuric areas. Both ecchymoses and purpura are a result of increased capillary fragility, by far the commonest cause of which is thrombocytopenia. Bruises are larger areas of bleeding, usually occurring subcutaneously. They may be found in thrombocytopenic patients, who may also have purpura. On the other hand, when there is a deficiency of a clotting factor, the capillaries are not unduly fragile and significant bruising may be found without purpura.

HISTORY

When taking the history the clinician should enquire closely into the length of time the patient has noticed the tendency to bleed: ask also about operations and tooth extractions, and about past attacks of joint swelling. Haemophiliacs usually begin to notice their symptoms when they are old enough to run about and hurt themselves. The onset of symptoms in thrombocytopenic purpura may be very abrupt, especially in children.

The extent of the bleeding should be ascertained. One should enquire whether the patient has noticed blood in the urine or stools. Visceral bleeding is of especial importance since, although it may occur in any patient with a bleeding tendency, it may equally well indicate underlying disease of the gut or urinary tract which the bleeding tendency has brought to light.

Conversely, although localized bleeding, for example from the gastrointestinal tract, will usually indicate a local disorder, the unexpected onset of bleeding from a local site may be the first sign of a generalized bleeding disorder.

Joint symptoms are of great importance for two reasons. Firstly, haemarthrosis is a very common feature of many bleeding disorders, especially haemophilia A and B. Secondly, polyarthritis may accompany diseases in which bleeding is a feature, such as allergic purpura, systemic lupus erythematosus and drug sensitivity.

Constitutional symptoms may be present. Fever is a common symptom in leukaemia, and may also occur as a result of infection in any condition where there is bone marrow depression. A febrile illness, sometimes viral, commonly precedes acute thrombocytopenia in children. Weight loss is an important symptom, often indicating an underlying neoplasm or lymphoma.

Drugs may cause thrombocytopenia alone, or a general bone marrow aplasia. The commonest are phenylbutazone, gold, chloramphenicol, thioureas, chlorothiazide and carbamazepine. Quinidine causes a selective thrombocytopenia due to an immune destruction of platelets. It is obvious that severe bleeding may result from anti-coagulant therapy, particularly if inadequately controlled. Similarly, most cytotoxic drugs will produce marrow depression as a direct toxic effect rather than due to idiosyncrasy.

Finally, a family history of any tendency to bruise or bleed should be sought. In haemophilia not only is there a family history, but the severity of the disorder tends to be similar in different members of the same family.

PHYSICAL EXAMINATION

Examination of the skin is very important. Purpura always suggests thrombocytopenia, although it also occurs in capillary disorders such as scurvy and von Willebrand's disease. 'Senile' purpura is often seen over the hands, forearms and shins of the elderly. The skin is usually smooth, atrophic and hairless, and there is no other abnormality.

The distribution and nature of the rash is characteristic in Henoch–Schönlein purpura. It is usually present over the legs and buttocks and around the elbows. The lesions are unusual because the bleeding is due to local vasculitis. They are often raised and accompanied by erythema, unlike thrombocytopenic purpura. While examining the skin, look for the facial, buccal and digital lesions of hereditary haemorrhagic telangiectasia, and the thickened lax skin of pseudoxanthoma elasticum which is often best seen around the neck. In scurvy, purpura mainly affects the legs, and is associated with a rough skin, due to follicular keratosis, and corkscrew hairs.

A number of important signs may be seen in the mouth. Bleeding gums suggests thrombocytopenia while loose teeth and bleeding gums suggest scurvy. Palatal and faucial ulceration are serious signs suggesting an associated neutropenia due to aplastic anaemia or leukaemia. Palatal ulceration also occurs in infectious mononucleosis, in which thrombocytopenia may sometimes occur. Oral thrush commonly complicates aplastic anaemia and leukaemia. Gum hypertrophy occurs in monocytic leukaemia, and palatal haemorrhages in thrombocytopenia from any cause.

The musculoskeletal system is important in both diagnosis and management. Recurrent haemarthroses often occur in haemophilia A and B. As a result, there may be loss of range of joint movement, fibrous ankylosis of joints, wasting of surrounding muscle groups and entrapment neuropathies. Sternal tenderness and pain in the bones are signs suggestive of acute leukaemia, or some other malignant process causing bone marrow infiltration. Subperiosteal haemorrhages may occur in a variety of bleeding disorders, especially scurvy, and may occasionally be misdiagnosed as bone tumours.

Enlargement of the spleen suggests lymphoma, leukaemia, or myeloproliferative disorders. However, splenomegaly, due for example to portal hypertension, may itself give rise to hypersplenism and pancytopenia.

In the central nervous system, any acute neurological disturbance in a patient on anticoagulants should raise the possibility of localized bleeding as a cause. The optic fundi may show retinal haemorrhages, especially in thrombocytopenia. They also occur in systemic infections such as subacute infective endocarditis. Retinal exudates may occur in systemic lupus erythematosus which is sometimes accompanied by thrombocytopenia. Occasionally the retinae may be infiltrated with leukaemic or lymphomatous deposits.

Generalized lymph node enlargement occurs in acute leukaemia, lymphoma and in chronic lymphatic leukaemia. Enlargement of cervical lymph nodes as a result of oral and pharyngeal inflammation is common in aplastic anaemia, acute leukaemia and infectious mononucleosis.

SIMPLE INVESTIGATIONS

In the majority of cases it will have been possible to decide on clinical grounds whether the bleeding ten-

dency is due to disturbance of clotting or of platelet function, and the cause which might underlie either. The following simple tests will usually confirm the diagnosis.

Full blood count

The diagnosis of thrombocytopenia is confirmed by the platelet count. The automated blood count must always be supplemented by examination of the peripheral blood film if thrombocytopenia is present. In general, the lower the platelet count the greater the risk and extent of bleeding. The presence of immature white cells with blast forms suggests an acute leukaemia, while the appearance of both immature red and white cells – a leucoerythroblastic blood picture – always suggests marrow infiltration, by carcinoma, lymphoma or myelofibrosis. Chronic myeloid leukaemia and chronic lymphatic leukaemia are easily recognized on a peripheral blood film. The atypical mononuclear cells of infectious mononucleosis may be seen.

THE CAUSES OF THROMBOCYTOPENIA
(see Box 19.1)

Bone marrow infiltration

Acute leukaemia must always be excluded in a thrombocytopenic patient. The peripheral white cell count may confirm the diagnosis, but in 'aleukaemic leukaemia' it may be normal or show a neutropenia. Chronic myeloid and lymphatic leukaemia, on the other hand, are accompanied by a characteristic white count and usually obvious physical signs. Secondary carcinoma, lymphoma and myeloma must be considered as possible causes.

The major physical sign in myelofibrosis is splenomegaly, which is usually gross. The disease may complicate polycythaemia rubra vera and myeloid metaplasia. It is usually accompanied by a leucoerythroblastic blood picture, and the platelet count is often reduced later in the disease. Occasionally the platelet count may be raised with large abnormal forms present.

Bone marrow depression

Aplastic anaemia is almost always accompanied by thrombocytopenia, and leucopenia is commonly present. Some drugs such as phenylbutazone may primarily affect platelet formation. Toxic depression of the marrow occurs as a direct effect of cytotoxic drugs and ionizing radiation. It may also occur in uraemia and in any severe systemic infection.

1. **Bone marrow infiltration**
   Leukaemias
   Lymphomas
   Myeloma
   Secondary carcinoma
   Myelofibrosis
   Infections such as tuberculosis
   Rare hereditary disorders (osteopetrosis, Gaucher's disease)

2. **Bone marrow depression**
   Drugs
   Metabolic (e.g. uraemia)
   Infection (severe systemic infection, e.g. septicaemia, typhoid)
   Megaloblastic anaemia
   Rare inherited disorders of platelet production (e.g. Wiskott–Aldrich syndrome)

3. **Increased platelet destruction**
   Antibody mediated:
   - idiopathic thrombocytopenic purpura
   - drugs
   - post-transfusion
   - viral infections (e.g. infectious mononucleosis, measles)

   Hypersplenism
   Disseminated intravascular coagulation
   Thrombotic thrombocytopenic purpura

4. **Intrinsic platelet defects**
   Myeloproliferative disorders (including thrombocythaemia)
   Hereditary disorders (e.g. Glanzmann's disease)

Increased platelet destruction

In some patients who have thrombocytopenia as a result of drugs, circulating antibodies can be found which are directed against the platelet-drug combination. In most cases of idiopathic thrombocytopenic purpura, antibodies against platelets can be demonstrated, but the techniques are difficult and the results variable.

In patients with a big spleen from any cause – lymphoma, tropical disease, portal hypertension – platelets may be destroyed excessively in the spleen. Often there is an accompanying neutropenia and anaemia. This is called hypersplenism.

Intrinsic platelet defects

In the myeloproliferative syndromes, although platelets may be produced in excessive quantities they do not

function normally, and the effect is as though there is thrombocytopenia. The platelets often assume bizarre and giant forms. This may occur in the myeloproliferative disorders such as polycythaemia rubra vera, chronic myeloid leukaemia and haemorrhagic thrombocythaemia. There is a rare congenital condition called Glanzmann's disease (or thromboaesthenia) in which the platelets are normal in number but do not aggregate properly in response to various agents including ADP.

Other causes of thrombocytopenia

Other causes of thrombocytopenia are shown in Box 19.1. In some of these the mechanism of production of the disorder is unclear.

FURTHER INVESTIGATION OF PLATELET DISORDERS

A wide variety of further investigations may be needed in order to define the cause of thrombocytopenia. The most important is examination of the marrow, since this may show leukaemia or cancer cells. The presence or absence of megakaryocytes in normal numbers will provide information as to whether there is defective production of platelets. If bone marrow aspiration is normal or a dry tap is obtained, a trephine biopsy should be done. It may show infiltration by carcinoma or lymphoma, or the appearances of myelofibrosis. It will also show the presence of aplasia.

Other investigations which may be indicated are blood urea, radiological skeletal survey, urine examination, protein electrophoresis and ANF tests.

CLOTTING DEFECTS

A simple but workable scheme of clotting is seen in Fig. 19.1. The simplest initial tests in determining the cause of a coagulation defect are as follows.

The prothrombin time

Tissue thromboplastin, in the form of brain extract, and calcium is added to the patient's plasma. The extrinsic system is activated and clotting will normally occur within 15 seconds. The intrinsic system is also activated, but takes longer to produce clotting, making the prothrombin time a test of the extrinsic system (Factor VII) and the common pathway. If Factors X, V, prothrombin and fibrinogen are reduced, then the prothrombin time will also be prolonged, but in this case tests of the intrinsic system will also be abnormal.

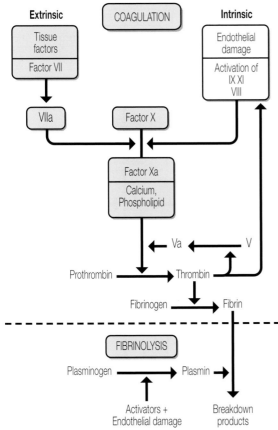

Fig. 19.1 A simplified scheme of coagulation.

Although it is called the prothrombin time and used to control anti-coagulant therapy, in practice prothrombin reduction is not the most important effect of these drugs.

Partial thromboplastin time and kaolin cephalin clotting time

These tests eliminate some of the variability of the whole blood clotting time. They provide a reliable surface for activation and an essential phospholipid. The intrinsic system (essentially Factors VIII and IX) is measured, since tissue juices are not added to the test system. The test normally produces clotting in about one minute. It will also be prolonged if the common Factors X, V, prothrombin and fibrinogen are deficient.

These tests will give a good idea of what kind of clotting defect is present. The thromboplastin generation test will define whether Factor VIII or IX is missing from the intrinsic system but specific assays are now available.

Thrombin time

A solution of thrombin is added to plasma and the time taken to clot is measured. Prolongation is seen in hypofibrinogenaemia and during heparin therapy.

CAUSES OF CLOTTING DEFECTS

A widely accepted current view is that coagulation is proceeding all the time, with fibrin deposition in blood vessels preserving the integrity of the vascular endothelium. Fibrinolytic mechanisms are also active, continuously removing excess fibrin and ensuring the patency of the vascular channels. Defects in coagulation can be considered under the following headings.

Inherited defects of specific clotting factors

The commonest deficiency states are haemophilia A, inherited as a sex-linked recessive, in which there is a deficiency of Factor VIII activity (AHG) and haemophilia B (Christmas disease, also a sex-linked recessive) where the deficiency is of Factor IX activity. (In some cases of haemophilia a form of Factor VIII is present which has no biological activity.) Many haemophiliacs know when they are bleeding even though there are no clinical signs of haemorrhage. Bleeding from any site may occur in either disease. The diagnosis is made on the history and nowadays by assay of the activity of the specific factor. The thromboplastin generation test is also used in the diagnosis of these two disorders.

In von Willebrand's disease (autosomal dominant) there is a deficiency of Factor VIII activity and an abnormality of platelet function in which the platelets do not aggregate in the presence of ristocetin. Factor VIII activity is dependent on von Willebrand's factor (VWF) for prolongation of its half-life, and VWF also binds platelets to the exposed endothelium. Absence of VWF thus causes deficient clotting and prolongation of the bleeding time.

Acquired defects in thrombin formation

The commonest cause by far is the use of anti-coagulants, but deficiency of vitamin K and liver disease both produce very similar effects. Production of Factor VII is mainly affected, but IX and X are also reduced in amount, as is prothrombin itself.

Disorders due to circulating coagulation inhibitors

A bleeding tendency may occur due to the formation of inhibitors of coagulation factors. These can develop in connective tissue diseases, in patients with malignancy, and in pemphigus. Occasionally they develop in elderly men without a predisposing cause. Usually the inhibitor is an antibody to AHG, but in systemic lupus erythematosus the inhibitors affect thrombin formation. Antifactor VIII antibodies may be produced in haemophiliacs undergoing prolonged treatment with cryoprecipitate or Factor VIII.

Disseminated intravascular coagulation

As a result of septicaemia, particularly Gram-negative septicaemia, a widespread intravascular coagulation can occur with generalized fibrin deposition. The whole clotting mechanism is activated and thus clotting factors and platelets are greatly reduced in amount. This acute defibrination is often called 'consumption coagulopathy'. There is a severe haemorrhagic disorder and often circulatory collapse. A similar state of affairs may occur as a result of antepartum haemorrhage or amniotic fluid embolism, probably as a result of autoinfusion of tissue thromboplastin. The disorder may also be found in association with some carcinomas, particularly of the prostate, although it is often less acute. A diagram of the sequence of events is shown (Fig. 19.2). A similar process occurs in the haemolytic uraemic syndrome. The haemolysis in this condition is caused by damage to erythrocytes in the fibrin mesh deposited in small vessels. In these cases treatment with fibrinogen may be harmful.

Release of plasminogen activator and excess fibrinolysis occurs in situations of tissue trauma and intravascular coagulation. Thus in all the disorders outlined as a cause of acquired fibrinogen deficiency, excess fibrinolysis is occurring too, and may aggravate the bleeding tendency. In addition, after prostatectomy, urokinase – which is an activator of fibrinolysis – may be liberated, and this may account for some cases of excessive bleeding after this opera-

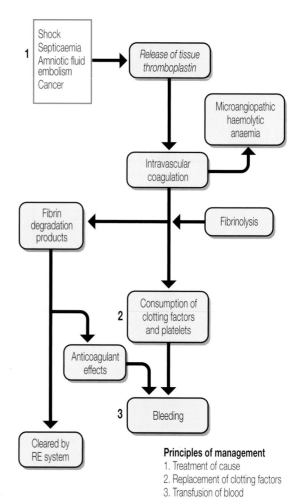

Principles of management
1. Treatment of cause
2. Replacement of clotting factors
3. Transfusion of blood

Fig. 19.2 Disseminated intravascular coagulation.

tion. Tests of fibrinolysis are not well standardized. In general they involve measurement of the time taken to lyse blood clot, and the detection of fibrin breakdown products.

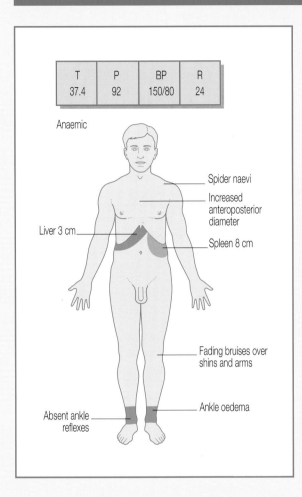

T	P	BP	R
37.4	92	150/80	24

Anaemic

Spider naevi

Increased anteroposterior diameter

Liver 3 cm

Spleen 8 cm

Fading bruises over shins and arms

Absent ankle reflexes

Ankle oedema

erate ankle oedema, and over the same period of time he had noticed that he was bruising easily. There had not been bleeding from other sites. He was a heavy smoker, having smoked 40 cigarettes a day for 35 years, and had a cough productive of mucoid sputum. He drank spirits regularly.

He had lived a solitary life abroad, in rural Nigeria. He had never married. There was no family history of any bleeding tendency.

On examination he looked unwell. He was clinically anaemic, but not jaundiced or cyanosed. There was moderate ankle oedema, but no other evidence of congestive cardiac failure. The heart was not enlarged. BP 150/80. Pulse 92 regular. In the chest there was an increased anteroposterior diameter, and occasional crackles in both lungs which cleared on coughing. In the abdomen the liver was palpable 3 cm below the costal margin, and was smooth. There was enlargement of the spleen, 8 cm below the costal margin. There were no abnormal abdominal wall veins and no ascites. The skin showed occasional purpuric areas over the backs of the hands, and fading bruises over the shins and arms. There were a few spider naevi over the shoulders. The central nervous system was normal apart from loss of both ankle reflexes.

Investigations Hb 8.1 g/dl; MCV 96 fl; WBC 2.4×10^9/l; neutrophils 1.0×10^9/l; lymphocytes 1.2×10^9/l; eosinophils 0.2×10^9/l; platelets 48×10^9/l; prothrombin time 17 s (control 13 s).

An oil company executive aged 55 returned home to England from Nigeria, having been dismissed from his job. He had been abroad for 15 years after demobilization from the army. He had been ill for the past year with weight loss and loss of appetite. There had been no alteration in bowel habit. For 2 months he had noticed mod-

Questions

1. What are the most likely diagnoses?
2. What further investigations should be undertaken?
3. What is the likely explanation of his bleeding tendency?

Discussion

This patient has chronic ill-health, enlargement of the liver and spleen, ankle oedema and absent ankle reflexes. Cirrhosis of the liver is a strong possibility, the ankle oedema being due to hypoalbuminaemia. The possibility of an alcoholic aetiology should be borne in mind because of the social circumstances, and because the ankle reflexes are absent which may indicate alcoholic peripheral neuropathy.

Lymphomas can cause hepatosplenomegaly, and the differential diagnosis from cirrhosis of the liver can sometimes be difficult. There is often lymph-node enlargement, but this is not always the case. Lymphosarcoma confined to the spleen can be especially difficult in this respect. Signs of hepatocellular failure such as spider naevi, palmar erythema and leuconychia are common in cirrhosis but are not found in lymphomas.

Massive splenomegaly is usual in myelofibrosis, but the absence of a leucoerythroblastic blood picture is against this diagnosis. Thrombocytopenia, neutropenia and anaemia can occur in splenomegaly from any cause due to 'hypersplenism', and these findings do not help in the differential diagnosis of the cause of a very large spleen.

Secondary carcinoma is rarely associated with splenomegaly although it may occur if there is portal vein thrombosis. Thrombocytopenia may also be caused by carcinoma if it invades the bone marrow although again a leucoerythroblastic blood picture might be expected.

Great enlargement of the spleen due to chronic malaria is uncommon in European adults in Africa. Kala-azar causes hepatosplenomegaly, and this is a possible diagnosis. It is however an uncommon disorder among Europeans in West Africa, and there is usually marked fever.

Further investigation will include liver function tests including transaminase, γGT and alkaline phosphatase estimations, serum protein determination and serum electrophoresis. An active cirrhosis will be suggested by raised transaminases and hypoalbuminaemia, and a raised gamma globulin. However, any diffuse infiltrative disorders involving the liver may lower the serum albumin and cause a rise in alkaline phosphatase.

An upper GI endoscopy or barium swallow is an important investigation, since the presence of varices would greatly strengthen the diagnosis of portal hypertension due to cirrhosis: their absence would not, however, exclude it. In cirrhosis a liver scan would show a patchy hepatic uptake of isotope and an increased uptake in the spleen. A similar patchy uptake can be observed in any diffuse infiltrative process in the liver.

Liver biopsy is contraindicated because of the bleeding tendency. A bone marrow aspiration may show infiltration with lymphoma and is also of value in the diagnosis of Kala-azar. A marrow biopsy may be needed to exclude myelofibrosis, but this is not a probable diagnosis.

The likely explanation of the bleeding tendency is a combination of thrombocytopenia due to hypersplenism, and hypoprothrombinaemia due to liver disease. Further studies of clotting are not appropriate, since the object of investigation is to establish the primary diagnosis.

This man was dismissed from his post because of alcoholism. It transpired that he had been a heavy drinker for many years and recently his work had begun to suffer. He had portal cirrhosis.

20

Fever of unknown origin

Fever (or pyrexia) of unknown origin (FUO) is a common problem. The improvement in imaging and diagnostic techniques, the AIDS epidemic and the increasing use of immunosuppressive and cytotoxic drugs, has changed the management of the condition. It is now useful to categorize the syndrome according to certain key clinical settings:

- arising in a previously healthy patient
- arising in a neutropenic patient
- arising in HIV-positive or in immunosuppressed patients.

FUO IN A PREVIOUSLY HEALTHY PATIENT

The causes of this classical form of FUO can be categorized as shown in Box 20.1 which also indicates the approximate frequency of the possible causes in the UK.

From this table it is apparent that infective and malignant causes constitute 55% of cases and 70% of cases where a diagnosis is made. The relative frequency of diagnoses changes according to the population in question. Widespread air travel means that diseases formerly rare in European countries are now becoming more frequent. Even within Europe the patterns are changing: for example, Leishmaniasis is very rare in northern Europe but less so in the south.

The multiplicity of causes means that the history and physical examination must be meticulous. The **pattern of the fever** is not usually helpful; although fever-free days may occur in diseases such as Hodgkin's disease (Pel–Ebstein) fever, this pattern is infrequent and has little diagnostic value. Under observation, factitious fever may disappear. In this condition the fever may not be real or be induced by self-injection or catheterization. The patient is often in an employment allied to medicine. An **intermittent fever** is one where the temperature rises for several hours and then returns to normal. Malaria is the classical example of this form of fever but it can occur in pyogenic infection. **Remittent fever**, in which the fever returns towards normal for a time but is always elevated, is often seen in abscess formation, tuberculosis and in carcinoma. The temperature more commonly shows an irregular pattern with no distinguishing features.

Drenching sweats occur in malignant and infective causes. Typically these occur between 1–3 a.m., the patient waking up drenched in sweat. **Rigors** are more common with bacterial infection, especially if there is abscess formation. **Joint and muscle pains** may suggest an underlying diagnosis of a connective tissue disease or vasculitis, such as polymyalgia rheumatica or SLE. **Skin rashes** may be transient in SLE (sometimes being induced by sunlight) or in bacterial infections such as infective endocarditis.

Physical examination must be comprehensive and, equally important, repeated. Signs may appear with time that will point to the diagnosis or indicate profitable routes of further investigation. Examples are: the development of a cardiac murmur, fundal haemorrhages, skin lesions and haematuria in infective endocarditis; choroidal tubercles in miliary tuberculosis; the appearance of an enlarged cervical lymph node in lymphoma or intra-abdominal carcinoma.

The presence of signs in several systems makes a diagnosis of a connective tissue disease such as polyarteritis or SLE, or of an infiltrative disease such as lymphoma or sarcoidosis, more likely. Examination of the retina with an ophthalmoscope is an essential routine and is repeated frequently. Retinal haemorrhages occur with leukaemia and lymphoma, arteritis and endocarditis. Uveitis may be found on slit-lamp examination in sarcoidosis and tuberculosis.

BASIC SCREENING INVESTIGATIONS

Certain simple investigations are performed as a routine in any patient with a fever because they often indicate the type of disease process which may be present, and which of the many possible more complex investigations are likely to be helpful in diagnosis.

The haemoglobin, red-cell indices and blood film

Anaemia is a common concomitant of many diseases but severe anaemia always suggests malignancy. If the blood film and indices show iron deficiency, then occult blood loss and gastrointestinal malignancy are highly probable. Normochromic normocytic anaemia is a common finding in infection, malignancy and most chronic diseases. It is therefore not of diagnostic help except that it makes a viral infection less likely.

Box 20.1 Causes of FUO in a previously healthy patient (% of all causes of FUO)

Infective (30%)

Abscess (usually intra-abdominal)	10%
Mycobacterial	8%
Infective endocarditis	4%
Viral (EBV, CMV)	3%
Urinary tract	3%
Tropical	2%*

*depending on country of origin of the patient

Cancer (25%)

Lymphoma	10%
Epithelial tumours	10%
Leukaemia*	5%

*including myeloproliferative diseases

Connective tissue diseases (15%)

SLE	4%
Polyarteritis	4%
Polymyalgia and temporal arteritis	4%
Juvenile Rheumatoid	3%

Miscellaneous causes (20%)**

Drug fever
Factitious fever
Mediterranean fever
Crohn's disease
Sarcoidosis

**examples of some of the main causes

Undiagnosed (20%)

The white blood count

The hallmark of pyogenic infection is neutrophil leucocytosis, with immature granulocytes and toxic granulation. However there may not be a leucocytosis, especially if the infection has been partially treated by the premature use of antibiotics. A rise in the neutrophil count can also occur in diseases such as Hodgkin's lymphoma and in cancer metastatic to the liver.

Some patients may have a neutrophil leucocytosis of great degree and this, with the presence of immature white cells, may lead to a mistaken diagnosis of leukaemia. **Leukaemoid reactions** of this type may be seen in any pyogenic infection. The differentiation from acute leukaemia may at times be difficult morphologically, but in acute leukaemia there is usually a high proportion of blast cells, together with thrombocytopenia and anaemia. Surface markers for leukaemia phenotypes will help to distinguish the uncommon cases where there is doubt.

Neutropenia is suggestive of viral infection although it is by no means always present and also occurs in typhoid fever and SLE. In many viral infections, but especially in infectious mononucleosis, atypical mononuclear cells may be seen.

A lymphocytosis sometimes occurs in tuberculosis and can occasionally be of such a degree as to be confused with lymphatic leukaemia. The presence of immature red and white cells in the blood – a leuco-erythroblastic blood picture – always suggests marrow replacement especially by disseminated malignancy. Lymphopenia, especially that due to a low T4 count, strongly suggests the diagnosis of HIV infection.

The erythrocyte sedimentation rate (ESR)

Although the ESR is raised in most causes of FUO, levels of 100 mm/h or more are suggestive of a connective tissue disease or malignancy.

The chest X-ray

Pyogenic infection in the lung, such as an abscess, pneumonia, bronchiectasis or empyema are usually symptomatic and the diagnosis can be made without difficulty. Pulmonary infiltrates occur in connective tissue disease, although they are often transient. In AIDS, pneumocystis carinii pneumonia typically presents with breathlessness and pulmonary infiltrates, although the X-ray may be normal. If suspected, bronchial lavage may be necessary for diagnosis. Secondary deposits may be seen in both the lung fields and as osteolytic or osteosclerotic lesions in ribs. Miliary mottling suggests tuberculosis, sarcoidosis or histoplasmosis. The hilar lymph nodes may be enlarged and if so, tuberculosis, lymphoma, sarcoidosis and secondary carcinoma are probable diagnoses.

Examination of the urine

Proteinuria is a non-specific finding in a febrile patient, but heavy proteinuria suggests renal disease, either inflammatory or neoplastic. All kidney infections including tuberculosis are commoner in diabetics, and glycosuria must be excluded. A fresh centrifuged urine must always be examined. Numerous white cells suggest infection, while granular or red-cell casts suggest renal inflammation of any cause such as connective tissue diseases and especially subacute infective endocarditis. The haematuria accompanying a hypernephroma may only be detectable on microscopy.

FURTHER INVESTIGATION

A common and most difficult problem is when there are no features in the history or physical examination to suggest the diagnosis and where no evidence is forthcoming in spite of repeated careful examination in hospital.

The problem is the distinction between infection either pyogenic or tuberculous, malignancy including lymphoma, and a connective tissue disease. The diagnosis of a connective tissue disease presenting as an FUO depends on histological evidence or on the later development of the distinguishing features of the disorder. The diagnosis is difficult to make but becomes more likely the longer the patient remains undiagnosed.

Repeated and careful bacteriological investigations are essential. Urine must be cultured in every case. A sterile pyuria suggests tuberculosis and is an indication for culture of the urine for *Mycobacterium tuberculosis*. It also occurs in inadequately treated pyelonephritis. Sputum, if present, must be cultured for *Mycobacterium tuberculosis* as well as pyogenic organisms. Blood cultures are an essential part of the examination and every attempt should be made to culture the blood on at least three occasions before treatment is started. The technique is important, care being taken to prevent skin contamination, and if possible to take the culture as the temperature begins to rise.

In addition to the standard cultures of urine and sputum in the search for tubercle bacilli, culture and animal inoculation of marrow aspirate, and lymph node and liver biopsy material may also be of value.

Serological tests are a useful adjunct to bacteriological investigation. If AIDS is suspected, the patient should be asked if an HIV test can be performed. Agglutination tests for the detection of *Salmonella* are an essential part of investigation, while brucellosis and Q fever endocarditis can often only be diagnosed in this way. An important point is that a rising titre is of great value in demonstrating active infection, and so the initial serology must always be done as early as possible in the investigation. In rheumatic fever, although a very high ASO titre is diagnostic of recent streptococcal infection, a rising titre is equally valuable. A Paul–Bunnell test for infectious mononucleosis should be performed if the diagnosis is at all likely. Cytomegalovirus infection and toxoplasmosis may closely resemble infectious mononucleosis, but the Paul–Bunnell test remains persistently negative.

Further investigations are undertaken as appropriate. The serum alkaline phosphatase and transaminases are often elevated in liver disease, and may suggest the need for more tests such as an ultrasound liver scan when abscess or carcinoma is suspected, or a liver biopsy when diffuse infiltration or carcinoma is a possibility. If the scan suggests a space-occupying lesion, more precise knowledge of its nature and site may be gained from a CT scan. If doubt persists then a fine-needle aspiration with culture and cytological examination of the specimen may be diagnostic. Low-grade fever may occur due to cirrhosis itself, or as a result of a complication such as hepatoma, Gram-negative septicaemia or tuberculosis. If there is a suspicion of disease in the bowel such as tuberculous enteritis, Crohn's disease or lymphoma then a barium follow-through may be helpful. The nature of the intestinal lesion can sometimes only be decided at laparotomy. Pyogenic abscesses and Crohn's disease can sometimes be demonstrated by scanning with the patient's [111]Indium-labelled leucocytes which localize at the infection.

Connective tissue diseases may cause great diagnostic difficulty. Antibodies to DNA are nearly always found in active SLE. The tests for rheumatoid factor may also be positive in any of the connective tissue diseases, but also in subacute infective endocarditis, chronic suppuration and sarcoidosis. In the case of polyarteritis the diagnosis is best established when necrotizing arteritis has been found in tissue such as muscle, skin, kidney or testis. Blind biopsies of these organs are seldom rewarding, but a biopsy should be undertaken if there is reason to suspect arteritis in a particular site. Coeliac angiography may reveal characteristic appearances of small vessel disease in polyarteritis. In an elderly patient with FUO and a high ESR a biopsy of the temporal artery, whether tender or not, may show giant-cell arthritis. The response to steroids is characteristically swift.

Ultrasound and CT scanning are of great value in the diagnosis of intra-abdominal tumours. If an abnormality is found but percutaneous biopsy does not give a diagnosis at laparotomy may occasionally be necessary, since occult cancers, especially Hodgkin's disease, may defy attempts at pre-operative diagnosis.

Ideally, treatment should never be started until the diagnosis is established. If this proves impossible, then a trial of a broad-spectrum antibiotic is a logical first step. Steroids are never given alone unless tuberculosis or pyogenic infection can be confidently excluded as a cause of the FUO and this is not often the case. If the probability of tuberculosis seems high, then a therapeutic trial of specific antituberculous drugs such as pyrazinamide, ethambutol and isoniazid must be seriously considered.

FEVER IN A NEUTROPENIC PATIENT

The use of intensive combination chemotherapy for the treatment of leukaemia, lymphoma and common solid tumours has meant that neutropenic infection is common. Although the use of haemopoetic growth factors such as GCSF has shortened the period of neutropenia, fever is still a frequent complication of chemotherapy and often occurs 5–10 days after the

Box 20.2 Causes of fever in a neutropenic patient

Bacterial
Staphylococcus aureus and epidermidis
E. coli
Intestinal anaerobes
Community acquired pneumonia
Mycobacterial

Fungal
Aspergillus
Candida

Viral
Herpes simplex
Cytomegalovirus
Herpes zoster

Protozoal
Toxoplasmosis

Recurrent tumour

cessation of treatment at a time when the patient has left hospital. It is a medical emergency demanding prompt investigation and treatment. In general neutropenia is more common, greater in degree and of longer duration the more cycles of chemotherapy that have been given. The incidence and severity of infection follows the same general rule.

The causes of FUO in a neutropenic patient are almost always infective (Box 20.2). The sites of entry are:

- The skin via in-dwelling subcutaneous catheters used for venous access. The organisms responsible are usually *Staph. epidermidis* and *Staph. aureus*. The organisms gain access through the puncture site and colonize the tip of the catheter, acting as a reservoir for repeated bouts of infection. The presence of organisms on the catheter can be suspected if there is a bout of fever or a rigor when the catheter is first opened and flushed with saline prior to treatment. Once infection is established the catheter must almost always be removed.
- The respiratory tract. Community acquired pneumonia is particularly dangerous in these patients. Pneumonia due to fungi, typically *Aspergillus* and *Candida*, is especially serious. It usually occurs in the context of profound neutropenia of more than 1 week's duration.
- The gastrointestinal tract. Many cytotoxic drugs damage the integrity of the intestinal mucosal barrier to infection leading to a susceptibility to infection with *E. coli* and other bowel commensals. Anal fissure and skin tags are other portals of entry. *Clostridium difficile* infection may occur in patients

treated with antibiotics and in those treated in hospital – as may other typical hospital-acquired (nosocomial) infections.
- Urinary tract. This is a less common source of infection unless the patient has been catheterized.

Management

This is a medical emergency, and treatment must begin without delay. For a general practitioner, seeing the patient at home, the important step is to move the patient to hospital for immediate investigation and to start treatment.

Investigation consists of a chest radiograph, a full blood count, blood urea and electrolytes and cultures of blood, urine and sputum.

Broad-spectrum antibiotic treatment should begin at once without waiting for the results of the cultures. The choice of antibiotic will be guided by hospital policy, the likely source of the infection and knowledge of previous antibiotics received by the patient.

If the chest radiograph shows pulmonary infiltrates, the possibility of a fungal pneumonia must be kept in mind, especially if there is a poor response to antibiotic treatment. Empirical treatment with antifungal antibiotics such as liposomal amphotericin and with anti-herpes virus agents (acyclovir, ganciclovir) may be necessary if the patient's condition is worsening.

Many centres will use GCSF in an attempt to stimulate recovery of the neutrophil count although the delay before the growth factor produces an effect means that its value is often marginal.

INFECTION ARISING IN HIV OR IN AN IMMUNOSUPPRESSED PATIENT

FUO frequently arises in patients infected with HIV or on long-term immunosuppressive treatment either for prevention of graft rejection or as treatment of a connective tissue or autoimmune disorder.

The diagnostic possibilities include all the causes of FUO found in a previously well patient (Box 20.1), but unusual opportunistic infections are far more likely than in the general population. Additionally, patients who are HIV-positive or immunosuppressed are more likely to develop certain specific malignancies which themselves may present as FUO. The most frequent diagnoses in this setting are shown in Box 20.3. Most of these infections, such as cerebral toxoplasmosis, pneumocystis and cryptococcal meningitis, present with characteristic symptoms that lead directly to the diagnosis. In other cases FUO is a frequent presentation as discussed below.

Pyogenic abscesses may form at any site. In AIDS these may be at unusual sites such as the prostate or

Box 20.3 Causes of FUO in HIV or in an immunosuppressed patient

Bacterial infection
Pyogenic bacterial infection (abscess formation)
Mycobacterium tuberculosis
Mycobacterium avium-intracellulare
Other atypical Mycobacteria

Fungal infection
Candida
Cryptococcus
Aspergillus

Protozoal
Toxoplasmosis
Pneumocystis

Malignancy
Lymphoma
Kaposi's sarcoma
Epithelial tumours

Persistent undiagnosed fever

paranasal sinuses. Physical examination and investigation must include these possibilities.

M. tuberculosis usually presents with fever associated with cough and weight loss. The chest radiograph shows pulmonary infiltrates. Extra-pulmonary disease is more common, however, and the X-ray appearances show less fibrosis and cavitation than in patients who are not immunosuppressed. Sputum culture is often negative.

M. avium-intracellulare complex (MAC) is a common cause of FUO in the advanced stages of AIDS, occurring in 10–20% of patients. The portal of entry is the gut. It disseminates widely through the blood and is found in the liver, bone marrow and lymph nodes. The presentation is with rigors and swinging fevers. The diagnosis is made by specialized blood culture and by culture of faeces, bone marrow and liver biopsy.

Non-Hodgkin's lymphoma is a frequent cause of FUO in advanced AIDS. It may present at almost any site. Patients with AIDS commonly have widespread lymph-node enlargement and this may create diagnostic difficulty on clinical grounds alone. Biopsy of enlarging nodes, CT scan of the abdomen and marrow biopsy may be needed to diagnose the tumour.

Persistent undiagnosed fever occurs in the late stages of AIDS and may continue for months. Trials of treatment for MAC and pyogenic infections are often made but are usually ineffective and treatment is symptomatic with some benefit from non-steroidal drugs and steroids.

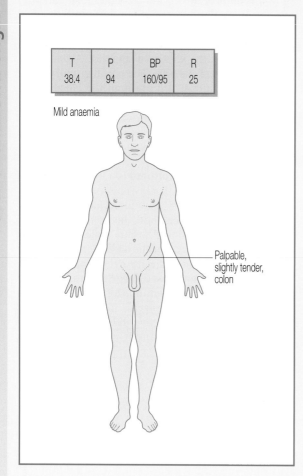

T	P	BP	R
38.4	94	160/95	25

Mild anaemia

Palpable, slightly tender, colon

A 65-year-old businessman presented with a 6-week history of rigors, weight loss and malaise. His wife had died 5 years earlier, and he had been very depressed and had been drinking heavily since that time. He had suffered from constipation for many years, for which he had regularly taken laxatives. On the advice of his family doctor he had gone on a recuperative holiday to southern Italy, and while there had had an episode of left iliac fossa pain and diarrhoea with some blood in the stool. He had received a 5-day course of a broad-spectrum antibiotic and the illness had subsided after 3 days. He had not had any recurrence of diarrhoea. Two weeks after his return he had begun to feel unwell, with fevers and vague upper abdominal discomfort.

On examination he was mildly anaemic, with a temperature of 38.4°C. There were no other abnormal physical signs except that the descending colon was palpable and slightly tender. Rectal examination was normal. Over the next few days in hospital he had an irregular continuous fever with temperatures varying between 37.5°C and 39.5°C.

Investigations Hb 10.2 g/dl; MCV 100 fl; MCH 31 pg; WBC $10.4 \times 10^9/1$ (80% neutrophils, 17% lymphocytes, 3% eosinophils); ESR 72 mm/h; chest X-ray showed a small right pleural effusion and fibrosis at the left apex. MSU – trace of protein, no other abnormality. Serological tests for Salmonella were negative with the exception of *Salmonella typhi* H antigen, which was positive at 1/10 on two occasions 10 days apart.

Questions

1. What do you consider to be the most likely diagnosis?
2. Which investigations would be most helpful in diagnosis?
3. What would be your immediate management?

Discussion

This patient had an episode of diarrhoea treated with broad-spectrum antibiotics before his present illness began. There is a strong possibility that his illness is related to this. There are no physical signs to suggest a local collection of pus in the abdomen or pelvis, but an hepatic or subphrenic abscess might well be present. The former is more likely, since his previous illness settled down quickly and it is unlikely that he perforated a viscus at that time. A liver abscess is more likely to occur in debilitated elderly patients, and when it does so it often produces few localizing signs. The small right pleural effusion would be compatible with either diagnosis. The slight neutrophil leucocytosis might occur in a partially treated infection of this kind.

An occult carcinoma is a possibility and the stomach, liver and intestine would be the likely primary sites. In Europeans hepatoma nearly always arises in a cirrhotic liver. It is difficult to explain his previous illness on this basis; the duration of his symptoms is only 6 weeks, and there is no evidence of metastases.

His chest X-ray shows apical fibrosis but there is little to suggest pulmonary tuberculosis in this patient. Abdominal tuberculosis causing diarrhoea would not resolve with broad-spectrum antibiotics. Involvement of retroperitoneal nodes is possible, but would not account for his previous episode of diarrhoea.

The course of the illness is too prolonged for typhoid fever. The serology is compatible with TAB immunization but not with infection. The high intermittent fever and rigors are not typical of brucellosis. A lymphoma involving retroperitoneal nodes can produce fever, but the illness is of short duration and the previous episode of diarrhoea would not be accounted for by this diagnosis. Despite the absence of signs of hepatic disease, this patient could have cirrhosis due to his heavy drinking which may cause low-grade fever, or be complicated by Gram-negative septicaemia.

On investigation, an ultrasound liver scan would be very valuable since it may show a filling defect if an hepatic abscess is present. If a filling defect was found, a CT scan might help to differentiate an abscess from a tumour. Blood cultures should be taken. A barium meal and follow-through and barium enema would be helpful, if the liver scan is normal, to look for a carcinoma of the stomach or intestine. A high alkaline phosphatase of liver origin with a low serum albumin would suggest an expanding intrahepatic lesion. If an intrahepatic lesion is found, a fine-needle aspirate should be considered for bacteriological and cytological examination.

If these investigations are normal, laparotomy should be considered. Before diagnosis, no treatment should be given. Immediate management is symptomatic.

This patient had a pyogenic liver abscess following an attack of diverticulitis. A liver scan showed a filling defect, and treatment with aspiration and antibiotics resulted in cure.

Polyarthritis

A common presenting complaint is swelling and pain in joints. One of the main difficulties is to establish whether or not a primary rheumatic disorder is present, or whether the symptom is part of another underlying disease. A precise diagnosis may be impossible at first, and only with time does the picture become clear. Nevertheless, every attempt must be made to reach a diagnosis quickly and here the clinical history and the pattern of joint involvement are the most valuable guides.

HISTORY

It is important to enquire very carefully about the true onset of the disorder. Sometimes patients will remember having had recurrent attacks of transient swelling or discomfort in a joint over periods of months or years. Such a history is often found in rheumatoid arthritis. An acute onset over a few weeks, involving many joints, frequently occurs in other connective tissue disorders, such as systemic lupus erythematosus (SLE) or polyarteritis nodosa, as well as in rheumatoid arthritis. A feature of rheumatoid arthritis is that the joint involvement is characteristically symmetrical, and the joints usually remain inflamed for a long period of time. This is in marked contrast to the flitting arthritis seen in rheumatic fever, and in subacute infective endocarditis. A history of morning stiffness, improving with exercise, is typical of rheumatoid arthritis, and may occur early in the disease. In contrast, pain rather than stiffness is common in osteoarthritis, and is often made worse by use of the joints.

The pattern of joint involvement is of great importance. Gout, which may involve more than one joint, nevertheless has a strong predilection for the metatarsophalangeal joints. The small joints of the hands are often involved in rheumatoid arthritis, but the distal interphalangeal joints are characteristically spared. This is not the case with psoriatic arthritis

in the hands, where the distal interphalangeal joints may be involved, often not symmetrically. The small joints of the hands may also be affected in systemic lupus erythematosus, which in the early stages, may be very difficult to distinguish from rheumatoid arthritis. Other characteristic sites of involvement in each disease will be discussed below. Arthralgia, which is pain in joints without swelling, may occur in any arthritic disorder and may herald the onset of true arthritis.

The onset, site and progression of the arthritis, and details of any associated systemic symptoms are of diagnostic importance. Fever, malaise and weight loss are found in many connective tissue diseases, and also occur with the arthropathy which may accompany malignant disease. Some systemic infections such as subacute infective endocarditis may be accompanied by polyarthritis even though the joints may not be directly invaded by the organism. When there is direct infection of a joint, for example with gonococcal arthritis, a monoarthritis is more usual. In both situations fever and rigors may occur. The exclusion of an infective cause is particularly important in a patient with a short history.

There may be a history of skin rash. Transient rashes are common in many connective tissue disorders, especially SLE and polyarteritis nodosa. They may also occur in rheumatic fever. The distribution of the rash may be characteristic, for example the facial 'butterfly' rash of SLE, or the erythema nodosum over the shins which may accompany sarcoidosis or rheumatic fever. Arthritis may accompany psoriasis, even when the primary skin disorder is not severe.

Pain and redness of the eyes may be due to the conjunctivitis and iritis accompanying Reiter's syndrome, or to the iritis of ankylosing spondylitis. Diarrhoea and abdominal pain suggest ulcerative colitis or Crohn's disease, where arthritis may be a prominent feature.

CAUSES OF POLYARTHRITIS

Rheumatoid arthritis

If a middle-aged woman complains of the gradual symmetrical involvement of joints, including the hands, with effusions and morning stiffness and without significant constitutional disturbance, the diagnosis of rheumatoid arthritis is very likely. Any large joint may be involved, but the small joints of the hands and feet and the cervical spine are characteristically affected. The temporomandibular and cricoarytenoid joints can also be involved. When arthritis appears suddenly, involving several joints, other diagnoses such as SLE will also have to be considered. In the early phases of the disease, with involvement of only one or two joints, a firm diagnosis may not be possible, even with X-rays and serological tests.

The essential feature of the arthritis is the destruction of particular cartilage and bones. Consequently joint deformity, including subluxation, and lateral and anteroposterior instability are very common. Capsular thickening is normally prominent and large joint effusions can occur. In the knee, these may form large cystic swellings, which may sometimes rupture into the calf, simulating deep venous thrombosis. Subcutaneous nodules over extensor surfaces of limbs and flexor and extensor tendons are characteristic of the condition.

Systemic features sometimes occur, such as pleural effusion, peripheral neuropathy and splenomegaly. When these features are present there may be some difficulty in distinguishing the disease from SLE. This is not usually a problem if it is remembered that the arthritis in SLE is not nearly so destructive, and that glomerulonephritis and CNS involvement, which are common in SLE, do not occur in rheumatoid arthritis. In rheumatoid arthritis, some degree of anaemia is common. Renal amyloidosis is not unusual in longstanding cases, occasionally giving rise to the nephrotic syndrome. Sjögren's syndrome is keratoconjunctivitis sicca and xerostomia in association with rheumatoid arthritis or another connective tissue disease.

Osteoarthritis (degenerative joint disease, osteoarthrosis)

The characteristic features of osteoarthritis are the involvement of only one or two joints, often asymmetrically, the very slow progression of the disorder in most patients, the advanced age at which it most commonly appears, and the lack of systemic complications. The commonest joints to be affected are the spine, hands, hips, knees and feet. It often arises in a single joint as a result of previous trauma, other joints being spared.

In some patients a history of trauma is lacking and the disease may affect several joints. In this form of the disorder the hands are often involved, especially distal interphalangeal joints and the metacarpo-phalangeal joint of the thumb. Heberden's nodes are a characteristic finding, related to the affected distal interphalangeal joints. In women the onset may be at the time of the menopause. Some patients with the generalized form may have a family history of the disease. In this form of the disorder distinction from rheumatoid arthritis can be difficult. Degenerative joint disease is a frequent sequel to rheumatoid arthritis whether active or not.

The main symptoms are pain, stiffness and decreased mobility. There is usually crepitus on moving

the affected joint, and joint effusions may be present which when aspirated show clear fluid with little cellular content.

Gout and pseudogout

Although usually presenting as a monoarthritis gout may affect more than one joint and is a diagnosis which must always be considered. Typically the first metatarsophalangeal joint is usually involved, but gout may affect any joint and occur in more than one joint at a time. Joint swelling may persist after the acute attack has subsided and this may create diagnostic difficulty. The onset of the attack is typically much more acute and painful than in any other form of arthritis, and often resembles pyogenic arthritis in the degree of inflammation present. Sometimes the onset is much milder and the disease may progress in a chronic fashion. The ears should be examined for tophi, which may also accumulate around the joints, especially in the hands. These may be confused with the synovial swelling commonly found in severely affected joints in rheumatoid arthritis. In primary gout there is often a family history of the disorder. Gout may be secondary to polycythaemia rubra vera and myeloid metaplasia in the elderly, and acute leukaemia in the young. An acute attack is sometimes provoked by treatment of these diseases and lymphoma by cytotoxic drugs. In primary gout trauma and operations may provoke an acute attack.

The serum urate is usually, but not always, raised in gout. Aspiration of the joint fluid and its examination under polarized light for the presence of the negatively birefringent urate crystals in polymorphonuclear leucocytes is the definitive diagnostic test. Aspiration will also exclude pyogenic arthritis which is the main differential diagnosis.

A clinically similar monoarthritis is 'pseudogout' or calcium pyrophosphate gout. This condition primarily affects large joints in which there is often chondrocalcinosis. It is the commonest form of monoarthritis in the elderly. The onset is abrupt, often following trauma. Calcium pyrophosphate crystals, which are weakly birefringent, can be seen in polymorphs in the joint fluid. The disease is sometimes a complication of hyperparathyroidism and haemochromatosis; it may become chronic, affecting more than one joint and difficult to distinguish from osteoarthritis.

Systemic lupus erythematosus (SLE)

This disease, with its diversity of symptoms and signs, may present as a polyarthritis, whose distribution can be identical to rheumatoid arthritis. Women are affected ten times more often than men. The onset of the disease is usually abrupt and constitutional upset is often severe. The disease may be precipitated by exposure to sunlight. A similar disease can be provoked by drugs such as hydralazine, procainamide, phenytoin and propanolol. Abdominal pain, pleurisy, neuropathy, pericarditis, fever, anaemia, CNS involvement, skin rashes of many types and glomerulonephritis are all common. The musculoskeletal manifestations are arthralgia, arthritis and tendon inflammation. Typically the arthritis is not erosive and deforming as in rheumatoid arthritis. A progressive glomerulonephritis occurs in approximately half of the patients with SLE. CNS disease includes mental confusion and psychotic symptoms, strokes and nerve palsies. Some patients have antibodies to phospholipids associated with a tendency to severe arterial and venous thrombosis. The skin manifestations take a variety of forms, the most typical of which are a butterfly rash over the nose and cheeks, photosensitivity and hair loss.

Polyarteritis nodosa

This disorder, like SLE, has numerous possible presentations apart from polyarthritis. These include asthma, skin rashes, mononeuritis multiplex, muscle pains, pericarditis, pulmonary infiltration, pleurisy, glomeruloneophritis and hypertension. The widespread vascular disturbance may cause acute inflammation of the gallbladder and testes, while cerebral arteritis is not uncommon.

This is very unlike the clinical picture found in rheumatoid arthritis. The arthritis of polyarteritis may have a similar distribution to rheumatoid arthritis, but has a predilection for large joints, is usually abrupt in onset, may move from joint to joint, and deformity and erosion of joints are not common. Approximately 30% of patients test positive for hepatitis B surface antigen.

Rheumatic fever

The classical history of arthritis, developing rapidly in one joint, and then moving from joint to joint, without causing any permanent damage, is usually all that is required to distinguish this disease from other forms of polyarthritis. An antecedent sore throat or the finding of a cardiac involvement further supports the diagnosis. The response to salicylates is not diagnostic, since many inflammatory polyarthritides will remit partially on large doses of aspirin. An interesting, albeit rare, sequel to rheumatic fever, especially if recurrent, is a form of chronic mild deformity of joints (often small joints of the hand) first described by Jaccoud. This is not likely to be a diagnostic problem since it occurs in the context of clearly established rheumatic fever.

Small nodules may appear over the elbows and knees. They are distinguished from those found in

> **Box 21.1** Causes of seronegative spondarthropathy
>
> - Ankylosing spondylitis
> - Enteropathic spondylitis
>   Ulcerative colitis
>   Crohn's disease
> - Reiter's syndrome
> - Psoriatic sacroiliitis
> - Whipple's disease

rheumatoid arthritis by their small size, their site over the joints rather than over the neighbouring bones and tendons, and by the fact that the nodules of rheumatoid arthritis accompany chronic joint deformity.

Ankylosing spondylitis

This disorder is the commonest of the heterogeneous group of diseases that are grouped together under the general term of sero-negative spondarthropathies (Box 21.1). The diseases are characterized by sacroiliitis and spondylitis, absence of rheumatoid factor in the serum and an association with HLA-B27.

Peripheral arthritis occurs in about 20% of patients with ankylosing spondylitis, and when it occurs usually involves proximal large joints, knees and feet. The diagnosis should be suspected if the arthritis occurs in a young man, and if there is a history of lumbar backache. There may be associated iritis, and aortitis causing aortic incompetence.

Polyarthritis is more likely to occur in adolescents, when it is more frequently associated with iritis and aortitis. In women the disease is rare, and may occur in association with ulcerative colitis and Crohn's disease (see below).

Reiter's syndrome and reactive arthritis

A syndrome of sacroiliitis, arthritis and dactylitis associated with oral and penile ulceration, uveitis and keratodermia blennorhagica, can follow urogenital and intestinal infection. The triad of arthritis, urethritis and conjunctivitis usually leads to early diagnosis. The onset is abrupt, often following sexual exposure, although bacillary dysentery may be a precipitating cause. Sometimes the urethritis can be mild and the conjunctivitis fleeting so that diagnostic difficulty can occur. Balanitis may be present and shallow painful ulcers can occur over the penis and in the mouth. A slit-lamp examination of the eyes is essential in all suspected cases, since iritis is often present and untreated can lead to blindness. Keratodermia blenorrhagica occurs over the soles of the feet and palms. It is characterized by small vesicles and brown scaly papules, and the rash may be indistinguishable from psoriasis.

Sacroiliitis is not uncommon and X-rays of the spine may show changes similar to those seen in ankylosing spondylitis, although they are more unevenly distributed. Plantar fasciitis and calcaneal spurs are characteristic of the syndrome. The arthritis is acute and destructive, often leading to deformity. It involves the hands, sometimes asymmetrically, and often only one or two fingers. Large joints in the legs are also affected, usually symmetrically. Aortitis may occur. The condition is relapsing and in some attacks symptoms of conjunctivitis and urethritis may be very mild or absent. A careful history will then reveal that these features were present in an earlier, initial episode (often with a long interval between attacks).

Ulcerative colitis and Crohn's disease

Both these diseases may be complicated by a form of joint disease which is not due to coincidental rheumatoid arthritis. The large joints are usually involved, and sometimes the arthritis may antedate the bowel symptoms. In both diseases sacroiliitis can occur, with changes indistinguishable from ankylosing spondylitis in the lumbar spine. These patients are often HLA-B27 positive. As in ankylosing spondylitis, aortitis and iritis are occasionally seen. The mechanism of the association between spondylitis, iritis and aortitis seen in these disorders and in Reiter's syndrome is not understood.

Although it is not likely to present diagnostic difficulty, the polyarthritis associated with these disorders should always be kept in mind, especially if the patient is a woman with sacroiliitis or spondylitis.

Psoriasis

Polyarthritis may complicate this disorder, and the skin eruption does not have to be severe for the joint complication to develop. There is usually a long history of psoriasis. The arthritis may involve the small joints of the hand. Here it may be asymmetrical, and involve distal interphalangeal joints, which help to distinguish it from rheumatoid arthritis.

When the hands are involved, a careful examination will often show pitting of the nails or subungual keratosis. Interestingly, this often occurs in the nail of the digit affected by arthritis. Any large joint may be involved and distinction from rheumatoid arthritis may be difficult unless a careful search for the skin lesions is made. The arthritis may be highly destructive, with erosion of bone and marked deformity. Further points of distinction from rheumatoid arthritis lie in the occa-

sional occurrence of sacroiliitis (20% of cases) and the negative serological tests.

Still's disease

This is a form of polyarthritis usually occurring in children but occasionally affecting young adults. Some cases have a severe systemic illness with fever, pericarditis, skin rash, polyserositis and anaemia. Glomerulonephritis does not occur. The distribution of joint disease is similar to rheumatoid arthritis. Tests for rheumatoid factor and antinuclear factors are negative. Progressive joint disease may occur and joints may become fused in the wrists, feet and spine after many years. The acute systemic disease may make the initial diagnosis difficult especially the distinction from SLE, polyarteritis and infective arthritis.

Sarcoidosis

Two forms of arthritis are seen in this condition. The first is an acute arthritis, which usually occurs in the context of erythema nodosum and constitutional upset. The knees and ankles are usually involved, and the arthritis settles without deformity. The second form is a chronic disorder seen in longstanding sarcoidosis. Joints which are adjacent to underlying bone disease are often involved. Both large and small joints may swell, and sarcoid granulomata can be found on synovial biopsy. Although the arthritis usually occurs in the presence of obvious disease, it should be borne in mind in any patient with a puzzling chronic polyarthritis.

Subacute infective endocarditis

Polyarthritis may occur in this condition and can be acute, resembling a septic arthritis, or subacute. The large joints are particularly affected, although any joint may be involved. The arthritis may move from joint to joint as in rheumatic fever. However, haematuria, a cardiac murmur, fever, anaemia and Osler's nodes are often present. The diagnosis of infective endocarditis should be considered in a patient with systemic upset, polyarthritis and a cardiac murmur. Under such circumstances, blood cultures must always be taken. A serious mistake is to treat such patients with corticosteroids on the presumption that they have a 'collagen' disease.

Other infective causes

Pyogenic arthritis usually affects one joint only. Staphylococci, gonococci, pneumococci, streptococci and pseudomonas are the commonest infecting organisms. It may, however, occur in a joint of a patient with rheumatoid arthritis, when it may be misdiagnosed as a relapse of the condition and treated with steroids. The joint is acutely inflamed and painful. Such a joint should always be aspirated and antibiotic treatment started at once. Gonococcal infection may present with an arthritis which moves from joint to joint, and is often accompanied by a rash. It is especially likely to present in this way in women, as opposed to men, in whom urethritis is a prominent symptom resulting in early treatment. After meningococcaemia a sterile polyarthritis may occur. Osteomyelitis may be accompanied by an effusion in an adjacent joint. Radiological changes in bone may occur late. Antibiotic therapy must not be delayed if the diagnosis is likely.

Virus diseases are being increasingly recognized as a cause of transient polyarthritis with a good prognosis; of these rubella is the commonest. The arthritis is not usually severe and is self-limiting. It may also follow rubella vaccine. Chickenpox, infective hepatitis, infectious mononucleosis and mumps are all recognized causes.

Malignant disease

A common accompaniment of carcinoma of the bronchus is hypertrophic pulmonary osteoarthropathy. Although this is not a true arthritis, it may occasionally be misdiagnosed as such. The presence of clubbing will point to the correct diagnosis, and the radiological appearance of symmetrical periosteal reaction at the ends of the long bones is characteristic.

Occasionally polyarthritis may be the first feature of an occult neoplasm. The association has been reported with a wide variety of malignant tumours. The arthritis may resemble rheumatoid arthritis and sometimes remits when the tumour is excised. Although rare, this form of polyarthritis should be borne in mind in a middle-aged or elderly person, especially if there is weight loss or anaemia.

Miscellaneous causes

Arthritis occurs as part of **Henoch–Schönlein purpura**, but the other features of this disorder will point to the correct diagnosis. Arthritis, similar to rheumatoid arthritis, may occur in **systemic sclerosis (scleroderma)**. Usually the skin changes are obvious but the joint symptoms may appear early in the disease before the other features (skin, lung and gut fibrosis, calcinosis, Raynaud's phenomenon and renal failure) occur, but occasionally only the visceral features of the disease are present. **Whipple's disease** may be accompanied by recurrent flitting polyarthritis.

The association with steatorrhoea and skin pigmentation will suggest the diagnosis. **Alkaptonuria** (ochronosis) predisposes to the development of osteoarthritis involving the knee and spine. The intervertebral discs become calcified and are visible on X-ray. In **Behçet's syndrome** oral and genital ulceration are combined with skin rashes, encephalitis, iridocyclitis and arthritis of one or two joints; venous and arterial thromboses and vascular involvement of the eye are the most serious complications. Acute arthritis, especially of the ankles and knees, commonly occurs in **erythema nodosum**. Although sarcoidosis is the commonest cause, drugs, streptococcal infection, fungal and tuberculous infections can also give rise to the syndrome.

RADIOLOGICAL INVESTIGATION

In the early stages of most of these disorders, X-rays of the affected joints often do not provide diagnostic information. In rheumatoid arthritis, for example, one of the earliest appearances is juxta-articular osteoporosis, and only later do the characteristic X-ray appearances develop.

Narrowing of the joint space signifies loss of articular cartilage; it occurs quite quickly in many inflammatory arthritides, especially in rheumatoid arthritis. It occurs after a longer period of time in degenerative joint disease, and by then the other signs of this disorder are usually present with sclerosis of underlying bone, and osteophyte formation at joint margins. Erosion of bone is typical of rheumatoid arthritis, and should be looked for carefully. The hands and feet, if involved, are good sites to observe these changes. The erosions appear as a ragged margin in the surface of the bone, usually seen first at the edge of the articular surface. The destruction extends and soon becomes obvious. In rheumatoid arthritis, if the wrists are involved clinically, X-ray often shows erosion of the ulnar styloid early on (Fig. 21.1).

In psoriasis, the destruction may be difficult to distinguish from rheumatoid arthritis. The heads of the metacarpals may be lost entirely and there is usually considerable deformity. Subluxation and gross deformity are typical of advanced rheumatoid arthritis, and secondary degenerative changes are usual.

The bones themselves may show lesions. In gout punched-out lytic areas are commonly seen, which are usually adjacent to the articular surface. Cystic areas in bone may also occur in rheumatoid arthritis, and sometimes in degenerative joint disease. In sarcoidosis granulomata may occur in bone, often in the metacarpals. The bone is often slightly expanded, and there are lytic areas.

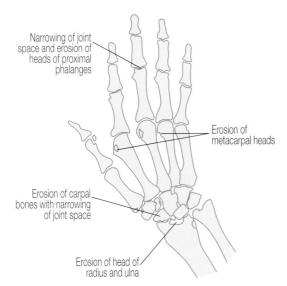

Narrowing of joint space and erosion of heads of proximal phalanges

Erosion of metacarpal heads

Erosion of carpal bones with narrowing of joint space

Erosion of head of radius and ulna

Fig. 21.1 Radiological changes in rheumatoid arthritis.

Periostitis is the hallmark of hypertrophic pulmonary osteoarthropathy, and is usually best seen along the ends of long bones. Appearances of damage to the joint itself do not occur. Local periostitis also occurs in many other conditions where there is true arthritis. For example, it is often seen near involved joints in Reiter's syndrome and in juvenile rheumatoid arthritis.

The sacroiliac joints are involved in many disorders and views of these joints may be helpful. There is narrowing of the joint space, often with sclerosis of the adjacent bone, and erosions may be seen at the joint margins. Ultimately these changes result in fusion of the joint. X-rays of the spine in ankylosing spondylitis initially may show 'squaring' of the vertebral bodies, the characteristic calcification of intervertebral ligaments occurring only later.

SEROLOGICAL TESTS

Too much emphasis should not be placed on the diagnostic value of serological tests in arthritis. Clinical criteria usually give the diagnosis, and serology may be only of marginal help. The serum factors which are being looked for are byproducts of the basic disease process and may be produced under a variety of other circumstances.

Rheumatoid factor

This is a large molecular weight antibody which is directed against altered human gamma globulin. It probably arises wherever altered gamma globulin is present in the blood, for example as circulating immune complexes, or adherent to bacteria. The antibody is found most consistently and in the highest titre in rheumatoid arthritis. The antibody is nearly always present if the patient has rheumatoid nodules or vascular lesions, and many believe that patients with rheumatoid arthritis who have rheumatoid factor (about 75–85%) have a more destructive disease than those who do not.

Rheumatoid factor is also found in some patients with SLE, polyarteritis, sarcoidosis, leprosy, subacute infective endocarditis and in 5–10% of normal elderly people. It is absent in ankylosing spondylitis, psoriasis and Reiter's syndrome. It is detected by the capacity of the patient's serum to agglutinate latex or bentonite particles coated with human gamma globulin.

Antinuclear antibodies

In SLE a variety of antibodies directed against various nuclear constituents may be found in the blood. They are usually detected by immunofluorescent techniques as a screening test. Anti-DNA antibodies can be measured by ELISA and are present in highest titre in active SLE. In active SLE, especially with nephritis, anti-DNA antibodies are almost always present and their absence is strongly against the diagnosis. However, they may be found in patients with rheumatoid arthritis and polyarteritis nodosa and occasionally seen in sarcoidosis, lepromatous leprosy and subacute infective endocarditis.

HLA typing

It is rarely necessary to tissue-type patients to make a diagnosis. A close association has been found between ankylosing spondylitis and the HLA-B27 type. Over 90% of patients have this histocompatibility antigen. A slightly less strong association exists between HLA-B27 and Reiter's syndrome although 10% of people who are HLA-B27 develop Reiter's syndrome after *Shigella* infection.

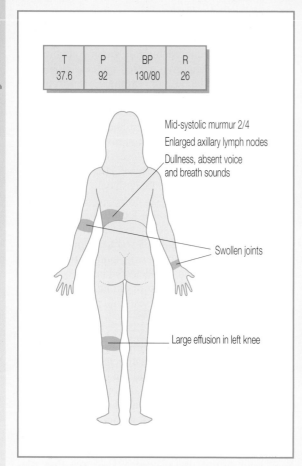

T	P	BP	R
37.6	92	130/80	26

Mid-systolic murmur 2/4
Enlarged axillary lymph nodes
Dullness, absent voice
and breath sounds

Swollen joints

Large effusion in left knee

A housewife of 54 was referred to the outpatients' clinic with the complaint that for the preceding 6 weeks she had had pain and swelling in the joints. She had noticed the rapid onset of arthritis in the left elbow, both knees and right wrist, and in the second and third proximal interphalangeal joints of both hands. She had started to feel unwell 8 weeks before being seen, while on a camping holiday in Portugal with her family. She had felt feverish, and had a poor appetite. During the course of the illness she had lost 5 kg in weight. Two weeks before being seen she had developed a persistent unproductive cough.

In the past she had been well, apart from menopausal symptoms which had started at the age of 48 and had lasted 4 years.

On examination she was clinically anaemic and had a slight fever. There was no evidence of heart failure but a mid-systolic murmur was present, heard best at the apex and left sternal edge, but not conducted to the neck or axilla. In the chest there was dullness to percussion with absent breath sounds and voice sounds at the left base posteriorly and in the left axilla. There was swelling of the left elbow and knee and right wrist, with pain and limitation of movement. There was a large effusion in the left knee. The affected joints in the hands showed swelling and limitation of movement. There was considerable soft-tissue swelling in the fingers of both hands and pain on flexion of the fingers. There were enlarged axillary lymph glands.

Questions

1. In what way may the signs in the chest be related to the arthritis?
2. What investigations would be of value?
3. What should be the immediate management?

Discussion

This patient has an acute onset of polyarthritis involving small and large joints. In addition she has signs of a pleural effusion, and there is a severe constitutional disturbance with weight loss, anaemia and fever. There is evidence of tendon sheath effusions in the fingers.

The pleural effusion may be part of the disease causing the arthritis or an unrelated finding. Pleural effusion is the commonest pulmonary manifestation of rheumatoid arthritis. It more commonly occurs in men who less commonly have rheumatoid arthritis. It may occur at the beginning of the illness or during its course. The effusion typically has a high protein content and low glucose concentration. A large pleural effusion without pleuritic pain is less common in systemic lupus erythematosus, and although this diagnosis should be considered, it is much less common than rheumatoid arthritis in post-menopausal women.

The pleural effusion may be caused by a coincidental disease. Primary or secondary cancer of the lung, or tuberculosis, are possible diagnoses in this case. A pulmonary neoplasm, either primary or secondary, may cause a pleural effusion, and can rarely cause a polyarthritis. Although lymph-node enlargement always suggests the possibility of malignancy, moderate local lymph-node enlargement is very common in acute arthritis from any cause, and is a usual finding in rheumatoid arthritis. There is nothing in the history to suggest that the effusion is post-pneumonic, or that it follows pulmonary infarction.

The acute arthritis will have a wider differential diagnosis if the effusion is not part of the disorder. Brucellosis in particular must be considered, since she has recently been on a camping holiday and may have drunk infected milk. Subacute infective endocarditis is a possibility, but her cardiac murmur is equally well explained by anaemia and fever and there are no other signs to support such a diagnosis.

Investigation must include a chest X-ray, which will confirm the presence of a pleural effusion and may show signs of a neoplasm or of pulmonary tuberculosis. A full blood count will confirm the presence of anaemia. A neutrophil leucocytosis would be in favour of an infective cause of the arthritis, but may occur to some degree in any acute inflammatory polyarthritis. The sedimentation rate will be raised whatever the diagnosis. The centrifuged urine must be examined microscopically. Haematuria is usually present in infective endocarditis but is also seen in nephritis due to SLE. It does not occur in rheumatoid arthritis. Blood cultures should be taken as infective endocarditis is a possible diagnosis, and they may also be positive in brucellosis. Aspiration of the pleural effusion is essential together with biopsy of the pleura. A straw-coloured effusion with a low glucose content will be found in rheumatoid arthritis. Pleural biopsy may show tuberculosis or secondary carcinoma. In rheumatoid arthritis diagnostic histological features are not usually found. If the effusion is haemorrhagic, this will strongly suggest carcinoma (see Ch. 8).

There is little to suggest direct invasion of the joints by pyogenic bacteria, but aspiration and culture of the fluid in the knees may be worthwhile if the diagnosis is still unclear after other investigations. Tests for rheumatoid factor will probably be positive if the pleural effusion is due to rheumatoid arthritis. A negative test has little diagnostic significance. Tests for antinuclear factors (especially anti-DNA antibodies) will be positive if there is active SLE, but may also be positive in rheumatoid arthritis. If negative, the tests make SLE highly unlikely.

Initial management must be with bed rest and salicylates. Steroids should be withheld until a diagnosis is reached. In particular an infective cause for the arthritis and pleural effusion must be firmly excluded.

The diagnosis was acute rheumatoid arthritis with pleural effusion. The patient was treated with steroid treatment and the disease remitted for a period of 6 months. Two years later, she had widespread rheumatoid arthritis with subcutaneous nodules.

22

Pruritus

Pruritus or itching may simply be defined as the desire to scratch. It is best regarded as a mild type of pain caused by tissue damage of a low order of magnitude. There is undoubtedly considerable variation between individuals in the threshold of stimulation at which the sensation is experienced. In the same way as one can describe one person as being more ticklish than another, so some are more susceptible to itching.

Itching is certainly the most important single dermatological symptom. It is usually a symptom of primary skin disease but diagnostic difficulty may occur when pruritus is the presenting symptom of a systemic disease. Although there may be skin lesions due to scratching, a rash may be a manifestation of an underlying disease.

Furthermore an erroneous primary dermatological diagnosis may be made if the secondary effects of scratching on the skin are not appreciated. There may be obvious scratch marks. When over a period of time they leave depigmented scars surrounded by an area of hyperpigmentation, the skin changes are called prurigo. Persistent rubbing gives rise to lichenification where the skin becomes thickened and raised in violet-brown lozenge-shaped patches between normal skin creases. This localized disorder is called neurodermatitis or lichen simplex. Other particularly troublesome localized forms are the closely related pruritus ani and pruritus vulvae. The diagnosis of general, senile or psychogenic (idiopathic) pruritus should not be made until all possible aetiological factors have been excluded.

GENERALIZED PRURITUS

Liver disease

Pruritus occurs commonly in all forms of obstructive jaundice. As such it is a helpful symptom in the differential diagnosis of jaundice, suggesting that it is due to cholestasis rather than hepatocellular damage or haemolysis. The cause of the pruritus is thought to be the retention of bile salts and it often precedes, or may not always be associated with, an elevated bilirubin. This seems borne out by the success of symptomatic oral treatment with the bile salt binding resin cholestyramine, used when the obstruction is not complete.

Obstructive jaundice due to gallstones, pancreatic carcinoma or drugs such as chlorpromazine will usually be easily detected. Likewise most patients with biliary cirrhosis will have jaundice, but pruritus without jaundice may be the presenting symptom of primary biliary cirrhosis. Itching may occur in other forms of non-icteric cirrhosis so that one should always look for signs of liver disease – hepatosplenomegaly, spider naevi, palmar erythema, leuconychia – in a patient presenting with pruritus.

Pregnancy

Pruritus may occur in the last trimester and disappear 2 or 3 days post-partum. It frequently recurs in subsequent pregnancies and may also be precipitated in such women by the taking of the contraceptive pill. Some, but not all, of these patients will have an obvious associated cholestatic jaundice. The syndrome is thought to be due to a disturbance of the liver metabolism of steroid hormones. Diagnostic difficulty may arise in some patients with pruritus who are not clinically jaundiced. There will, however, usually be biochemical abnormalities to suggest cholestasis such as a raised liver alkaline phosphatase. A similar benign recurrent intrahepatic cholestasis occurs rarely in males and, in one family at least, in females who have pregnancy- and contraceptive pill-associated jaundice.

Herpes gestationis is a rare condition occurring in pregnancy. There is a skin eruption resembling pemphigoid, which is accompanied by intense itching.

Renal failure

Pruritus may be an early feature of chronic renal failure from any cause but does not occur in acute renal failure. The mechanism by which pruritus occurs is not understood. In those patients who develop secondary hyperparathyroidism, and who have pruritus, rapid relief of itching may occur after parathyroidectomy, though the impairment of renal function remains unchanged. It is possible, in these cases, that the elevated calcium–phosphate product causes pruritus through its deposition in the skin. Pruritus does not occur with hypercalcaemia due to other causes which are not associated with a raised serum phosphate and where the calcium–phosphate product is not greatly elevated. Ultraviolet radiation (UVB) may also give relief by mechanisms which are not understood.

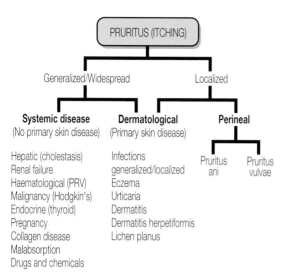

Fig. 22.1 A guide to the diagnosis of pruritus.

The figure shows:

PRURITUS (ITCHING)
- Generalized/Widespread
  - Systemic disease (No primary skin disease)
    - Hepatic (cholestasis)
    - Renal failure
    - Haematological (PRV)
    - Malignancy (Hodgkin's)
    - Endocrine (thyroid)
    - Pregnancy
    - Collagen disease
    - Malabsorption
    - Drugs and chemicals
- Localized
  - Dermatological (Primary skin disease)
    - Infections generalized/localized
    - Eczema
    - Urticaria
    - Dermatitis
    - Dermatitis herpetiformis
    - Lichen planus
  - Perineal
    - Pruritus ani
    - Pruritus vulvae

Diabetes mellitus

Hyperglycaemia and glycosuria predispose to infection, especially with yeasts. Candida infection, particularly of the anogenital region, is a common complication causing pruritus. There is also a form of generalized pruritus of unknown cause that may rarely occur particularly at the onset of diabetes. In these patients other paraesthesiae may also occur, suggesting that there is a metabolic disturbance of the peripheral nerves.

Malignant disease

There are many paraneoplastic skin manifestations of internal malignancy. Pruritus can be a presentation of a remote cancer. Pruritus is a feature of Hodgkin's disease in some patients. When it occurs it may ante-date the diagnosis by years. The itching may be intense and is often worse at night, and often affects the palms of the hands and soles of the feet. It is a most distressing, intractable and untreatable symptom and is only relieved by treatment of the underlying disease. Curiously it is a very uncommon symptom in non-Hodgkin's lymphoma when it affects lymph nodes. In chronic cutaneous T cell lymphoma, formerly known as mycosis fungoides, the mycotic phase of ulcerating skin tumours is often preceded for many years by a variety of premycotic lesions. These may be eczematous or psoriasiform and are sometimes associated with intense pruritus. The erythrodermic form is known as Sezary's syndrome.

Disorders of blood

Pruritus may be a presenting symptom of leukaemia. It occurs, in the form of erythroderma, in some patients with chronic lymphatic leukaemia. In the rare monocytic leukaemia pruritus and rash may be present for some time before blood abnormalities. At this early stage skin biopsy will show infiltration with monocytes.

Pruritus is a common symptom in primary (PRV) but not secondary polycythaemia and, as with some of the other causes of itching, it may be precipitated by taking a hot bath or shower. Using this 'provocative test' an incidence of 20–50% has been described. Usually, however, other symptoms of headache, dizziness, dyspnoea or thrombotic episodes in the heart or brain will predominate. On rare occasions pruritus may be a symptom of a severe anaemia, especially pernicious anaemia; it also occurs with iron deficiency, even in the absence of anaemia, when it can be corrected with oral iron.

Malabsorption syndrome

In steatorrhoea, especially that associated with gluten sensitivity, a variety of non-specific skin disorders may occur. For example, pruritus may thus be associated with eczema-like lesions or pigmentation.

Collagen diseases

In systemic sclerosis, where there is scleroderma together with involvement of the oesophagus, gut, lungs and kidneys, pruritus may occur. Dermatomyositis is an uncommon condition in which pruritus may also rarely occur. There is proximal limb girdle muscle weakness, together with skin involvement often affecting the upper eyelids or knuckles.

Thyroid disorders

Pruritus can be a symptom of both thyrotoxicosis and myxoedema. It occurs so rarely as to be more of a curiosity than of diagnostic value, and in the latter, may be another manifestation of dryness of the skin.

Drugs and chemicals

Drug eruptions frequently itch and do not cause too much diagnostic difficulty. Occasionally pruritus may be the only manifestation of an otherwise subclinical sensitivity reaction. Cocaine characteristically causes itching. Another agent whose effect on the skin is not clinically visible is fibreglass used for insulation purposes.

LOCALIZED PRURITUS

Itching is a feature of many skin disorders. In these cases a dermatological diagnosis can be made from the appearance and distribution of the lesion or the demonstration of the causative agent. Pruritus is prominent in infections such as scabies, pediculosis and can occur with HIV including a widespread folliculitis. It is also a prominent symptom of urticaria, eczema and dermatitis herpetiformis, and the prodrome of shingles (Herpes zoster).

Proctologists and gynaecologists are frequently consulted because of pruritus. In pruritus ani and pruritus vulvae there are numerous local disorders which may be responsible, some being common to both conditions.

Pruritus vulvae

Perspiration and lack of hygiene predispose to pruritus vulvae, as may previous gynaecological operations. It may also complicate incorrect treatment with locally irritant or sensitizing preparations, such as topical antihistamines or deodorants. Topical steroids or broad-spectrum antibiotics may predispose to *Candida* infection. The glycosuria of uncontrolled or undetected diabetes mellitus may give rise to candidiasis and thus present as pruritus vulvae. This complication has also been described in users of the contraceptive pill.

Pruritus ani

Pruritus may be confined to the anus in the diseases which can cause generalized pruritus mentioned above. Similarly, primary dermatological disorders such as psoriasis, contact dermatitis, lichen planus, lichen sclerosis, leucoplakia or local neoplasms may cause pruritus ani and pruritus vulvae.

Many local anorectal conditions have pruritus as a presenting symptom, along with soreness, bleeding and discharge. The commonest, of course, is haemorrhoids but fissure, fistula, condylomata, polyps and even carcinoma of the rectum can be responsible. Faecal soiling may be a factor common to these conditions. Treatment of the underlying disease should, of course, cure the pruritus.

Infections are a common cause of pruritus ani. Candidiasis due to the yeast, *Candida albicans*, is as important here as in pruritus vulvae and has the same predisposing causes. Fungal infection with epidermophyton is the cause of tinea cruris (Dhobi itch). This may spread from the groin to involve the anus. Another infection of intertriginous areas, which may involve the anus, is erythrasma due to *Corynebacterium minutissimum* which can be identified using fluorescence in ultraviolet light since the organism produces a porphyrin. The threadworm, *Oxyuris*, may cause nocturnal pruritus ani, especially in children, and when the worms are seen in the stool, there is great alarm in the parents. The diagnosis is best confirmed by applying Scotch tape to the perianal skin on waking and microscopically identifying the ova that adhere to it.

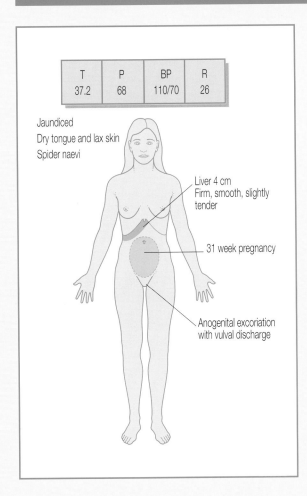

T	P	BP	R
37.2	68	110/70	26

Jaundiced
Dry tongue and lax skin
Spider naevi

Liver 4 cm
Firm, smooth, slightly tender

31 week pregnancy

Anogenital excoriation
with vulval discharge

became worse gave her a 10-day course of cotrimoxazole. This relieved the dysuria but her frequency persisted. Two weeks after treatment the dysuria recurred, and associated with it, she developed intense pruritus of the perineum involving both the anus and vulva. Ten days before admission she was started on ampicillin 500 mg 6 hourly in an effort to control her presumed urinary infection. Again the dysuria improved within a few days, but her other symptoms persisted. Five days before admission she developed nausea and vomiting. She noticed her urine becoming darker followed by yellowness of her eyes and skin. Her pruritus and frequency continued.

There was no relevant past or family history. Apart from the drugs already mentioned she had been taking ferrous sulphate during pregnancy. Although she had been greatly upset when pregnancy had been confirmed, she had apparently accepted the fact but was planning to have her baby adopted. She strongly denied the suggestion that she might have been taking any other drugs.

On examination, she had a dry tongue and lax skin. She was moderately jaundiced but not anaemic and spider naevi were present on the arms, shoulders and face. In the abdomen, the uterus was enlarged corresponding to 31 weeks of pregnancy. The liver was palpable 4 cm below the costal margin; it was firm, smooth and slightly tender. The skin of the vulva and around the anus was excoriated and inflamed, and there was a whitish vulval discharge. On rectal examination and proctoscopy she had haemorrhoids which did not prolapse. The remainder of the examination was normal and she was afebrile.

A 25-year-old unmarried hairdresser was admitted to hospital because of jaundice. She was 31 weeks pregnant and had been well for the first 20 weeks of her pregnancy, without nausea, vomiting or heartburn. She had suffered from haemorrhoids for some years which had recently become worse. She had developed frequency of micturition at 24 weeks which, a week later, was associated with dysuria. Her own doctor initially advised her to drink more fluids but when her symptoms

Questions

1. What are the probable causes of her jaundice?
2. What are the probable causes of her pruritus?
3. What is the connection, if any, between these two symptoms?
4. What immediate investigations would be of value?

In addition to the various causes of jaundice in a young woman, certain causes specifically related to pregnancy will have to be considered.

Viral hepatitis occurs predominantly in young adults and carries a worse prognosis in pregnancy. The prodromal illness of 5 days in this patient would be unusually short, though it is somewhat difficult to separate from her symptoms of urinary tract infection. Hepatomegaly with some tenderness and spider naevi could both be features of hepatitis. However, spider naevi are also a common finding in pregnancy, and palmar erythema may also occur.

Although gallstones are also more common in pregnancy, no doubt related to the hypercholesterolaemia that occurs, the absence of pain makes this an unlikely cause for her jaundice.

Drug-induced jaundice is an important cause to be considered. It may give rise to either a cholestatic or hepatocellular jaundice or to a mixed pattern. Drug jaundice may either be due to a hypersensitivity reaction or a direct toxic effect on the liver which is dose related. The only three drugs this patient has had are ferrous sulphate, cotrimoxazole and ampicillin, and the first two can cause jaundice under certain circumstances. Ferrous sulphate has a toxic effect on the liver only if taken in considerable overdose, when abdominal pain, vomiting and diarrhoea would occur. Sulphonamides cause jaundice very rarely; when it occurs it may be purely cholestatic or of a mixed cholestatic–hepatocellular type.

Other causes of jaundice in pregnancy usually occur in the third trimester. They include acute fatty liver and HELLP syndrome, the latter being associated with pre-eclampsia. HELLP is **H**aemolysis (microangiopathic), **E**levated **L**iver enzymes and **L**ow **P**latelets. The clinical picture is of vomiting, jaundice, bleeding and renal failure. Both conditions carry a bad prognosis and one would expect the patient to be more severely ill. In contrast, intrahepatic cholestasis of late pregnancy is a benign condition, and generalized pruritus is a very common feature in this disorder.

Pruritus confined to the vulva and anus is very unlikely to be due to a systemic disorder such as cholestasis and a local cause must be sought.

Although haemorrhoids may cause irritation of the anus, this would not explain pruritus vulvae. Broad-spectrum antibiotics predispose to candidiasis which is a common cause of pruritus ani and vulvae. However, the pruritus in this patient antedated the use of ampicillin.

The glycosuria of uncontrolled diabetes mellitus is another common cause of itching and pruritus may be the presenting symptom of this disease. This patient had frequency of micturition followed by dysuria; when the presumed infection was treated the dysuria improved but the frequency persisted. It is unlikely that the frequency was due to a high fluid intake alone as the patient showed signs of dehydration on admission. Diabetes beginning in mid-pregnancy, complicated by urinary infections and candidiasis, is very likely in this patient. It is therefore unlikely that there is any connection between the jaundice and the localized itching.

The investigations in this patient should be directed towards establishing the diagnosis of diabetes and the presence of candidiasis as both these conditions require treatment. Attempts to establish the cause of the jaundice from liver function tests are likely to be unrewarding, particularly as the advanced pregnancy precludes liver biopsy unless it is considered to be of vital importance.

The urine should therefore be tested for glucose, and a random and fasting blood sugar obtained, probably followed by a glucose tolerance test or measurement of glycosylated haemoglobin in case there is a lowered renal threshold for glucose, as may occur in pregnancy. The vulval discharge must be examined microscopically and cultured for *Candida albicans*, and the patient started on treatment with nystatin pessaries and ointment. A blood count may show a leucocytosis due to the recent urinary infection, and the presence of a lymphocytosis or viral lymphocytes might suggest hepatitis; hepatitis viral antigen and antibody screen is required. Liver function tests would be performed to establish the pattern of jaundice but are unlikely to reveal the underlying cause. There may be a purely cholestatic pattern with bilirubinuria and urobilinogen absent from the urine, together with markedly raised alkaline phosphatase but moderate elevation of transaminase. This would favour a diagnosis of sulphonamide hypersensitivity or the cholestasis of pregnancy. Hepatocellular jaundice with bilirubinuria and excess urobilinogen in the urine, high transaminases and slight elevation of alkaline phosphatase would be more suggestive of viral hepatitis.

> Glycosuria and an abnormal glucose tolerance test confirmed the presence of diabetes. *Candida* was easily seen on smear. The jaundice faded over the next 10 days and the investigations showed a mixed hepatocellular and obstructive jaundice. The IgM antibody to hepatitis A was positive suggesting recent infection.

23

Confusion and dementia

A wide variety of organic brain syndromes occur in which psychiatric symptoms are prominent and may constitute the initial presentation. It is usual to divide them into acute and chronic syndromes, but this is by no means a sharp distinction and there is very considerable overlap.

Acute brain syndromes develop quickly and are usually associated with clouding of consciousness and impairment of orientation. Memory is affected, there is often marked distractibility and as a result concentration is poor. The severity of the condition varies greatly, from delirium to coma. Frequently the syndrome is completely reversible. An example is delirium tremens as a result of alcoholism.

In contrast the term **chronic brain syndrome** is used very similarly to the older diagnosis of dementia. Here the onset is more gradual, and the clinical course usually more steadily progressive. There is much less clouding of consciousness and confusion, and orientation may be reasonably good. Memory impairment is variable, but is usually present and particularly affects recent memory. In chronic brain syndrome or dementia, it is intellectual failure which predominates. In the past this diagnosis was commonly thought to imply an irreversible deterioration in mental function, but this is not now an essential part of the definition, even though it is still true in the majority of cases. As a result of advances in treatment considerable improvement may be obtained in some dementias, for example those due to neurosyphilis, vitamin B_{12} deficiency and low-pressure hydrocephalus.

An important differential diagnosis is between dementia and depression. These two conditions are both common and increase in frequency with advancing years. They therefore constitute an increasingly frequent problem in diagnosis and management. In their early stages both are easily missed. Although both are often regarded as psychiatric diagnoses, their very frequency and the multitudinous guises under which they can present, means that all clinicians must be expert in establishing an initial diagnosis, even if the later management is more specialized.

In practice many mistakes are made because early in the disease the conventional medical history and physical examination often fail to suggest any abnormality. Only by a conscious evaluation of the mental state of the patient both directly and on the basis of information from friends, relatives and employers, will a diagnosis be reached. This analysis of the mental state must be done formally, as is the examination of the various visceral systems, otherwise no meaningful assessment will be arrived at. It cannot be emphasized too strongly that to rely on simple social conversation and the patient's spontaneous complaints is, in the majority of cases, totally inadequate. Tests should include recent and past memory, abstract reasoning and calculation, assessment of affect, insight and orientation. There may be physical signs of a fronto-parietal lesion such as a grasp reflex.

In dementia the very nature of the condition, with its progressive loss of intellectual capacity, often results in loss of insight, so that the patient commonly is unaware of his own deterioration and remains well satisfied by the level of his performance. This is the reason for the sound aphorism of the neurologist – 'always suspect dementia in the patient who has no complaints.'

In the future, computerized psychometric testing may form part of screening protocols for the elderly, allowing semi-automatic recognition of early cognitive failure.

PRESENTATION

In the confusional states any history will, at best, be fragmentary and unreliable. This is usually immediately obvious and every effort must be made to obtain an account of the patient's illness from some reliable informant. Without this information it may well be impossible to establish the reason for a confusional episode in some cases. The circumstances under which the patient has been found may be suggestive of the cause, and the police and social agencies can be of considerable help on occasion. The patient's belongings should be carefully searched, particularly for evidence of drugs. He may carry a card or bracelet if he suffers from a common disease such as diabetes mellitus.

THE ACUTE CONFUSIONAL STATE – THE CLINICAL APPROACH

Presentations

The first step is to recognize that a patient has developed an acute confusional state. This is usually

Box 23.1 Causes of acute confusional state (acute brain syndrome)

Drugs	e.g. anti-depressants, neuroleptics, dopamine agonists, anti-convulsants, anti-cholinergics, benzodiazapines
Alcohol	acute ingestion, acute withdrawal (delirium tremens), Wernicke's encephalopathy
Infections	systemic: bacterial, viral, fungal intracranial: meningitis, encephalitis, cerebral abscess
Trauma	head injury
Intracranial tumour	primary or secondary
Epilepsy	post-ictal state or non-convulsive status epilepticus
Vascular	subdural, extradural, intracerebral or subarachnoid haemorrhage, venous sinus thrombosis
Metabolic	electrolyte disturbances (e.g. severe hyponatraemia, acute hypercalcaemia) liver, renal, cardiac or respiratory failure, hypoxia, hypercapnia anaemia
Endocrine	hyperthyroid, hypothyroid, Addison's disease, diabetic pre-coma, hypoglycaemia

straightforward. There are a number of typical features whatever the underlying cause.

The patient usually exhibits **clouding of consciousness**. This is an important distinction from chronic brain syndromes (dementia) in which the patient's conscious level is normal. Typically, in acute confusional states the patient's level of consciousness fluctuates and they may have a reversal of the sleep–wake cycle, being more alert in the night and drowsy in the day. In severe cases it may be impossible to interact with the patient at all. The patient may be preoccupied by **hallucinatory experiences**: this is particularly common in alcohol withdrawal states.

The patient is usually **disorientated in time**. In more severe cases disorientation in space and even person may be present. It will be evident that the patient's thinking is impaired and often it is impossible to have any conversation. The patient may exhibit impairment of registration and recall if tested.

Having established that the patient is in an acute confusional state, as much information as possible must be obtained about the events leading up to the presentation. This will usually be from relatives. The circumstance in which the patient was found may be relevant. For example if it appeared that they had fallen or sustained external injury this raises the possibility of intracranial haemorrhage. A history of excessive alcohol consumption should be sought. Alcohol withdrawal symptoms may develop after admission to hospital for an unrelated illness, e.g. elective surgery. A detailed account of any previous medical illnesses, such as renal impairment or endocrine disorder, might be relevant. Some patients with chronic medical disorders such as diabetes wear medical bracelets indicating this. A drug history might be important because a patient might have inadvertently, or intentionally, taken an overdose. A previous history of epilepsy raises the possibility of anti-convulsant toxicity or even non-convulsive status epilepticus. In the latter there is usually a previous history of generalized or partial seizures.

EXAMINATION

The general and neurological examination are equally important and in cases where the patient has no accompanying informant the examination is often the only information available.

In the acutely confused patient there may be obvious motor restlessness and distractibility. Indeed the overactivity can be so marked as to constitute a major problem in management. Sometimes hallucinations are prominent and if present these are often visual in nature. A typical example are the small animals commonly seen in delirium tremens. Such experiences merge into those of an illusionary nature, and sensory misinterpretations are particularly likely if the lighting is poor, as occurs at night. The presence of confusion and agitation may make any systematic examination very difficult, and certain aspects such as neurological sensory testing will usually be impossible.

Many general medical conditions can produce a chronic confusional state and this is a common feature of terminal liver and renal failure. It may also be seen in severe cardiac and respiratory failure. However, consciousness is usually impaired and there is not usually any diagnostic difficulty.

Evidence of sepsis should be sought. Signs of external injury might be relevant, for example bruising to the head may suggest intracranial pathology such as a subdural haematoma. General physical examination may reveal evidence of respiratory, cardiac, renal or liver failure. The patient may exhibit a flapping tremor (asterixis) in liver failure and with CO_2 retention.

Careful neurological examination should be undertaken. Focal neurological signs in the limbs (e.g. hemiparesis) might indicate intracranial pathology such as an abscess or other mass lesion causing raised intracranial pressure. In the latter there may be papilloedema. There may be neck stiffness associated with intracranial infection. It is important to be aware that most patients who have ischaemic or intracerebral haemorrhagic strokes are not in an acute confusional state, unless the area of damaged brain is very large and is promoting cerebral oedema and therefore raised intracranial pressure. Dysphasia or dysarthria which commonly follow strokes should not be misinterpreted as an acute confusional state. If an acute confusional state does appear to be present in a stroke patient then an additional process should be considered. For example, the patient may have developed sepsis such as a chest or urinary infection. In Wernicke's encephalopathy due to acute alcoholism, ataxia and nystagmus are prominent features.

INVESTIGATION

In the acutely confused patient the approach to investigation will be determined by information obtained from the history and examination. The investigations will therefore differ in different situations. When there is uncertainty, simple tests should be done first. This will include blood glucose, electrolytes, full blood count, arterial blood gases, urine microscopy, chest X-ray and ECG. Further investigations depending on the presentations might include brain imaging; EEG; a detailed search for sepsis – for example cardiac echo in suspected endocarditis; tests of endocrine function and plasma drug levels (for example anti-depressants, anti-convulsants). Treatment will obviously be guided by the investigation findings. If there is a possibility of Wernicke's encephalopathy the patient should be given glucose and thiamine urgently to prevent the development of a severe permanent amnesic syndrome (Korsakoff's psychosis), even if there is no certainty about the diagnosis.

DEMENTIA

Presentation

Dementias present in various ways but generally symptoms evolve over weeks and months. There is usually deterioration in one or more of the brain cortical functions (known as higher cognitive functions). While the specific cortical functions which are impaired differ, particularly among the different types of cortical degenerative dementias, one feature in common is that consciousness is generally preserved. The cortical functions which are commonly impaired, in varying combinations, may include memory, thinking, orientation, comprehension, calculation, learning capacity and judgement. Patients may even present complaining of an awareness of decline in cognitive performance such as memory. Alternatively friends, family or work colleagues may report such a decline. Sometimes there is a marked change in personality and behaviour which distresses relatives. In other situations there may be associated neurological features which provoke the clinical presentation such as chorea in Huntington's disease or gait disturbance in normal pressure hydrocephalus.

Alzheimer's disease

Alzheimer's disease is the commonest neurodegenerative dementia and tends to begin in the temporoparietal cortex. Patients experience an early decline in memory recall and recognition. Recall disturbance tends to affect recent events first and distant events may be well recalled in the early stages of the disease. Language difficulties are common at the onset and there may be difficulty with calculation. In contrast **frontal dementias** (e.g. Pick's disease) tend to present with different symptoms reflecting frontal lobe dysfunction. Early change in personality is typical, often with loss of feelings and disinhibited behaviour. This combination of presenting features is often particularly distressing for close relatives who may be rejected by the patient. Patients with Pick's disease may lack insight into their symptoms.

One of the most important aspects in considering the differential diagnosis of dementia is to exclude a treatable cause. Many of the causes, such as the degenerative dementias, are currently incurable and supportive care is the mainstay. However, important treatable causes account for approximately 15% of patients with dementia. These include certain space-occupying lesions, endocrine and vitamin alterations, normal pressure hydrocephalus and certain infections.

Depressive pseudodementia

Depressive pseudodementia is an important differential diagnosis and should always be considered as a cause of decline in cognitive function. There may be a preceding history that might have triggered a depressive illness such as bereavement or other personal problem. In addition to the cognitive disturbance the patient may exhibit prominent affective symptoms from the outset such as sadness, loss of interest in activities and

Box 23.2 Causes of dementia (chronic brain syndrome)

Psychiatric disease
Depressive pseudodementias

Neurodegenerative dementias
Alzheimer's disease
Frontal dementia (Pick's disease)
Lewy body dementia
Huntington's disease

Vascular disease
Multi-infarct dementia

Trauma
Boxer's dementia (dementia pugilistica)

Space-occupying lesions
Chronic subdural haematomas
Primary or metastatic intracranial tumour

Infections/inflammatory
AIDS-dementia complex
Creutzfeldt–Jakob disease
Neurosyphilis
Progressive multifocal leukoencephalopathy
CNS vasculitis

Metabolic/endocrine
Vitamin B12 deficiency
Hypothyroidism
Folate deficiency

Other causes
Normal pressure hydrocephalus

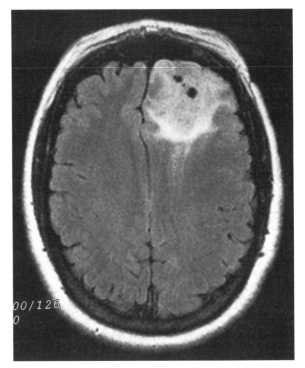

Fig. 23.1 MRI brain scan showing high-signal mass lesion with some cystic change in the left frontal lobe. Brain biopsy confirmed this to be a glioma. The 62-year-old patient presented with a six-month history of change in personality, confusion and morning headaches.

thoughts about death. The patient may be very slow to answer questions, seem disinterested, may be unkempt and will often look depressed. They may appear to simply lack interest in co-operating with the doctor or with the psychologist. There may be a previous history of depressive illness. If there is any doubt then it is wise to treat with anti-depressant medication and assess the response.

Benign tumours, such as meningiomas, may present with clinical picture similar to dementia. Frontal lobe meningiomas may grow to a very large size before they cause focal neurological signs and may mimic the behavioural changes seen in Pick's disease. **Chronic subdural haematomas** may similarly produce a slowly progressive dementia.

Hypothyroidism, vitamin B$_{12}$ deficiency and folate deficiency must always be excluded in a patient suspected to have dementia. *Chronic infection* with syphilis may cause a dementia and is a diagnosis to be considered particularly in HIV-positive patients. *Normal pressure hydrocephalus* is a somewhat enigmatic disorder. Although the clinical presentation is well character-

ized, the underlying pathophysiology is unclear and the name is probably misleading since the pressure is often intermittently raised. Patients present with a triad of dementia, urinary incontinence and gait disturbance. The gait is usually slow and shuffling. These patients have a communicating hydrocephalus which is confirmed on brain imaging and they respond to therapeutic lumbar puncture or insertion of a ventriculo-peritoneal shunt.

EXAMINATION

In dementia, physical examination is commonly normal. It is important to look for the signs of vascular disease, both arteriosclerotic and hypertensive, paying particular attention to the fundi. Bilateral cerebrovascular disease may be evident in the form of pseudobulbar palsy with emotional lability, difficulty in swallowing, dysarthria, jaw jerk and bilateral pyramidal signs. Evidence of a primary neoplasm should be sought, as multiple cerebral secondaries may first present with a rapidly developing dementia. Occasionally, such dementia may turn out to be a non-metastatic complication of malignancy. Usually the primary neoplasm will be a carcinoma of the bronchus, while occasionally multifocal leucoencephalopathy may occur with a lymphoma. The presence of adenoma sebaceum will lead to a diagnosis of tuberose sclerosis, in which the mental deterioration can occur quite late on in childhood, after a period of normal or even high intelligence.

Chronic alcoholism may be suspected if there are signs of peripheral neuropathy or portal cirrhosis. Severe dementia may occur in hepatolenticular degeneration (Wilson's disease). The presence of a Kayser–Fleischer ring is pathognomonic, and there may be choreiform movements and cirrhosis.

In the central nervous system there may be focal signs indicating vascular disease or tumour. The presence of papilloedema will indicate raised intracranial pressure, which may have been completely unsuspected. The visual fields must always be tested and they may provide the first evidence of a tumour such as basal meningioma. The signs of vitamin deficiency, which may present great diagnostic difficulty, are important. In our society the deficiency most likely to cause dementia is vitamin B_{12}. The picture of subacute combined degeneration of the cord is often very typical but early on the signs may be minimal (see Ch. 30). There is usually an associated peripheral neuropathy, and a combination which must always arouse suspicion is paraesthesiae with depression of the ankle jerks and extensor plantar responses.

The association of dementia with evidence of damage in the pyramidal, extrapyramidal, or lower motor neurones will suggest the possibility of a presenile dementia, a group of disorders consisting of Pick's, Alzheimer's and Creutzfeldt–Jakob's diseases.

INVESTIGATIONS

All patients presenting with dementia must have the appropriate blood tests to rule out treatable causes. This must include haemoglobin indices, blood film, thyroid function, calcium, urea, electrolytes and serum B_{12}. Serological tests for syphilis and HIV should be considered. A chest X-ray will help diagnose bronchial carcinoma or metastasis. Lumbar puncture and CSF examination is appropriate if chronic CNS infections, inflammation or malignant meningeal involvement is suspected. An EEG may be helpful by showing generalized slow waves in cases of chronic metabolic encephalopathy. In the primary cortical dementias loss of alpha rhythm may be an early EEG change. Brain imaging should be regarded as mandatory in all cases of dementia. MRI is the imaging modality of choice. Brain imaging will help to rule out a space-occupying lesion or hydrocephalus. It may provide evidence of small vessel arterial disease or strokes. Alternatively brain imaging may reveal specific patterns of cortical atrophy in the different cortical dementias; e.g. temporal lobe atrophy in Alzheimer's or frontal lobe atrophy in Pick's disease (Fig. 23.1).

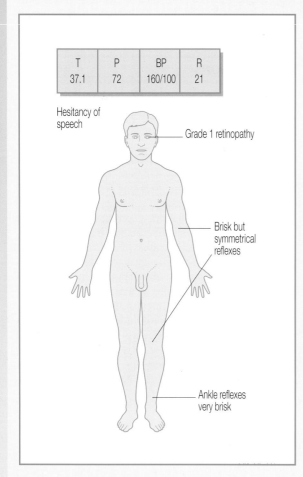

T	P	BP	R
37.1	72	160/100	21

Hesitancy of speech

Grade 1 retinopathy

Brisk but symmetrical reflexes

Ankle reflexes very brisk

A 50-year-old accountant was seen in the outpatients' clinic at the request of his general practitioner. The patient had originally consulted his doctor only because of the anxiety of his wife, who felt that his health had deteriorated recently. She complained that for the past 6 months he had seemed nervous and a little depressed. He had increasingly brought work home from the office to complete and she believed that there had been some dissatisfaction with him in his firm. He had worked in his present job for the past 12 years and had always appeared to cope without difficulty. He had not been especially successful in his career, and his present post was not one of very great responsibility. The patient had told the GP that he thought his wife was being unreasonably concerned. He felt perfectly fit, although he admitted that he had been under some pressure recently in his job. He explained this by the greatly increased volume of work which had developed over the last few years.

He had been found to be moderately hypertensive (170/110) at a routine insurance examination 3 years previously, and had been taking a small dose of a diuretic regularly ever since. Otherwise he had been well except for an inguinal hernia that had been successfully repaired 2 years earlier. There was no relevant family history.

The GP found no abnormality except that his blood pressure was still raised at 170/105 but he referred the patient to hospital mainly to reassure his wife.

On direct questioning the patient did say that one thing had bothered him recently. For the last few months he had had some difficulty with his walking and on several occasions had tripped and fallen. He tended to catch the toe of his right shoe particularly on the edges of carpets and kerb stones.

On examination there was a slight hesitancy of speech. His fundi showed Grade I changes and the BP was a little raised at 160/100. He was right-handed. The cranial nerves were normal, but in the limbs it was noted that all the tendon reflexes were very brisk. While taking the history and talking to the patient no abnormality was apparent in his appearance, personality or in his use of language. Simple tests of mental arithmetic such as serial 7s revealed, however, a surprising number of mistakes for a man of his occupation and background.

Questions

1. What are the main diagnoses that must be considered?
2. What investigations should be done immediately?

Discussion

The diagnosis in this man is uncertain at this stage. He has no complaints, and the explanation he offers of his recent behaviour is rational and may well be true. There are, however, a number of disturbing points. Until recently he had always been able to cope with his responsibilities and his job is apparently not especially arduous. He has had difficulty in walking, and its nature raises the possibility of a pyramidal lesion involving particularly the right leg. His hesitancy of speech may also have an organic basis. He is known to be hypertensive, and this must increase the likelihood that cerebrovascular disease is present.

An alternative explanation which would also be reasonable would be a psychiatric one. He is a man never of outstanding talent and of mediocre achievement. He is now aged 50, a time when depressive illnesses become increasingly common. There may well be more work than he can comfortably cope with and this may have triggered a depressive reaction. Depression is commonly associated with some degree of anxiety and agitation, and in itself will impair his work performance, thus putting increasing stress upon him. Any affective disturbance is often denied by the patient, who may have no insight into his condition. Anxiety is the commonest cause of increased tendon reflexes, and there are no unequivocally abnormal signs present on examination. The impaired concentration so often produced by emotional distress could also explain his poor performance on tests of arithmetic ability.

At this point, therefore, the two main alternative diagnoses are of a mixed anxiety depressive state, or some diffuse organic disease of the nervous system, as yet in an early stage of development, but already impairing higher mental functions, speech and gait.

If there is the possibility of an affective illness it is always worthwhile trying the effect of an antidepressant such as imipramine. This will not influence organic disease but may completely reverse any depressive mood change. In the past when the only effective treatment available for depression was ECT, such a diagnostic trial was not possible, for ECT may produce considerable deterioration in the presence of organic brain disease.

Immediate investigation need only be quite simple. The chest should be X-rayed, mainly to exclude a carcinoma of the bronchus, dementia being a feature of cerebral metastases or of the much rarer non-metastatic complications of this tumour. Examination of the blood will reveal any anaemia, which may be a reflection of some other underlying disease such as carcinoma of the stomach or vitamin B_{12} deficiency. At the same time a normal blood picture in no way removes the necessity to estimate the serum B_{12}, as dementia can occur without either anaemia or the typical findings of subacute combined degeneration of the cord. Syphilis is rare, but it would still be wise to check the VDRL, even though a negative blood VDRL does not completely exclude this diagnosis. If neurosyphilis is ever seriously suspected a lumbar puncture must be done and the serology of the CSF examined. Straight X-rays of the skull are a simple investigation although they are unlikely to provide much useful information. If the pineal is calcified, a midline shift might be detected, while a rise in intracranial pressure might show itself by erosion of the clinoid processes. Some cerebral tumours, such as craniopharyngiomas and oligodendrogliomas, may be calcified and thus reveal themselves. In the past a very common screening test at this stage was an EEG. This is now been replaced in this clinical context by one or other of the various imaging techniques.

MRI brain scan is a powerful investigation in this situation and can give additional information concerning ventricular dilatation and cortical atrophy. If available, SPECT scanning to visualize blood flow may allow even more diagnostic information; patients with Alzheimer's typically show symmetrical bilateral reduction in flow to both parietal and frontal lobes, even at a stage when the MRI scan is still normal.

All these investigations except SPECT were done in this patient and revealed no abnormality. Cerebral biopsy was considered, but rejected as being unlikely to show any treatable abnormality.

Over the next 2 years he showed continued intellectual deterioration to the level of profound dementia. His speech difficulty increased and he became completely mute. Over this time the tendon reflexes became more exaggerated, and ankle clonus with extensor plantar reflexes developed. His walking difficulty increased and on examination both upper and lower limbs showed generalized wasting with widespread fasciculation. At no time was there evidence of any sensory loss and there were never any cerebellar signs. Autopsy revealed generalized depletion of neurones in the cerebral cortex, with degeneration of both upper and lower motor neurones. A diagnosis had been made in life of Creutzfeldt–Jakob syndrome and a subsequent CT scan showed ventricular dilatation and diffuse cerebral atrophy. This was confirmed by the histological findings.

Blackouts, fits and faints

The patient presenting with a history of recurrent blackouts has an important and common problem. The two principal causes are syncope and epilepsy. In syncope the symptoms experienced by the patient are entirely due to reduced cerebral and brain-stem perfusion leading to hypoxia of neurones. In epilepsy the symptoms are caused by abnormal cerebral cortical–neuronal electrical discharge. Achieving a precise diagnosis is essential, not only because this will allow appropriate management, but also because there are often important social consequences following a diagnosis of epilepsy, including implications for employment and for driving.

Since the patient is unaware during a blackout the account of an eye-witness is critically important. The patient should be asked about any warning symptoms and also about the recovery period. However, it is the eye-witness who can give crucial information about the period of unconsciousness. In making a diagnosis it is more useful to bring the patient back to the clinic with a witness or to telephone a witness, than to start investigation without a clear history. It should also be noted that in-between attacks of blackout, whatever the cause, all investigations (including ECG, EEG and brain imaging) are often normal.

SYNCOPE

Syncope is the commonest cause of a blackout. **Vasovagal syncope** is the commonest form of syncope, frequently occurring in otherwise healthy young people. In response to triggers such as pain and emotion there is a reflex increase in vagal nerve activity. This results in a decrease in heart rate. The resulting reduced cardiac output impairs cerebral perfusion.

Cough syncope may occur in patients with chronic lung diseases such as chronic bronchitis. Typically a bout of coughing may culminate in syncope. A combination of decreased venous return, due to a

Vasalva manoeuvre during coughing, and a reflex increase in vagal output combine to reduce cardiac output and therefore cerebral perfusion. **Micturition syncope** typically occurs in elderly males with prostatic hypertrophy who have difficulty micturating and who get up in the night to pass urine. Straining at micturition leads to a Valsalva manoeuvre, decreased cardiac output and therefore reduced cerebral perfusion. In **carotid sinus syncope** the sensitivity of the carotid baroreceptors may be increased. Light touch in this region may result in excessive baroreceptor-mediated vagal discharge and therefore syncope. Syncope may be an important feature of certain cardiac disorders. Arrythmias such as complete heart block may cause sudden syncope. The restriction in cardiac output in valvular disease such as aortic stenosis may result in **exertional syncope**, as a result of falling blood pressure due to arteriolar vasodilation without an increase in cardiac output.

EPILEPSY

Epilepsy is the major differential diagnosis to consider in the patient with a blackout. Epilepsy is a disorder characterized by episodes of aberrant neuronal cortical electrical activity. The clinical consequences of such abnormal electrical activity vary but one of the commonest is a generalized tonic–clonic seizure (a convulsion). One of the simplest classifications of epilepsy is based on the clinical and EEG features. The two main divisions are partial epilepsy and generalized epilepsy.

Partial epilepsy

In partial epilepsy there is a focal (or partial) abnormal electrical discharge in one part of the brain. Partial epilepsy is subdivided into **simple partial** and **complex partial** on the basis of the patient's awareness during the attack. In simple partial attacks the patient is fully aware of their surroundings, but in complex partial attacks the patient's awareness is reduced (they seem to go blank). Typical simple partial seizures include focal motor seizures due to focal electrical discharge in one part of the motor cortex. In such attacks the patient experiences involuntary jerking of one limb in a state of clear consciousness. A typical complex partial seizure may originate in the temporal lobe. In such temporal lobe attacks the patient usually has a warning known as an aura. Typical auras include a sense of *déjà vu* or a strong smell or taste. Following the aura the patient's awareness is reduced and they become blank although do not usually lose tone. During the blank phase in a complex partial seizure of temporal lobe origin the patient may have an automatism: an automatism is a purposeless motor act which

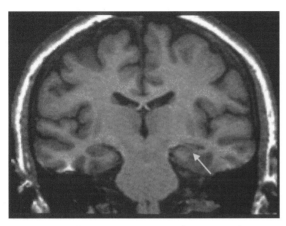

Fig. 24.1 MRI brain scan in coronal section. The arrow shows a small atrophic hippocampus compared to the other normal side. This is the typical appearance in hippocampal sclerosis which is a common cause of partial epilepsy (temporal lobe epilepsy). (Courtesy of Dr S. Sisodyia.)

is often repetitive. For example, the patient may open and close the mouth repetitively (known as lip-smacking) or may fiddle with their hands in a purposeless repetitive fashion (Fig. 24.1).

Generalized epilepsy

In generalized epilepsy there is a widespread abnormal electrical discharge throughout the cerebral cortex. The commonest clinical consequence is a generalized tonic–clonic seizure (a convulsion). Typically the patient has no warning. All voluntary muscle suddenly becomes rigid (the tonic phase) causing the patient to fall to the floor. Increased tone in the jaw muscles often causes tongue biting in this phase. The clonic phase follows in which the patient has symmetrical jerking movements of all four limbs usually lasting 1–2 minutes. Injury and urinary incontinence are common in the clonic phase.

HISTORY

It is important to take a careful and detailed history from the patient and the eyewitness. Ask the patient to describe exactly where they were, the date and the time of day. Each phase of the blackout should then be considered in sequence as outlined below.

Precipitating factors

Were there any precipitating factors? In epilepsy, lack of sleep, intercurrent illness (such as infection), emo-tional or physical stress, excessive alcohol or ingestion of drugs should be specifically considered as factors that may precipitate a seizure. In syncope the situation in which the blackout occurred may be important. For example vasovagal syncope may occur in response to emotional stress, or sudden shock such as the sight of blood. Prolonged standing, particularly in a hot environment, might be the trigger. There are certain forms of syncope which are confined to very specific circumstances. These include cough syncope and micturition syncope. Generally, vasovagal syncope is more likely to occur when the patient is standing up. In contrast the onset of abnormal cortical electrical activity which characterizes epilepsy is not influenced by body position.

Warning symptoms

The patient may remember specific warning symptoms. In vasovagal syncope common symptoms may include light-headedness, dizziness, nausea, ringing in the ears and sweating. Visual disturbance may be prominent: usually described as a 'blackening out' of vision. The warning may be less specific and the patient may simply describe a more general feeling that they are going to collapse: 'I felt like I was going to go'. They may describe a feeling that their legs 'turned to jelly'. Patients do not usually have all of these warning symptoms, but a combination of a few of them is very suggestive that syncope has occurred.

Patients with cardiac arrythmias leading to syncope may have a warning feeling of palpitations in their chest. However, it is important to note that in some forms of syncope associated with cardiac disease, such as complete heart block, there may be no warning phase. This is likely to be because in such cardiac disorders there is a sudden loss of cardiac output and therefore of cerebral and brain-stem perfusion. This contrasts with the situation in vasovagal syncope in which there is generally a progressive fall in heart rate over a period of seconds. This results in a progressive fall in cardiac output and cerebral perfusion and brain-stem perfusion. It is this more gradual reduction in perfusion which accounts for the warning symptoms – most of which are caused by hypoxia of brain-stem structures.

Patients with epilepsy may or may not have a warning which, in this context, is referred to as an aura. When an epileptic discharge in the brain is focal (also referred to as partial) the patient may experience a warning. In contrast, if the patient has primary generalized epilepsy (in which the epileptic discharge begins throughout the cerebral cortex synchronously) a warning is not present. Patients with vasovagal syncope often remember falling to the floor. Patients with epilepsy usually do not.

The unconscious phase

The details of the unconscious phase will be obtained from the witness. In a syncopal attack the patient will often appear pale. The witness may recall that the patient was complaining of some of the warning symptoms described above. Typically the patient, if standing, will slump down to the ground in a slow, semi-controlled, fashion as postural tone is lost. Once on the ground the syncopal patient will be motionless and appear pale. The pulse, if palpated, may be undetectable or very slow. It is important to note that some syncopal patients exhibit small twitching movements of the limbs. These are usually of low amplitude and are random and assymetric, flitting from one part of the body to another. They are quite different from the more violent synchronized symmetrical limb jerking exhibited by the epileptic patient. It is very important to interrogate the witness carefully about the features of any such twitching or jerking to avoid an erroneous diagnosis of epilepsy. Injury, tongue biting and incontinence are unusual in syncopal attacks.

In a generalized tonic–clonic seizure (a grand mal seizure) the witness describes a quite different sequence of events. In the initial, tonic, phase there is sudden generalized increase in muscle tone. The arms and legs stiffen and the neck may extend. Rapid contraction of the respiratory muscles may produce a forced exhalation resulting in a loud grunt. The sudden increase in lower limb tone usually results in the patient being thrown forcefully to the ground, and injury may occur at this point. Tonic contraction of the jaw muscles may result in tongue biting. The clonic phase follows and is characterized by symmetrical jerking of all four limbs. Initially the clonic jerking is of low amplitude and high frequency; however, as the seizure proceeds the clonic jerks become of lower frequency and higher amplitude until they finally terminate. Incontinence, tongue biting and injury are common in the clonic phase. Typically a generalized tonic–clonic seizure terminates in less than 2 minutes. The patient then enters the post-ictal phase.

The recovery phase

Recovery is usually rapid following the unconscious phase in vasovagal syncope. Once cerebral perfusion is restored the patient regains consciousness and is usually fully orientated within a few minutes. In contrast, the recovery phase (also termed the post-ictal phase) is often more prolonged following a generalized convulsion. The patient may be disorientated and confused. There may be a headache, muscle aches or pains related to any injury sustained during the convulsion. The tongue may be sore due to tongue biting, usually during the tonic phase of a generalized tonic–clonic seizure. Indeed, some patients with nocturnal generalized tonic–clonic seizures only know they had a seizure during the night because on waking they have a sore tongue. For many patients with epilepsy these post-ictal symptoms may only fully resolve when the patient has slept for some hours.

THE DIFFERENTIAL DIAGNOSIS OF BLACKOUTS

Although the majority of patients presenting with blackouts will have either syncope or epilepsy there are other disorders which enter the differential diagnosis. Often there will be clues in the history pointing to the correct diagnosis. The main possibilities to consider are hypoglycaemia, transient cerebral ischaemia, microsleeps, panic attacks, transient global amnesia and non-epileptic attack disorder (previously known as pseudo-seizures).

Hypoglycaemia

Hypoglycaemia can prove difficult (Table 24.1). In the known diabetic the situation is straightforward, but recurrent hypoglycaemia may occur at the stage of pre-diabetes. Hypoglycaemia in the diabetic does not only occur in the patient receiving insulin but is a well-recognized hazard with the long-acting sulphonyl ureas, particularly in the elderly patient with cerebral arteriosclerosis. Another common cause of hypoglycaemia is the condition of functional reactive hypoglycaemia, where there is thought to be an excessive insulin response to a glucose load. The hypoglycaemia comes on some 3 hours after a meal, but is not usually severe enough to cause loss of consciousness. A similar syndrome can occur after partial gastrectomy. In both situations the glucose tolerance curve shows a lag

---

> **Box 24.1** Causes of hypoglycaemia
>
> - Insulinoma
> - Large non-pancreatic tumours; retroperitoneal sarcoma, hepatoma
> - Hypopituitarism
> - Hypoadrenalism
> - Liver disease: inherited glycogen storage disorders, cirrhosis, acute liver failure, alcohol
> - Drugs: insulin, sulphonylureas
> - Reactive hypoglycaemia (only occurring after a meal), pre-diabetes, thyrotoxicosis, post-gastrectomy, anxiety

storage pattern. Treatment is by reducing the carbohydrate content of the diet. A very important, though rare, cause is an insulinoma of the pancreas. The majority of these tumours are benign, only 10% being malignant. Most occur in late middle age and about a quarter of patients give a family history of diabetes. Presentation is very varied and may be bizarre. Recurrent loss of consciousness, recurrent fits both focal and general, and recurrent psychiatric disturbances are all common, and frequently occur before breakfast as a result of the overnight fast. In the investigation of this group of patients the prolonged glucose tolerance test (6 h) and the prolonged fast test (up to 72 h) are of value. Every effort should also be made to obtain a blood glucose during an attack. The plasma glucose measurement is of greater value if it can be related to simultaneous plasma insulin levels. A low plasma glucose will, in a patient with insulinoma, be associated with an inappropriately high plasma insulin level.

Certain other diseases have also to be considered when investigating the cause of recurrent blackouts. Tetany, due to a low ionized calcium, does not usually present much difficulty. Paraesthesiae and carpopedal spasm may occur, and Chvostek's and Trousseau's signs should be looked for. An important cause of transient lowering of the ionized calcium is hysterical hyperventilation which can be confused with epilepsy.

Transient ischaemic attacks (TIAs)

Transient ischaemic attacks are commonly caused by occlusion of intracerebral arterial vessels either by in situ thrombosis or by emboli. Typically a patient develops sudden onset focal neurological features which resolve within 24 hours. The particular neurological features depend upon which blood vessel is occluded. TIAs may be broadly divided into those affecting the anterior cerebral circulation (supplied by the anterior and middle cerebral arteries) and those affecting the posterior circulation (supplied by the vertebral and basilar arteries). Since global cerebral ischaemia is required to cause loss of consciousness and anterior TIAs generally result in focal ischaemia, anterior circulation TIAs do not result in blackouts. In contrast, it is possible that a posterior circulation TIA can result in a blackout. This is because ischaemia of the reticular activating system in the brain stem can result in loss of consciousness. However, posterior circulation TIAs are a rare cause of blackouts and are overdiagnosed. Unless there is additional clear evidence of brain-stem ischaemia (diplopia, ataxia, facial motor and sensory disturbance or nausea) it is unlikely that a blackout is due to posterior circulation TIA. It is also unlikely that

kinking of the vertebral arteries by cervical spondylitic osteophytes is a common cause of vertebrobasilar ischaemia.

Microsleeps

Patients who are sleep deprived from whatever cause may be prone to brief daytime naps which may occasionally be confused with syncope or epilepsy. Obstructive sleep apnoea is the most important cause. This is most common in obese males with short fat necks and a reduced oropharyngeal space. Such patients often give a history of poor sleep quality and loud snoring. These patients experience episodes of severe airflow limitation during sleep culminating in apnoea. The resulting chronic daytime hypersomnolence makes them prone to sudden daytime naps, often in inappropriate settings, such as during a meal or driving.

Narcolepsy. Narcolepsy is uncommon and often missed. It may be confused with epilepsy, fainting and psychiatric disturbance. This is particularly unfortunate as simple and effective treatment is available. The sleepiness of narcolepsy is in every way comparable with normal sleep except that it is excessive and occurs under inappropriate circumstances. The patient can always be easily awakened, and the response to amphetamine is usually good. The frequent association with cataplexy, sleep paralysis and hypnogogic hallucinations is often of help in the diagnosis.

Panic attacks

In some patients certain situations may result in acute attacks of anxiety known as panic attacks. Some of these patients also have a chronic anxiety state or they may have a specific phobia which precipitates panic attacks. In an attack the patient is consumed by an overwhelming fear that something terrible is going to befall them. Typically they hyperventilate, which results in alkalosis and hypocalcaemia. Hypocalcaemia causes tingling and may lead to tetany which may be confused with a convulsion. Generally the patient remains conscious, although in severe cases a vasovagal syncope may be precipitated.

Transient global amnesia

This condition usually occurs in patients over the age of 40 and may be confused with a complex partial epileptic seizure. Typically patients suddenly lose the ability to acquire new information and they appear confused. They characteristically ask the same questions repeatedly, but are unable to register the answer. They do not lose the ability to remember information

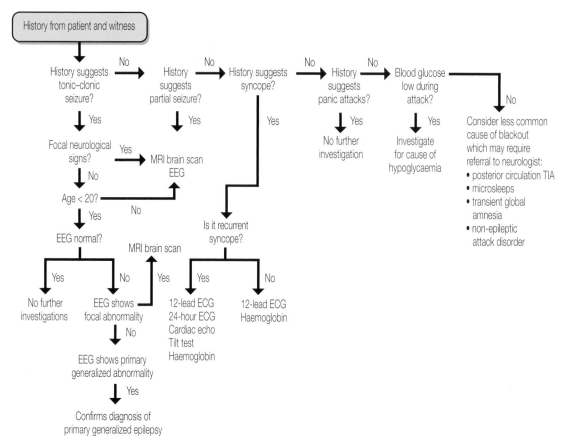

Fig. 24.2 An approach to the investigation of a patient with blackouts. The two commonest causes of blackouts are syncope and seizures. Less frequent causes may need referral to a neurologist.

acquired before the attack, such as their identity. The ability to perform previously learned complex tasks is not affected. For example, the patient may be able to continue driving a car. Episodes may be precipitated by physical exertion. Attacks last 2–6 h and may recur. The attacks are believed to be caused by transient medial temporal lobe dysfunction. Patients often have a history of migraine. The attacks are not caused by epilepsy and there is no increased risk of stroke in this group of patients.

Non-epileptic attack disorder (pseudoseizures)

This group of patients are prone to blackouts that may have similarities to either syncope or generalized tonic–clonic seizures. However, the mechanisms leading to such attacks are not cerebral hypoperfusion or abnormal neuronal electrical activity. Generally they have a psychological basis. Such attacks are commoner in females and patients may have a history of

abnormal illness behaviour (in some cases amounting to Munchhausen's syndrome) or may have a history of other psychiatric disorders. Sometimes there is secondary gain. Distinguishing such attacks from true syncope or true epilepsy can be difficult and normally requires specialist assessment.

Investigation and management

Investigations are guided by the history and examination findings (see Fig. 24.2). If a patient has had a single episode with features to suggest syncope and the neurological and cardiological examination is normal it is reasonable to perform a standard 12-lead ECG and to check the haemoglobin. If these tests are normal no further investigations are required. If the patient has a history to suggest recurrent syncopal attacks more detailed cardiological assessment is usually required. This should include standard ECG, haemoglobin, echocardiogram and continuous ambulatory ECG monitoring. If these are unremarkable during an episode tilt table testing should be considered.

Following a single tonic–clonic seizure, if the neurological examination is normal, further investigations are dictated by the age of the patient. Under the age of 20 an EEG should be performed. If this is normal or shows evidence of primary generalized abnormality a brain scan is not necessary. If there is a focal EEG abnormality a brain scan (preferably MRI) should be done. Patients who have had a single generalized seizure who are over the age of 20 should all have a brain scan (preferably MRI) in addition to an EEG. All patients who are suspected to have had partial epileptic seizures should have brain imaging since they are more likely to have focal cerebral pathology. In patients with normal brain scans, irrespective of the EEG findings, treatment with anticonvulsant medication is generally not commenced unless the patient has a second seizure. This is because a significant proportion of patients will not progress to a second seizure.

Blackouts, fits and faints

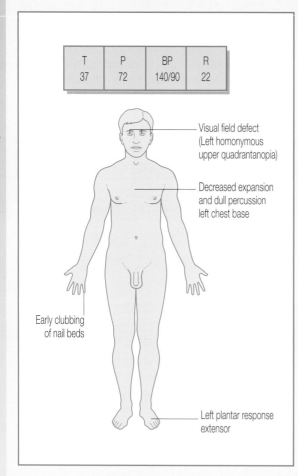

T	P	BP	R
37	72	140/90	22

Visual field defect
(Left homonymous
upper quadrantanopia)

Decreased expansion
and dull percussion
left chest base

Early clubbing
of nail beds

Left plantar response
extensor

A 45-year-old bus driver gave a 6-month history of morning headaches and, more recently, blackouts which were occurring 2–3 times per week without obvious precipitant. Immediately before some of the blackouts he experienced a warning characterized by a strong rising sensation beginning in his epigastrium and spreading up to his neck. It was similar to indigestion although he did not normally suffer from this. The next thing he remembers is coming round having lost track of time. The previous week this had resulted in a minor road traffic accident and he had stopped driving awaiting his urgent hospital appointment. His wife had witnessed an attack. She described having a conversation with him at breakfast one day. He was sitting talking normally when he suddenly put his hand to his chest and complained of heartburn. He then became blank and stopped talking. He did not fall off his chair but his wife couldn't get through to him; she noticed he began to fiddle with his hands in his lap for no reason. After about 1 minute he regained his senses and was able to continue the conversation. He had no memory of the event except for the feeling in his chest at the onset. On two occasions he had woken in the morning with a sore tongue and a stiffness in the muscles of his arms and legs.

He had not suffered from headaches very much in the past. However, over the previous 6 months morning headaches often accompanied by nausea were a common occurrence. He found they were marked for the first hour or two but they generally subsided by the middle of the day. If they did not, paracetamol was usually effective. He had smoked 20 cigarettes a day for 20 years but did not drink alcohol. There was no family history of neurological disease.

On examination he was alert and orientated. His left optic disc was normal but the medial margin of the right disc was indistinct. Visual field testing was abnormal revealing a left homonymous upper quadrantanopia. The rest of the cranial nerves were normal. In his limbs tone, power and coordination were normal in arms and legs. His tendon reflexes were symmetrical and normal. His left plantar response was extensor and his right plantar was flexor. General physical examination revealed nicotine staining of his fingers and early clubbing. Chest examinations revealed reduced expansion of the left side and dullness to percussion at the left lung base. Tactile and vocal fremitus were reduced at the left base as were breath sounds. The rest of the general physical examination was normal.

Questions

1. What is the nature of the blackouts?
2. What investigations should be done?
3. What are the probable diagnoses?

Discussion

This 45-year-old bus driver gives a history of blackouts which have typical features of complex partial seizures. He has an epigastric aura characterized by a rising sensation from the epigastrium to the neck. He then goes blank and has an automatism characterized by purposeless fiddling with his hands. He is amnesic for the episode and describes losing track of time which is typical. The commonest site in the brain from which such partial seizures arise is the temporal lobe. There is evidence from the neurological examination that there may be structural pathology in the temporal lobe. A homonymous upper quadrantanopia is usually caused by temporal lobe pathology. In addition to partial seizures there is a suspicion that he may have had secondarily generalized nocturnal seizures. This should always be suspected when a patient gives a history of waking up with a sore, bitten, tongue. There are other features in the history that indicate one should be con-cerned about structural pathology. First he has morning headaches sometimes accompanied by nausea: such headaches raise the possibility of raised intracranial pressure and should always prompt a search for an intracranial space-occupying lesion, even in the absence of definite papilloedema as in this case. The findings on general examination suggest a left pleural effusion. In a smoker with early clubbing this raises the possibility of a bronchogenic carcinoma.

> The patient's chest X-ray confirmed a left pleural effusion. Cytology of the pleural fluid confirmed a non-small cell lung cancer. The MRI brain scan revealed multiple metastases throughout both hemispheres including the right temporal lobe. Phenytoin controlled the seizures. The patient received cytotoxic chemotherapy and cranial radiotherapy but died 12 months after his first symptoms had developed.

which result in raised intracranial pressure. Such raised pressure causes downward displacement of supratentorial structures and pressure on the brain stem and therefore disrupts reticular activating system activity. Processes in the infratentorial space (that is, the posterior fossa) may directly interfere with the reticular activating system (for example, a cerebellar haemorrhage will press on the brain-stem). It is therefore logical to consider the causes of coma on the basis of whether the causative insult is acting diffusely at the level of the cerebral cortex or is acting by disrupting reticular activating system function (see Box 25.1).

PRESENTATION

The history from relatives or other witnesses is critical for diagnosis and every attempt must be made to identify such individuals. The account of the ambulance staff who may have found the patient is often useful. If no such witnesses or accounts are available assessment relies purely on the examination of the patient.

When witness information is available it is important to establish the rate at which the coma developed and the exact circumstances in which the patient became comatose. In addition, a detailed past medical history is often invaluable. Patients with depression who are on treatment may take overdoses of their medication. This suspicion may be supported by the finding of empty bottles where the patient was found or even a suicide note. Such overdose-induced coma is the commonest cause of coma seen in accident and emergency departments. There may be a history of diabetes in the patient with hyper- or hypoglycaemic coma. A history of hypertension might be relevant to the patient presenting with a brain haemorrhage causing coma.

Sudden onset coma may follow hypoxic ischaemic events such as cardiac arrest. Patients who experience cardiac arrest out of hospital, and who receive prolonged or inefficient resuscitation, frequently remain comatose even following restoration of cardiac output. If cardiac arrest is not the cause, sudden onset of coma usually indicates major intracranial pathology or epilepsy. For example, a large subarachnoid haemorrhage may cause sudden coma in a previously well patient. Sudden coma may also occur with posterior fossa haemorrhage (e.g. cerebellar haemorrhage). In epilepsy there may be a clear history of a generalized seizure and the comatose patient may be post-ictal (see Ch. 24). Occasionally sudden onset coma may be due to non-convulsive epileptic status. In this situation there are no visible convulsive movements. There may be a history of generalized convulsive attacks at other times but non-convulsive status may sometimes be the first presentation of epilepsy. Coma as a result of raised intracranial pressure may be sudden but often there is

PATHOPHYSIOLOGY AND CAUSES OF THE COMATOSE STATE

The assessment and diagnosis of the patient presenting in a comatose state is a common challenge for physicians, both in the casualty department and on the wards. There is a large differential diagnosis for this clinical presentation but, by careful history-taking from witnesses, and by examination of the patient, this can usually be narrowed down to a few possibilities even before any investigations are performed. The pathophysiological basis and causes of coma will be considered first; the clinical approach to the comatose patient is then discussed.

PATHOPHYSIOLOGY AND CAUSES OF THE COMATOSE STATE

Although a fundamental understanding of the neural basis of human consciousness remains to be established there are certain principles that are useful in considering the causes of coma. Consciousness depends upon normal activity in the reticular activating system (located in the brain stem) and in the neurones of both cerebral cortices. The reticular activating system is a complex neural network ascending through the brain stem and, via connections to the thalamus, projects widely to all parts of the cerebral cortex. Normal neuronal activity in both the reticular activating system and the cerebral cortex must be present in order for the patient to be in the normal conscious state. Unconsciousness may result from disruption of the reticular activating system or from disruption of cortical neuronal function. Since the cortical component of consciousness is not localized to one part of the cerebral cortex it follows that consciousness will not be disrupted by a focal cortical lesion; rather, if the basis of coma is at the cortical level, the insult must diffusely affect cortical neuronal function.

Reticular activating system dysfunction may result from supratentorial or infratentorial processes. Supratentorial processes include space-occupying lesions,

Box 25.1 The causes of coma

Disorders resulting in diffuse cortical neuronal dysfunction

Metabolic
  diabetic hyperglycaemic coma
  hypoglycaemia
  hypothyroidism
  hepatic failure (increased ammonia levels)
  renal failure (uraemia)
  severe electrolyte derangement e.g.
    hyponatraemia
  alcohol (acute intoxication or Wernicke's
    encephalopathy)
  respiratory failure (hypercapnia)
  hypothermia

Self-poisoning
  drugs (especially tricyclic anti-depressants,
    benzodiazepines and neuroleptics)
  alcohol (often taken with drugs overdose)
  accidental in children

Hypoxic/ischaemic
  following cardiorespiratory arrest or other low
    cardiac output state
  carbon monoxide poisoning

Infective
  advanced meningitis, encephalitis, septicaemia

Vascular
  subarachnoid haemorrhage, cerebral vasculitis,
    hypertensive encephalopathy, cerebral venous
    sinus thrombosis

Trauma
  head injury leading to concussion

Epilepsy
  non-convulsive epileptic status
  post-ictal state

Insults resulting in dysfunction of the reticular activating system

Supratentorial focal lesions
  haemorrhage (extradural, subdural or
    intraparenchymal)
  tumour
  abscess
  large infarct
  obstructive hydrocephalus

Infratentorial focal lesions
  intraparenchymal haemorrhage (e.g. cerebellar
    haemorrhage)
  abscess
  tumour
  infarct

a preceding history of headaches, which suggests raised intracranial pressure, or even of focal neurological features such as an evolving hemiparesis in a patient with a supratentorial brain tumour.

Coma of slower onset may be due to infective or metabolic causes. Intracranial infections such as encephalitis or brain abscess usually evolve over hours or even days and there may be symptoms to suggest infection such as fever. Patients with encephalitis often experience seizures, or changes in behaviour or memory prior to coma. Patients with abscesses may have a history of focal neurological features. Coma may occur in meningitis, but since the infecting process begins in the meninges it is usually only in advanced untreated cases that coma supervenes. The exception to this is in very young children with meningococcal meningitis as part of a septicaemia when coma may rapidly develop. The majority of the other causes of coma such as metabolic disorders or self-poisoning usually evolve over hours or longer rather than being sudden. It should be noted that supratentorial infarcts do not usually result in coma unless they are very large and behave like a mass lesion.

PHYSICAL EXAMINATION

Many patients on regular therapy with potent drugs such as steroids, insulin, or anti-coagulants, carry a card saying so. Similarly if they suffer from a rare disease such as porphyria or even a common condition like epilepsy there may well be a statement to this effect in their wallets or on a bracelet. This is a habit to be encouraged and can be of great value in helping one to arrive quickly at the correct diagnosis and treatment. In the future 'smart cards' (data storage cards), which can be read by computer, are likely to be available and will be able to contain unlimited information about an individual.

On occasion systematic clinical examination may have to be delayed to allow for urgent resuscitative measures, such as the establishment of a clear airway. A careful examination of all the body systems must be carried out scrupulously as soon as possible however, and this must include the back as well as the front of the patient! All findings should be carefully recorded with the date and time so that changes in the physical state and in particular in the level of consciousness can be easily assessed, if necessary by other observers. Such notes will also be of the greatest value if medicolegal complications arise.

General observation

The patient's colour should be observed, remembering that minor degrees of jaundice are easily missed in artificial light. Cyanosis will be of obvious importance, and the physician should also look for any abnormal pinkness suggestive of carbon monoxide poisoning. The pigmentation of Addison's disease must also be looked for. Any movements of face or limbs must be noted, paying especial attention to asymmetry. Focal epileptic discharge is of the greatest value in establishing the site of the lesion as well as narrowing down the list of possible causes of the coma. The rate, rhythm and depth of respiration are all of importance. Cheyne–Stokes respiration or other forms of periodic breathing usually indicate severe cortical or medullary damage and a less good prognosis. Respiration is often shallow, with marked reduction in tidal volume in barbiturate-induced coma. If there is the slightest doubt as to the adequacy of ventilation the question of urgent mechanical ventilation must be considered and blood gas estimations are of the greatest value in making the decision. Continuous non-invasive monitoring of oxygen saturation (oximetry) of the blood can be of great assistance. These tests frequently demonstrate the inadequacy of a purely clinical assessment of the effectiveness of respiration.

Respiratory failure due to lung disease, when severe, can be a cause of coma. There is disturbance of cerebral function, the high $paCO_2$ causing increased cerebral blood flow, and this, together with the anoxia, leads to cerebral oedema. Brain swelling will cause a rise in intracranial pressure and dilated retinal veins and papilloedema may be seen. Although most patients with respiratory failure will present only with confusion, coma can develop rapidly at any time, particularly after ill-advised therapy with a high concentration of oxygen.

The typical sighing respiration of diabetic acidosis will usually be obvious and the breath should always be smelt for acetone. Hepatic or uraemic fetor are signs which may be of value but their detection is often difficult.

Examination of the skin can be helpful. The scars of the mainliner drug addict may be found, while diabetics on insulin may show areas of fat atrophy. Loss of body hair, pallor and thinning of the skin will suggest hypopituitarism. The various stigmata of liver disease must also be carefully sought, including spider naevi, clubbing, palmar erythema and Dupuytren's contractures. In the abdomen the discovery of polycystic kidneys or the enlarged bladder of chronic prostatic obstruction may point to uraemia as the underlying cause of the coma.

Temperature

One important measurement is usually left to the nurse: the patient's temperature. Although error is less likely in the detection of fever, hypothermia is easily missed. Hyperpyrexial coma is very rare in Britain but hypothermic coma has been increasingly recognized. If the temperature is low, even if the reading of the routine clinical thermometer is still above the minimum, it is worth checking using a low-reading thermometer inserted rectally. Hypothermia is mainly a disease of the newborn and the elderly, and the likelihood of it developing will obviously be related to the prevailing weather. At these extremes of age, the homeostatic mechanisms which maintain normal body temperature may be impaired. Drugs such as phenothiazines further impair the shivering response to cold. Intercurrent infection may lead to elderly people feeling too ill to keep themselves warm. Myxoedema is not a common cause of hypothermic coma, although hypothermia itself may produce a state resembling myxoedema.

The blood pressure

The blood pressure should be carefully checked, although it can on occasion be misleading. In the hypertensive patient, cerebral haemorrhage is more common, both from congenital anomalies and also from the intracerebral rupture of an arteriosclerotic vessel. A rise in blood pressure may, however, occur as a response to the cerebral catastrophe of haemorrhage, both subarachnoid and intracerebral, and can also occur with extensive cerebral infarction. Indeed anything which produces a rapid rise in intracranial tension seems capable of producing this response, the exact underlying mechanism remaining controversial. Usually the rise in pressure is modest but the blood pressure can occasionally be dramatically high. It will normally settle over the next few days and if continued for more than a week will usually turn out to be long-standing, and not due to the recent neurological damage. The finding of hypertensive fundal changes, together with the signs of left ventricular hypertrophy, will also support the latter interpretation. Hypertension is common in the older age groups and its presence must not weigh too heavily in the making of a diagnosis.

A rare condition to consider if the blood pressure is high and the fundi show Grade III or IV changes is hypertensive encephalopathy. This is sometimes loosely diagnosed whenever neurological signs occur in association with a raised blood pressure. It is however much more than this, being characterized by spasm of the cerebral vessels and widespread cerebral oedema. These changes fluctuate and the neurological signs may vary from hour to hour. Consciousness is impaired and convulsions are common. Sometimes, particularly in association with the renal failure of acute nephritis, the whole clinical picture may occur at levels of blood pressure which are not markedly raised. This probably reflects the widespread damage to small blood vessels seen in acute nephritis. Treatment in hypertensive encephalopathy is a matter of urgency, as disastrous cerebral haemorrhage or infarction can occur at any time. Lowering of the blood pressure in other situations of neurological deficit has aroused considerable controversy. In general all one can say is that firstly the higher the diastolic pressure, whatever the cause, the stronger the indication for treatment, and secondly that in the presence of neurological damage the pressure should be lowered slowly. Marked fluctuation in the pressure is to be avoided.

The pulse

A slow full-volume pulse may occur in raised intracranial tension from any cause. If this is due to respiratory failure then other features may be noted, such as the generalized vasodilation associated with hypercapnia. The presence of an arrhythmia should lead one to suspect a recent myocardial infarction, in which mural thrombosis may develop. This may cause cerebral embolism. However, consciousness is less often lost in embolism in comparison with cerebral thrombosis or haemorrhage. The presence of atrial fibrillation, with or without other evidence of heart disease, will also suggest this possibility. Cardiac arrhythmia of any origin, if it gives rise to profound tachycardia or bradycardia, may cause such a drop in cardiac output that, particularly in the elderly, cerebral perfusion is impaired and confusion results. Syncope may occur but coma is unlikely.

Trauma

Evidence of trauma must always be carefully sought. It may be the cause of the coma or have resulted from the abruptness of the patient's collapse. The temporal fossa should be felt for the boggy swelling due to a haematoma, which would suggest an underlying fracture and possible extradural collection of blood from a torn middle meningeal artery. Bruising about the head in an elderly person will raise the possibility of a chronic subdural haematoma. The skull itself should be carefully felt for depressed fracture and at the same time the nose and ears should be looked at for the bleeding or leakage of CSF which may indicate a fracture of the skull base. Usually with head injury the circumstances under which the patient has been found will indicate the diagnosis. The error is still made of regarding the confused and aggressive man smelling of alcohol as yet another drunk and his gradual lapse into coma as extradural blood collects is missed for want of careful neurological observation.

The nervous system

Examination of the nervous system is obviously limited in the comatose patient. Its main aims will be to establish the level of coma and to look for asymmetry or signs which may suggest the site of a lesion. The fundi may show papilloedema, hypertensive retinopathy, diabetic changes, or the subhyaloid haemorrhages of subarachnoid bleeding. Pupillary abnormalities must be noted and are often a sensitive index to change in the patient's level of consciousness. The constricted pupils of brain-stem haemorrhage or morphine poisoning are well known. Facial weakness can often be detected both by appearance and the way the face blows out on respiration. Neck stiffness should be looked for, but may be absent in deep coma, even in the presence of meningitis. In the limbs, posture, tone, spontaneous movement and reflex pattern should all be noted, together with any features suggestive of long-standing neurological disease. Sensory testing will usually be impossible but the response to deep and superficial pain should be assessed on each side.

INVESTIGATIONS

In the majority of cases initial investigations will not need to be extensive. Diabetic coma will usually be suggested by the clinical picture and easily confirmed by examination of the urine and blood. Measurement of blood sugar, even with modern techniques, should not be left to the most inexperienced nurse! If hypoglycaemia is suspected an instant rough estimation of blood glucose can be done at the bedside, but because the test is inaccurate at low concentrations a therapeutic trial of intravenous glucose may be necessary. Blood should be taken first so that later a glucose estimation by the laboratory will confirm the diagnosis. If poisoning by drug or chemical is a possibility, blood and, if available, gastric contents should be taken and stored, even if immediate analysis of the sample is not possible locally. Later analysis may prove of value and occasionally in forensic problems the presence of such samples will prove of the greatest help. Rapid analysis, both qualitative and quantitative, for common causes of drug coma, such as salicylates and benzodiazepines can be of the greatest assistance. Not only can the precise diagnosis be established, but an assessment can be made of the vigour with which treatment must be pursued.

Suspected subarachnoid haemorrhage or meningitis must usually be confirmed by lumbar puncture. Provided there is nothing which suggests the presence of raised intracranial pressure the risk is negligible. Intracerebral haemorrhage commonly leads to blood in the subarachnoid space and lumbar puncture does not differentiate between the two types of haemorrhage. In subarachnoid haemorrhage, X-ray CT examination may be of great value, but if negative does not exclude the diagnosis.

In the patient where trauma has occurred or may reasonably be suspected, skull X-rays should be obtained. With the widespread availability of CT scanning of the brain, quick, reliable, non-invasive investigation can be undertaken, making other techniques such as angiography, ultrasound and isotope scanning obsolete. In selecting cases for investigation careful and repeated assessment of the level of coma is of the greatest importance in guiding management.

Commonly in cases of coma the cause is initially in doubt. Provided the patient is properly cared for so that deterioration does not pass unnoticed, he is unlikely to come to any harm, and with the passage of time the diagnosis will usually become clear. Deepening coma in an undiagnosed patient is an emergency requiring active investigation and the fullest possible consultation with other specialists, particularly neurosurgeons. The patient should be supported, if necessary by mechanical ventilation, while this is being done.

It remains true that many cases of coma are misdiagnosed or not diagnosed at all in the first few hours, because the patient has taken an overdose of one of the less obvious drugs under circumstances which do not suggest this diagnosis.

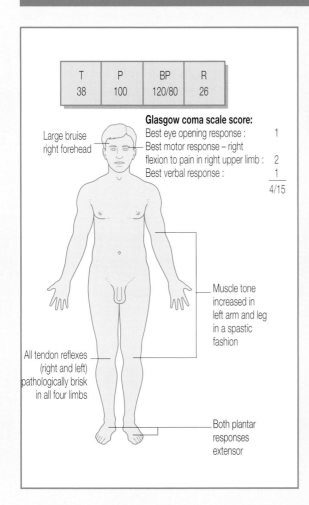

T	P	BP	R
38	100	120/80	26

Glasgow coma scale score:

Large bruise right forehead

Best eye opening response : 1
Best motor response – right flexion to pain in right upper limb : 2
Best verbal response : 1

4/15

Muscle tone increased in left arm and leg in a spastic fashion

All tendon reflexes (right and left) pathologically brisk in all four limbs

Both plantar responses extensor

A 22-year-old medical student was in his first clinical term. He was found in an unconscious state in his room in the hall of residence by a friend at 9 a.m. on a Monday morning. He was lying on the floor beside his bed with a large bruise on his right forehead. His friend had last seen him the night before, when he had been complaining of feeling tired and feverish with a headache and went to bed early. His friend also reported that the day before he had been behaving somewhat strangely. He had been withdrawn, which was uncharacteristic. In addition his friend reported that the day before while talking to him he suddenly went blank for a few moments 'like a zombie' and opened and closed his mouth repetitively during this blank state. It lasted less than 1 minute.

His friend explained that they occasionally used cannabis but no other illicit drugs. As far as the friend knew, the patient had apparently been fit and well in the past. However, none of the patient's relatives were available to confirm this.

On arrival in hospital the patient was comatose. There was no verbal response or eye opening response to pain. His motor responses to pain were asymmetrical. There was flexion to pain in his right upper and lower limbs but extension to pain in the left limbs. On general examination his temperature was 38°C, BP 120/80, pulse 100 regular. There was no skin rash or visible needle puncture marks. Examination of his heart, lungs and abdomen was normal. The optic discs were normal. Tone was increased in a spastic fashion in his left limbs but normal on the right side. All deep tendon reflexes were pathologically brisk. Both plantar responses were extensor. Soon after arriving he had a witnessed generalized tonic–clonic seizure which was terminated with diazepam.

Questions

1. What are the possible causes of this presentation?
2. What investigations should be done?

This 22-year-old medical student appears to have been fit and well in the past. He presents in a deeply comatose state with a fever, focal neurological signs in the limbs and has a witnessed generalized seizure. The prodrome leading up to this presentation is relatively short. His friend had made a number of observations in the preceding 48 hours. The patient had been somewhat withdrawn, he had had a blank spell with possible lip smacking and the night before he had been complaining of a headache and feeling feverish. The blank spell is suggestive of a complex partial seizure.

The suspicion that seizure activity is at least part of the process leading to coma is substantiated by two further observations. First, the patient was found beside his bed with a bruised forehead which might suggest he had had a seizure during the night. Second, he went on to have a witnessed generalized seizure after arrival. There are additional features to suggest that there may be an infective pathology and also focal brain process, possibly in the right hemisphere. The evidence to support infection is that he had been complaining of fever and that a pyrexia was confirmed on arrival in hospital.

It is important to remember that although fever may associate with infection other brain processes such as subarachnoid haemorrhage and the post-ictal state itself may be associated with fever. The presence of neck stiffness would suggest meningeal irritation and may be caused by both infective processes and subarachnoid haemorrhage. Although subarachnoid haemorrhage does need to be considered, the prodrome of 48 hours would not be usual. Subarachnoid haemorrhage is generally a sudden event. Although there is a history of cannabis use – and drugs always need to be considered as a cause of coma – the focal signs present in this patient would not be expected in drug overdose. Patients who abuse drugs intravenously are at risk of infective endocarditis. The latter can be complicated by septic cerebral emboli which could lead to a cerebral abscess. The absence of skin puncture marks would argue against regular intravenous drug abuse. However, a cerebral abscess needs to be seriously considered. A subdural abscess, for example, could explain the prodrome with infective features, the focal signs and the signs of meningeal irritation. It could also explain the seizures. The other infective process which could explain the observations is a viral encephalitis. The commonest viral encephalitis is due to herpes simplex virus. There is inflammation of grey and white matter, and this often begins in the temporal lobes before spreading to other regions. Because grey matter is affected early in the disease process seizures and behavioural changes may be prominent initial symptoms. Focal brain signs and meningeal irritation are also common.

A further possibility is that the patient may have dual pathology. He could have been ill from an infective process such as early encephalitis, and then sustained a head injury during the night in his room resulting, for example, in a right-sided extradural or subdural haemorrhage.

In conclusion, the main conditions which would best explain the history and signs would be an infective process particularly affecting the right hemisphere. The overriding priority in this patient is first to protect his airway following the seizure and then to obtain urgent brain imaging. Even in the absence of papilloedema it is certainly possible he may have a space-occupying lesion (e.g. an abscess or a haematoma) which needs immediate neurosurgical decompression.

In this patient an urgent MRI brain scan was abnormal. There were scattered high signal areas on the T2 weighted images particularly in the right hemisphere and the right temporal lobe. There was a mild degree of generalized brain oedema. The appearances were typical of an acute viral encephalitis. An EEG confirmed epileptiform activity originating in his right temporal lobe. It was considered unsafe to obtain CSF because of the presence of brain oedema. CSF examination, when safe, is useful to confirm a viral infective process. Typical CSF changes would be a normal glucose, a raised protein (usually above 1 g/dl), and a raised white cell count (predominantly or exclusively lymphocytes – usually a few hundred). Examination of the CSF using the polymerase chain reaction (PCR) allows detection of viral DNA. In this patient the presumptive diagnosis was of herpes simplex encephalitis. He was treated with intravenous acyclovir and regained consciousness over the next few days. His ultimate recovery was good and he was able to return to his medical studies, but he required long-term anti-convulsant medication to prevent complex partial seizures.

26

Stroke

A stroke is an acute focal neurological deficit which is the result of a disturbance in the cerebral circulation. Stroke is a common cause of death and morbidity in the western world and all physicians are likely to be involved in the diagnosis and care of stroke patients. The majority of strokes are ischaemic (80%) and 20% are due to haemorrhage.

The diagnosis of an acute completed (ischaemic or haemorrhagic) stroke is usually straightforward on clinical grounds alone. However, it is not possible to determine reliably if a stroke is haemorrhagic or ischaemic solely on clinical features. It is necessary to confirm the type of stroke by imaging. It is particularly important to rule out haemorrhagic stroke if thrombolytic therapy is being considered, although at present the place of thrombolytic therapy in ischaemic stroke treatment is not established. On occasions, space-occupying lesions such as tumours or abscesses may present with what appears to be an acute focal neurological event, for example a hemiparesis. If all stroke patients have a brain scan these possibilities will not be overlooked.

While a completed stroke may be a relatively straightforward diagnosis, other related disorders may produce diagnostic difficulties. For example symptoms produced by transient ischaemic attacks (TIA) may be mimicked by other neurological conditions such as migraine or multiple sclerosis. Cerebral venous sinus thrombosis may result in stroke but there are often additional neurological features, such as focal seizures, which may cause diagnostic difficulty.

ISCHAEMIC STROKE

The main risk factors for an ischaemic stroke are hypertension, increasing age, smoking, heart diseases which lead to embolism (such as atrial fibrillation and mitral valve disease), hypercholesterolaemia and diabetes. There is evidence that the oral contraceptive slightly increases the risk while HRT may lower the risk slightly. In young patients with stroke, rarer causes need to be considered and excluded. These include arterial dissection, fibromuscular dysplasia, Fabry's disease, mitochondrial diseases and haematological disorders.

Arterial dissection is usually caused by trauma to the neck and most commonly involves the carotid or vertebral arteries. The trauma leads to breach in the endothelium allowing blood to enter the wall. The resulting haematoma splits the arterial wall and the true lumen of the artery becomes narrowed. Thrombosis within the true lumen may form and subsequently embolize resulting in a TIA or stroke. The neck trauma may be relatively trivial and may sometimes not be remembered. In carotid dissection, damage to the sympathetic nerve fibres in the carotid sheath may result in a painful Horner's syndrome. Some patients with dissections have a disease of the arterial wall called fibromuscular dysplasia. In this group of patients, dissection of other arteries, such as the renal arteries, may occur. Aortic arch dissection usually occurs on the basis of atheromatous disease of the aorta. Patients present with a sharp central chest pain which often radiates into the back. If the dissection extends into the common carotid arteries, local thrombosis may form. Subsequent embolization may result in TIA or stroke.

Four patterns of ischaemic stroke are recognized which depend on the affected arterial territory.

Infarction in the middle cerebral artery territory

If the proximal trunk of the middle cerebral artery is occluded its entire territory will be infarcted. There will be hemiplegia, hemisensory loss, hemianopia and global dysphasia. The large volume of infarcted brain tissue may induce surrounding oedema and the patient may develop features of raised intracranial pressure. Occlusion of more distal branches produces some but not all of these features.

Infarction in the anterior cerebral artery territory

This is less common than middle cerebral artery involvement. The anterior cerebral artery supplies the medial aspect of the frontal lobe. The principal consequence is contralateral hemiplegia and hemisensory disturbance mainly affecting the leg. Apathy and incontinence are also common. There may also be an expressive dysphasia.

Infarction in the posterior cerebral artery territory

The commonest consequence is an isolated hemianopia. Often the macular is spared since the occipital

Box 26.1 Types of stroke

Cerebral haemorrhage	• lobar
	• posterior fossa
	• intraparenchymal
Cerebral infarction	• within an arterial territory (e.g. middle cerebral artery)
	• watershed (usually follows systemic hypertension)
	• lacunar
Subarachnoid haemorrhage	• usually from berry aneurysm on circle of Willis*
Venous	• usually associated with venous sinus thrombosis

*subarachnoid haemorrhage is described in detail in Ch. 29

Box 26.2 Causes of ischaemic stroke

Common causes of ischaemic stroke
• In-situ thrombosis
• Embolism:
  artery to artery
  cardiogenic

Rarer causes of ischaemic stroke*
• Arterial dissection (carotid, vertebral or aortic)
• Coagulopathies:
  protein C and Protein S deficiency
  anti-thrombin III deficiency
  lupus anti-coagulant
• Sickle cell disease
• Homocysteinuria
• Polycythemia
• Leukaemia
• Thrombotic thrombocytopenic purpura
• Fibromuscular dysplasia
• Fabry's disease
• Drug abuse
• Mitochondrial disease
• AIDS

*rare causes of stroke should be considered particularly in young-onset strokes

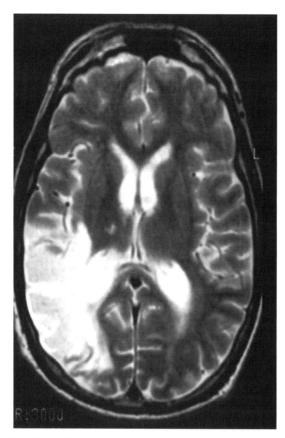

Fig. 26.1 MRI brain scan showing an ischaemic stroke in the territory of the right middle cerebral artery.

pole may receive an arterial blood supply from a branch of the middle cerebral artery. There may be additional features such as visual neglect and inattention.

Infarction in vertebral artery territory

Occlusion of one vertebral artery does not usually cause symptoms since there is adequate collateral circulation. If the collateral circulation is inadequate brain-stem infarction may follow. Various sites of infarction within the brain stem may occur but most commonly infarction occurs in the distribution of the posterior inferior cerebellar artery which supplies the lateral medulla (known as Wallenberg's syndrome). Typically the patient has an ispilateral Horner's syndrome (due to involvement of the sympathetic pathway), ipsilateral cerebellar ataxia (due to involvement of the cerebellar connections), ipsilateral facial pain and temperature loss and contralateral loss to these modalities in the limbs (due to spinothalamic tract involvement) and nystagmus often to either side (due to cerebellar and vestibular nucleii involvement).

TRANSIENT ISCHAEMIC ATTACKS (TIAs)

A transient ischaemic attack is a sudden onset focal neurological deficit lasting less than 24 hours. It is

Box 26.3 Common symptoms in transient ischaemic attacks

Anterior circulation
- Contralateral limb weakness
- Dysphasia
- Monocular visual loss (amaurosis fugax)
- Hemisensory loss*
- Dysarthria*
- Hemianopia*

Posterior circulation
- Diplopia
- Vertigo (usually with other brain-stem symptoms)
- Bilateral visual loss
- Bilateral or unilateral limb weakness
- Hemisensory loss*
- Dysarthria*
- Hemianopia*
- Cerebellar ataxia

*indicate symptoms which do not reliably distinguish between anterior and posterior circulation

Box 26.4 Differential diagnosis of transient ischaemic attacks

- Migraine
- Hypoglycaemia
- Multiple sclerosis
- Epilepsy
- Space-occupying lesions eg meningioma

Box 26.5 Common lacunar syndromes

	Anatomical localization
Ataxia hemiparesis	Internal capsule
Dysarthria/clumsy hand	Pons, internal capsule
Pure motor	Internal capsule, pons, cerebral peduncle or medullary pyramid
Pure sensory	Thalamus

caused by embolic occlusion of a retinal or cerebral artery.

The symptoms depend entirely on the vascular territory involved. The main symptoms are outlined in Box 26.3. The importance of TIAs is that they act as warning signals that the patient is at risk of a completed ischaemic stroke. Such patients should be investigated as a matter of urgency for a potential source of emboli. The main sources to consider are the carotid and vertebral arteries or the heart.

Differential diagnosis of TIAs

A number of disorders may mimic transient ischaemic attacks (Box 26.4). Sometimes there are other clues in the history or on the examination that point to the cause. On other occasions the cause may only be revealed by specific investigations such as measuring the blood glucose or brain imaging.

Hypoglycaemia, usually due to treatment in known diabetics, may cause temporary focal neurological symptoms which can be difficult to distinguish from TIAs on clinical grounds alone. The timing of attacks in relation to meals or to medication may be a clue.

Patients with **focal motor epilepsy** may have a period of paralysis after a jerking episode (known as Todd's paresis). This is sometimes confused with a TIA, although a careful history usually reveals the correct diagnosis. The visual aura of **migraine** is usually easily distinguished from transient visual loss (amaurosis fugax) due to a TIA, but on occasions there may

be diagnostic difficulty. Occasionally **mass lesions** in the brain may present with temporary focal neurological deficits e.g. meningioma. Patients with **multiple sclerosis** can experience transient neurological symptoms: for example brain-stem demyelination may produce transient vertigo and ataxia which might be confused with posterior circulation TIA. It is generally advisable to obtain an MRI scan of the brain of all cases of suspected TIAs to exclude structural pathology or demyelination.

LACUNAR STROKES

Patients with hypertension frequently develop what is known as 'small vessel disease'. This is usually most marked in the lenticulostriate arterioles (arising from the circle of Willis) which supply deep structures in the brain such as the basal ganglia and the internal capsule. It is characterized by a degeneration of the walls of these small vessels termed lipohyalinosis. Such patients may have small deep infarcts known as **lacunar infarcts**. Patients may experience a preceding TIA before a completed infarct develops. Since only deep brain structures are involved, the infarcts in these patients do not produce cortical defects such as dysphasia or hemianopia. The internal capsule is commonly involved and therefore patients may present with pure motor or sensory strokes. A similar process may occur in the pons and may result in a combination of dysarthria and clumsy hand due to damage to cerebellar and pyramidal fibres in this region. Often such lacunar syndromes slowly recover over weeks. Control of blood pressure is important. Since patients with

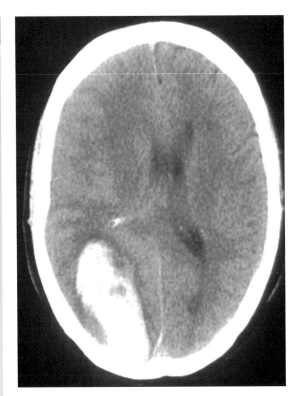

Fig. 26.2 CT brain scan showing an acute haemorrhagic stroke in the right occipital region.

- Hypertension (Charcot–Bouchard microscopic aneurysms)
- Arteriovenous malformations and aneurysms
- Anti-coagulant therapy
- Venous thrombosis
- Disseminated intravascular coagulation
- Amphetamine abuse
- Amyloid angiopathy

embolic infarcts described above can also sometimes present with pure motor or sensory strokes it is advisable to investigate patients who might on clinical grounds be thought to have lacunar infarcts for embolic sources (i.e. carotid arteries and heart).

HAEMORRHAGIC STROKE

Approximately 20% of strokes are due to cerebral haemorrhage. There are a number of potential causes of such strokes (see Box 26.6). The commonest setting is in the patient with chronic hypertension. Hypertension predisposes to the formation of microaneurysms particularly on small deep penetrating arterioles (e.g. the lenticulostriate arterioles). The rupture of such an aneurysm results in the sudden development of a haematoma. The main consequences are a sudden headache and focal neurological deficit. Blood may escape from within the brain tissue into the ventricular system. If the haemorrhage is large there may be a rapid rise in intracranial pressure causing loss of consciousness and even death from pressure coning.

Since microaneurysms are mainly found in vessels located deep within the brain supplying the basal ganglia and internal capsule, these are the commonest locations for such haemorrhages. The majority of haemorrhages remain inside the brain substance and are readily visualized by CT or MR imaging. A putamenal haemorrhage is the most common site. Typically the patient presents with sudden onset hemiparesis and hemisensory loss.

There is sometimes a primary intracerebellar haemorrhage. This is less common than haemorrhage into the deep structures of the cerebrum but it is important to recognize since unlike the other haemorrhages described, urgent surgical intervention is often life saving. The patient develops sudden onset cerebellar ataxia. However, since the posterior fossa is a small confined space, there is a rapid rise in pressure, compressing the brain stem and resulting in reduction and loss of consciousness. Hydrocephalus due to obstruction of the aqueduct will cause further pressure on brain-stem structures. Without rapid surgical decompression, death is inevitable.

CEREBRAL VENOUS SINUS THROMBOSIS

This unusual cause of stroke develops in hypercoagulable states such as dehydration and in patients with sickle-cell anaemia. It is more common in the puerperium and in women taking the oral contraceptive. There is also an increased incidence in patients with inflammatory bowel disease such as ulcerative colitis.

Typically, patients develop headache which has the features of raised intracranial pressure; they frequently become drowsy and may have focal and generalized seizures. Focal neurological signs such as a hemiparesis may develop. These clinical features are consequent upon thrombus developing in one of the major cerebral venous sinuses. Raised pressure ensues because of impaired reabsorption of CSF by the arachnoid villi which normally project into the venous sinuses. There is impaired venous return from cortical veins into the thrombosed sinus. This leads to venous cortical haemorrhage. Such cortical haemorrhage is very irritative which is why seizures may be prominent. The focal neurological signs are a consequence of the cortical damage. The diagnosis is confirmed by urgent brain imaging. MR is the modality of choice with venous phase MR angiography. If confirmed the treatment is urgent anti-coagulation with i.v. heparin and sometimes thrombolysis.

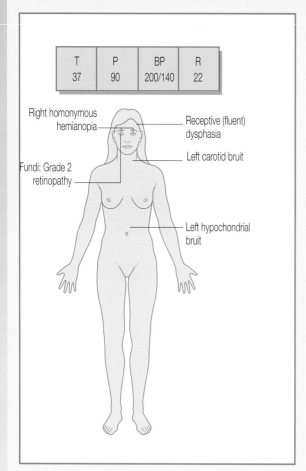

T	P	BP	R
37	90	200/140	22

Right homonymous hemianopia

Fundi: Grade 2 retinopathy

Receptive (fluent) dysphasia

Left carotid bruit

Left hypochondrial bruit

A 32-year-old right-handed female media agent developed sudden onset difficulty with speech 24 hours before seeking medical attention. Three days before she had been at a night club and got fairly drunk. She remembered being pushed over awkwardly and straining her neck. It was then sore for 24 hours but resolved.

Her past medical history included frequent migraine headaches with aura. The normal aura comprised bright flashing flights for 10–15 minutes before the onset of a throbbing unilateral headache. There was also a history of two blackouts two years previously which were not investigated. She remembered experiencing a sudden onset vertigo and nausea while seated. There was associated double vision and she then lost consciousness. Her partner who accompanied her said that she was unconscious only briefly, with no convulsive movements. There were no precipitants.

In her family history her father had hypertension from the age of 40 years.

On examination she was alert and seemed to be orientated. She did not complain of headache or nausea and there was no neck stiffness. She had a receptive (also termed fluent) dysphasia and a right homonymous hemianopia. The rest of the neurological examination was normal apart from the fundi showing grade 2 retinopathy. Her blood pressure was noted to be elevated on admission at 200/140 and remained elevated at 200/130 the next morning. There was a soft left carotid bruit. A soft bruit could also be heard over the left hypochondrium. Cardiovascular examination was otherwise normal. The rest of the general examination was normal.

Questions

1. What are the possible diagnoses?
2. What investigations are needed?

Discussion

Any patient who presents with a sudden onset dysphasia should be considered to have had a stroke until proved otherwise. In this patient there is a past history of migraine with aura. This might lead one to consider whether her dysphasia could represent a migrainous phenomenon. While it is true that the nature of an aura in a given patient may change and that patients may on occasion develop an aura that does not proceed to a headache there are strong indications that this patient's dysphasia is not migrainous in basis. Firstly, the duration of dysphasia is too long. Migraine auras should not last longer than 30 minutes and in this patient it had not resolved after 24 hours. In addition, there is evidence of a visual defect (a right homonymous hemianopia) which, in combination with the dysphasia, points to a lesion in the left hemisphere in the region of the temporal lobe. The only way in which her migraine could be implicated is if the attack had progressed to a migrainous infarction in this region. While this is a possibility, in the absence of headache it would be very unusual.

Other causes of stroke in a young patient must be considered. There are potentially a large number of possible causes, but there are some additional clues in the history and examination which might help the investigative process. The patient had marked hypertension on admission. This is unlikely to be related to the stress of coming into hospital since the blood pressure was still greatly elevated the next morning. The cause of this hypertension must be determined. She is young to have essential hypertension and therefore a secondary cause of hypertension should be investigated. It is possible that the presence of hypertension, particularly if chronic, may have predisposed to the stroke. The other observation on examination is that she has a soft carotid bruit on the left side. This may indicate that she has a carotid stenosis. She would be rather young to have atheromatous carotid stenosis (unless she has a genetic disorder elevating cholesterol such as familial hypercholesterolaemia). However, in the context of a possible neck injury, the possibility of a carotid artery dissection must be considered.

Carotid artery dissection is an important cause of stroke in young adults. There may be a history of a neck injury or strain. This can be relatively trivial, as was the case here. Usually a tear occurs in the intima of the artery which is then the site of thrombus formation. The formed thrombus may detach and embolize distally to cause an ischaemic stroke. The treatment for such dissections is anti-coagulation although the exact duration for such treatment is unclear. Patients with fibromuscular dysplasia (an inherited disorder of vascular connective tissue) of the carotid arteries are at increased risk of dissection and stroke. The soft bruit in the abdomen raises the question of fibromuscular dysplasia of the renal arteries which could lead to hypertension.

In summary, the sudden onset of dysphasia with a right homonymous hemianopia in a right-handed person strongly suggests that a stroke may have occurred in the territory of the left middle cerebral artery. The presence of a stroke should be established by brain imaging. Occasionally structural lesions such as gliomas can present with sudden onset focal symptoms, but this will be excluded by imaging. If an ischaemic stroke is confirmed the cause of the stroke must be determined. In view of the young age of the patient the cause of the stroke is unlikely to be atheromatous arterial disease. A search for the rarer causes of stroke should therefore be initiated. In this case there is some clinical evidence that the patient may have had a carotid dissection and this should guide clinical investigations. If this turned out to be incorrect then a systematic search of all the causes of young stroke should be undertaken.

Brain imaging in this patient confirmed middle cerebral territory infarct. MR angiography confirmed a left internal carotid artery dissection and showed changes of fibromuscular dysplasia. Renal angiography revealed a left renal artery stenosis also caused by fibromuscular dysplasia. She underwent renal artery angioplasty successfully and her blood pressure came under control. She was anti-coagulated with warfarin for 1 year. Her dysphasia and field defect resolved fully after 1 month.

Visual failure

Visual failure is a common symptom and one that is often frightening, especially when it develops rapidly. It is caused by many disease processes which may be intraocular, intracranial or systemic. These range from simple cataracts through to occipital lobe strokes. The commonest causes of blindness in the UK are cataracts, senile macular degeneration, glaucoma, retinal detachment and diabetic retinopathy. A careful history and systematic examination of the visual system will reveal the cause of visual failure in most cases.

HISTORY

The presence of a scotoma or photopsias may be established from the history. **Scotoma** is the term used to refer to a defect in the field of vision. If a patient loses central vision this is usually noticed very quickly. In contrast peripheral field defects, such as a homonymous hemianopia, may not be immediately apparent to the patient. Generally, the presence of a central scotoma indicates disease of the retina or of the optic nerve along its path. Scotomas caused by disease of the macular are usually noticed as blackness or greyness by the patient (e.g. a retinal transient ischaemic attack). In contrast lesions behind the retina, in the optic nerve, optic tract, optic radiation or visual cortex usually produce an absence of vision rather than blackness. **Photopsias** are bright momentary flashes of light. They usually indicate the presence of an 'irritative' lesion of the retina or optic nerve. Retinal migraine is one example. Occasionally they can arise in the visual cortex when the cause is usually migrainous although sometimes an occipital epileptic focus can produce this effect. The pattern of visual field loss may be suspected from the history but will need to be confirmed on examination. For example patients with right hemisphere lesions, interrupting the optic radiation, may report that they are aware of difficulty in seeing to the left.

An additional important point to establish is the rate of onset of visual failure. This is because visual failure can be classified into different possible causes simply on this basis.

UNILATERAL TRANSIENT VISUAL LOSS

Amaurosis fugax

Amaurosis fugax is the term used to describe the monocular visual loss which occurs as a consequence of emboli to the retinal circulation, usually from carotid atheromatous disease. Attacks are sudden in onset. The patient notices a greying or blackening of vision. Sometimes this is described as a 'curtain coming down'. The attacks rarely last more than 20 minutes and typically resolve more slowly than their sudden onset. Such patients should be investigated for carotid arterial disease by an imaging technique such as carotid ultrasound Doppler blood flow studies.

Retinal migraine

Transient monocular visual loss may be caused by retinal migraine. It is presumed to be caused by vasospasm of retinal blood vessels. Typically the vision is lost in a concentric pattern and there may be photopsias. Blindness is usually longer than in amaurosis fugax. It occurs in a younger population than those with amaurosis fugax without risk factors for atheromatous disease.

Multiple sclerosis

Temporary monocular visual loss lasting a few hours with elevated temperature may be seen in the setting of optic neuritis associated with multiple sclerosis.

Papilloedema

Patients with papilloedema may experience transient monocular darkening of vision. This may particularly occur with manoeuvres that increase intracranial pressure, such as cough, sneezing or moving the head rapidly. This symptom is thought to be due to transient hypoperfusion of the swollen optic nerve head.

BILATERAL TRANSIENT VISUAL LOSS

This symptom almost always indicates bilateral visual cortex dysfunction. The commonest causes of this are migraine and cerebral hypoperfusion. Epilepsy is a less common cause. Patients with migraine and aura frequently experience a visual aura prior to the onset of the headache. This frequently includes bright flashing lights, which may be coloured. Scintillating scotomas are described which frequently expand and migrate within the visual field. Such migraine with aura typically develops for the first time before the age of 40 years. Onset after this age may occur but should prompt a search, ideally by an MRI brain scan, to exclude pathology in the occipital cortex. Occasionally elderly patients present with isolated typical migrainous aura that causes visual loss but in whom headache does not develop. Furthermore there is usually no prior history of migraine headache. Once again a careful search for structural pathology should be made. However, often no abnormality is found and this group of symptoms have been termed 'migraine equivalents'. The occipital cortex is particularly sensitive to cerebral hypoperfusion. Patients typically describe sudden onset loss of vision. Causes include systemic hypotension, thromboembolism to basilar artery (in posterior circulation TIA) hyperviscosity syndromes, vascular compression and vasospasm.

SUDDEN ONSET UNILATERAL VISUAL LOSS WITHOUT RECOVERY

A number of disorders cause sudden onset monocular visual loss without recovery or progression. These processes are all confined to the orbit and can usually be diagnosed by careful ophthalmoscopic examination. Of these, anterior ischaemic optic neuropathy is the most common to present to the non-ophthalmologist. The patient is aware of sudden onset monocular visual loss without recovery. It is commoner over the age of 60 years and is associated with atherosclerosis affecting the microcirculation of the optic nerve. It is important to note this can be a presentation of temporal arteritis and the ESR should be checked urgently. Direct ophthalmoscopic examination usually reveals pallor of the retina with a cherry red spot at the macular. An altitudinal field defect (a field defect which is below the horizontal axis of the visual field) is usually present.

SUDDEN ONSET BILATERAL VISUAL LOSS

This is uncommon but may be caused by bilateral occipital lobe infarctions or pituitary infarction (apoplexy). It can be a functional disorder but then there is usually other evidence of psychological distress.

PROGRESSIVE VISUAL LOSS

There are a large number of causes of progressive visual loss (Box 27.4). The majority of them act on the anterior visual pathway (i.e. anterior to the chiasm). The majority of patients develop slowly progressive bilateral visual failure and optic atrophy is usually present on examination.

Optic neuritis. One of the commonest visual manifestations of multiple sclerosis. It is caused by acute demyelination within the optic nerve. It is usually unilateral. The patient may become aware of pain in the affected eye. There follows a progressive loss of vision over hours to days. The degree of visual loss can be marked. Recovery then begins and most patients return to normal or near-normal acuity. At its peak there is swelling of the optic nerve head, which can have appearances not dissimilar to papilloedema. The major difference is that visual acuity loss is an early feature of optic neuritis and only a very late feature of chronic papilloedema. The commonest visual manifestations of papilloedema are transient visual obscurations and an enlarged blind spot.

Compressive lesions of the optic nerve. An important cause of progressive visual loss. Depending on the site of the lesion this can be monocular or binocular. Examples include mass lesion in one orbit such as granulomas or optic nerve gliomas. Retro-orbital meningiomas may spread 'en-plaque' into the orbit causing progressive optic nerve compression. Such lesions can spread to the opposite side. Patients with compressive lesions complain of progressive decrease in visual acuity and examination shown optic atrophy.

Toxic and nutritional disorders may result in progressive bilateral visual failure. Vitamin B deficiencies have been implicated, usually in individuals with poor nutrition (e.g. alcoholic smokers); the term tobacco–alcohol amblyopia is used.

EXAMINATION OF THE EYE

It is as well to begin with the eyes, both to confirm and measure the patient's disability and also because the diagnosis may be immediately apparent and thus allow the remainder of the examination to be both more appropriate and rapid. Fortunately the diagnostic aids need only be very simple. The highest plus lens of the ophthalmoscope gives a good view of the front of the eye, of the anterior structures such as cornea, aqueous, iris and lens. The retina is examined in the usual way. Visual fields and blind spots can be usefully assessed by the traditional whiteheaded pin, even though the precise delineation of field defects and central scotomas will require formal perimetry and the use of a Bjerrum screen. These latter techniques, although simple, require some practice and are time-consuming. Undoubtedly in the future increasing use will be made of the newer methods of automatic screening.

A measurement which is commonly ignored by the general physician is a precise evaluation of visual acuity. Although the use of a Snellen chart is difficult unless the ward or clinic has been properly equipped, a reasonable idea of the acuity can be obtained by the use

of a set of test types, such as Jaeger's Test Card. It can be surprising on occasion how poor is the correlation – in either direction – between the complaint by the patient and the degree of defect found. Measurement of acuity also allows the progress of the patient to be followed and for treatment to be initiated at an early stage. Although acuity is important it only reflects macular function and if normal does not exclude other defects. Gross reduction in visual field may occur with complete preservation of central vision.

As in the other areas of the body examination of the eye must be systematic. Proptosis is displacement of the eyeball forwards. It may be caused by primary or secondary tumour, granulomas such as histiocytosis X, and leukaemic infiltrations. It is also a characteristic feature of Graves' disease. Occasionally it may be combined with pulsation of the globe and a bruit, due to an aneurysm in the cavernous sinus or a vascular tumour. In all these situations there may be pressure on the optic nerve with visual failure. Apparent proptosis may occur when the large eyeball of high myopia is misinterpreted.

Ptosis can occur as a result of sympathetic or third nerve damage. It is a feature of neurosyphilis where there may also be optic atrophy. It may be a feature of myasthenia, and in younger patients as a congenital abnormality.

The ocular movements must be checked and the pupillary reflexes elicited both directly and consensually. In optic atrophy there may be a fixed dilated pupil which will only react to consensual stimulation. The pupil may also be fixed after previous iritis with adhesions. If visual impairment is due to damage to the optic radiation or occipital cortex the pupillary reflexes will be normal. Cortical blindness is not common and is often misdiagnosed, for there are no physical signs other than a failure to blink on menace. The pupillary reflexes are retained and the differential diagnosis is from hysterical blindness.

Cataract occurs commonly in diabetic patients. In juvenile diabetes a specific type of cataract may rapidly develop which has a characteristic snowflake appearance. In addition senile cataract occurs more frequently and at an earlier age but does not differ otherwise from that seen in the non-diabetic. Impairment of vision is also seen if the blood sugar is varying widely, probably due to osmotic changes altering the curvature of the lens. It responds quickly to control of the diabetes.

The cornea is examined for inflammation or ulceration or the presence of a foreign body. Cloudiness and oedema occur in acute glaucoma and the tension of the eyeball must always be carefully assessed, certainly by palpation and ideally by tonometry. The surrounding conjunctiva may show the generalized hyperaemia of conjunctivitis or the circumcorneal injection of iritis. Exudation of pus or blood may be seen in the anterior chamber, and keratic precipitates may be present on the back of the cornea due to an underlying iridocyclitis. The iris may be tremulous, due to lack of support by the lens because of dislocation, as seen in Marfan's syndrome or homocystinuria. Adhesions may be present from the iris to the back of the cornea or to the lens due to inflammation, with associated deformation of the pupil.

In the older age group, senile cataract becomes an increasingly important reason for visual impairment. Commonly, in the early stages, the opacification begins as streaks spreading in from the periphery of the lens like the spokes of a wheel. Later, without surgery, after a period of swelling the lens shrinks, losing fluid, and becomes generally opaque; this is the stage of hypermaturity when it is ripe for operation.

Knowledge of the anatomy of the visual system allows classification of visual defects into three groups. These are prechiasmal, chiasmal and retrochiasmal. Prechiasmal lesions such as in the retina or the optic nerve produce visual defects in one eye (monocular field defects); chiasmal lesions, such as a pituitary tumour, produce field defects in both eyes in a non-homonymous fashion (e.g. bitemporal hemianopia); retrochiasmal lesions, such as a stroke in the left visual cortex produce homonymous field defects (e.g. a right homonymous hemianopia). Homonymous quadrantic field defects may be caused by lesions in different parts of the optic radiation. Lesions in the superior parts of the optic radiation tend to produce contralateral inferior homonymous quadrantinopias. Lesions in the inferior parts of the optic radiation tend to produce contralateral superior homonymous quadrantinopias.

Ophthalmoscopic examination

When looking at the fundus, adequate illumination is essential and exhausted batteries and blackened bulbs remain the commonest reason for failure in diagnosis. Ideally the room should be darkened. If the pupil is small a suitable mydriatic should be used to allow adequate examination. Although mydriatics such as atropine have no effect on the tension of the normal eye they may precipitate an attack of glaucoma if the angle of the anterior chamber is narrow. For this reason the depth of the anterior chamber should be assessed before they are instilled. The usual diagnostic mydriatic is tropicamide, which is mild and short-acting and does not need to be reversed. An alternative is to use cocaine, which lowers the intraocular tension. The action of other mydriatics should be reversed after use. It is important not to be confused by normal variations such as opaque nerve fibres spreading out from the margins of the disc, or by choroidal pigments surrounding the disc. The nasal margin may be indistinct

normally, and the disc generally may be less sharply seen in young long-sighted individuals. The physiological cup is usually a little paler than the rest of the disc and may occupy up to one-half of its area. It never occupies the whole disc.

Examination may reveal a wide variety of abnormal conditions, but the commoner changes are those of papilloedema, optic atrophy, retinopathy, retinal detachment, choroiditis and senile macular degeneration. Among the more important types of retinopathy are diabetic and hypertensive.

Papilloedema is an important finding and typically visual acuity is not greatly impaired early except for transient obscurations. Later on however, severe failure may occur very rapidly. When present bilaterally the commonest cause is cerebral tumour, particularly of the posterior fossa. It is unusual in cerebrovascular accidents, although it may occur transiently in subarachnoid haemorrhage. Viral encephalitis, toxic encephalopathy or trauma can also produce the necessary cerebral swelling and rise in intracranial pressure. Sometimes when there is marked CO_2 retention due to respiratory failure, papilloedema develops. An important although rare cause is benign intracranial hypertension, and sometimes surgical decompression is necessary in this condition to prevent visual loss. Its occurrence almost entirely in females, and the common relationship between the onset of the disorder and menstrual disturbances will help in the diagnosis (see Ch. 29). Unilateral papilloedema may occasionally occur on the side opposite to a frontal lobe neoplasm, but more often it reflects local disease of the eye or orbit. Central retinal vein thrombosis may give rise to blindness and is usually obvious on ophthalmoscopic examination. The optic disc is swollen and the retinal veins overfilled, with A-V nipping. Scattered large and small haemorrhages and exudates are seen. This condition may occur as a complication of hypertension, diabetes, atheroma, various clotting disorders and polycythaemia.

In contrast to papilloedema, optic neuritis usually produces marked impairment of visual acuity with little evidence of change in the optic discs and fundi. If inflammatory change occurs immediately behind the eye some swelling of the disc may occur but this is not usually marked, nor is it associated with other retinal changes. Demyelination is the most important cause and when unilateral is usually due to multiple sclerosis. Central vision is impaired with a central or paracentral scotoma. The eyeball is commonly tender, and there is retro-orbital or temporal pain. If bilateral it may be due to neuromyelitis optica where transverse myelitis occurs in association with bilateral optic neuritis. Nutritional deficiency, particularly of vitamin B_{12}, can cause an optic neuritis, as may drugs such as tobacco or methyl alcohol.

Optic atrophy can follow any of the above conditions and if it has been preceded by any degree of swelling of the disc there may be evidence of this. One may see sheathing of the disc with connective tissue, hiding the lamina cribrosa, while the veins will be tortuous and may be partially surrounded by fibrous tissue. Although optic atrophy can be diagnosed ophthalmoscopically little information will usually be gained as to its cause. Frequently it will be due to pressure on the optic nerve, chiasma or tract. Visual field and Bjerrum screen examination can provide most valuable data as to the site of the lesion in the optic nerve.

GENERAL EXAMINATION

Severe anaemia from any cause can occasionally lead to visual failure, with retinal haemorrhages and exudates. Impairment of vision may occur rapidly if there has been severe blood loss, probably due to a failure of perfusion of the retina and occipital cortex. Impairment is especially likely in severe pernicious anaemia, as in this case deficiency of B_{12} may lead directly to damage to the optic nerves. A plethoric colour suggests the possibility of polycythaemia with its tendency to both arterial and venous thromboses. The skin should also be examined for evidence of any bleeding tendency such as petechiae or ecchymoses, and for the septic emboli that may occur, especially in the finger pulps, from infective endocarditis. The peripheral pulses, if absent, will suggest vascular disease or perhaps embolization from endocarditis.

The blood pressure must always be measured. If the patient is on hypotensive drugs any postural drop must be noted, and always the effect of exercise on the blood pressure. When examining the head and neck the temporal arteries should be felt, as sudden blindness and also diplopia and field defects may occur abruptly, without warning, in the presence of cranial arteritis. Cortical blindness may also occur from this condition. In association with arteritis the muscles of the neck may be tender and some degree of cervical lymphadenopathy can occur.

The carotid and vertebral arteries should be felt and auscultated. Recurrent microembolization of the retina producing transient episodes of blindness may be caused by atheromatous ulceration of a carotid artery and effective treatment by surgical disobliteration or anticoagulation is effective in some patients.

Examination of the heart may reveal rheumatic or congenital disease which predispose to endocarditis. Cortical blindness can occur in acute nephritis, probably due to cerebral oedema resulting from vasoconstriction and damage to small vessels. There may be few

signs pointing towards renal disease, so the urine should always be examined and the blood urea measured in any such case. Visual loss in the end stages of chronic renal disease may also occur but is unlikely to cause diagnostic difficulty.

Pituitary tumours producing compression of the visual pathways can lead to marked visual field defects which are often diagnosed late. They can also lead to endocrine failure and this may be clinically obvious. Skin texture and hair distribution should be noted particularly.

The examination of the nervous system is most important. A wide variety of diseases can affect any part of the visual pathway from the back of the eyeball to the occipital cortex. As well as the visual changes they will often produce symptoms and signs resulting from damage to other parts of the brain and spinal cord, which will commonly lead more easily to the diagnosis. An obvious example of this is multiple sclerosis, but it is also true for arterial aneurysm compressing the visual pathway in the region of the chiasma, and for tumours and areas of infarction within the cerebral hemisphere. The localization of the visual cortical areas posteriorly at the occipital poles means that they may be specifically damaged by localized trauma in this region, and also, since they are supplied by the posterior cerebral arteries, that they may be affected by ischaemic disturbances of the vertebrobasilar system.

The underlying diagnosis will usually be obvious in such conditions as meningitis, encephalitis and neurosyphilis. It is often obscure in chronic granulomatous disorders like sarcoidosis, and may only become established when lesions develop elsewhere, more accessible to biopsy.

SPECIAL INVESTIGATIONS

In the majority of the above diseases the diagnosis is reached on clinical grounds alone. Biochemical tests will be needed to establish the presence of diabetes and renal disease, and may be of value in identifying chemical toxins. Assay of vitamin B_{12} may show a deficiency despite a normal haemoglobin and the absence of the classical signs of subacute combined degeneration. Neuroradiology is essential to exclude neoplasm, if this is suspected, for example: glioma of the optic nerve, chromophobe adenoma of the pituitary, or meningioma of the base of the skull. While the diagnosis can sometimes be obvious from straight skull films, special views of the optic foramina, CT scan, MRI scan and angiography may all be needed. In diseases of the carotid arteries Doppler ultrasound imaging will be required.

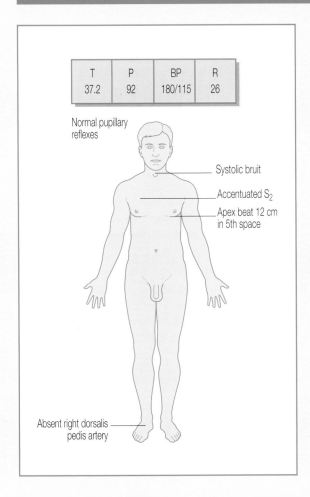

T	P	BP	R
37.2	92	180/115	26

Normal pupillary reflexes

Systolic bruit

Accentuated S$_2$

Apex beat 12 cm in 5th space

Absent right dorsalis pedis artery

A man of 72 years, a retired publisher, was admitted to hospital because of the abrupt onset of total blindness. His vision had been completely normal and he had felt quite well until the morning of admission, when on standing up after cleaning the bath he became blind. He had rested for several hours but his vision did not improve.

In the previous few months he had been under some stress at home because of the illness of his wife with an inoperable carcinoma of the breast. Five years previously he had been found to have a raised blood pressure when he had consulted his GP because of recurrent episodes of dizziness. He had been treated since that time with a thiazide diuretic. He had smoked 20 cigarettes daily for many years, and had taken only moderate quantities of alcohol. There was nothing of relevance in his family history.

On examination he was distressed and agitated and said he could see nothing. The pupillary reflexes were normal, the pupils responding to both direct and consensual stimulation. His pupils constricted when he was asked to look towards the end of his nose. There was, however, a failure to blink on menace, in both eyes. The fundi showed minimal arteriosclerotic changes only. Pulse 92 regular. Blood pressure 180/115. Neck movements were full and pain-free. There was cardiac enlargement with a forceful cardiac impulse. The second sound was accentuated, but no murmurs were present in the heart. A systolic bruit however could be heard over the left carotid artery. The right dorsalis pedis artery could not be felt. There were no signs of heart failure and the lungs were clear.

No abnormality was otherwise present in the cranial nerves. Examination of the limbs was quite normal, there being no long tract signs. He appeared to be appropriately concerned about his sudden disability and there was no evidence of any gross psychiatric disturbance.

Initial investigations included chest and skull X-rays which were normal. There was no anaemia and no abnormality was seen in the peripheral blood film. The urine contained no sugar, but there was a trace of protein.

Questions

1. What is the most likely cause of this patient's blindness?
2. What further investigation would be of value?
3. What do you imagine will be the eventual outcome?

This patient's presenting complaint is straightforward: he had suddenly become blind. It is always important in such a case to analyse carefully the degree of visual loss, the speed with which it came on, and the circumstances under which it developed. Any past history of visual disturbance however transitory should also be sought. The rapidity of onset of symptoms in this case suggests a vascular cause, although a similar story is also commonly given by patients with hysterical blindness. The continuation of the blindness for at least several hours would indicate that there is probably some degree of structural damage and not simply a reversible functional impairment.

The patient's past history of hypertension and of heavy cigarette smoking also increase the likelihood of cerebrovascular disease. Furthermore when his hypertension was first diagnosed he was complaining of recurrent episodes of dizziness, presumably occurring on a basis of impaired cerebral perfusion, and suggesting that there was some degree of cerebrovascular disease already present. The drug treatment he is receiving for his blood pressure is unlikely to be relevant in this respect as it does not produce postural hypotension.

The recent illness of his wife with carcinoma of the breast can reasonably be supposed to be a cause of considerable stress and the possibility of a psychogenic reaction must be seriously considered. Gross hysterical symptoms such as blindness or paralysis are much less common now than in the past. They were particularly well described in battle casualties during the Second World War. They still occur occasionally, and are usually a response to some situation which the patient finds intolerable. Such a reaction is more common in those of low intelligence or poor education, and is undoubtedly predisposed to by previous head injury. The likelihood of the diagnosis of an hysterical illness being correct would be greatly increased if there had been previous reactions of an hysterical nature or some other evidence of a neurotic personality structure in the past. It is rare for an hysterical reaction to occur for the first time at the age of 72 years and the absence of any previous psychiatric history must therefore throw doubt on this diagnosis. However any form of organic cerebral disease may lead to the appearance of hysterical or affective symptoms for the first time at any age. It could therefore be argued that a background of developing cerebrovascular disease has predisposed this man to an hysterical response to his wife's illness. It is important in this type of case, both when taking the history and when examining the patient, to evaluate the mental state and to try and assess whether the patient's reaction to his symptom is appropriate. A lack of emotional response may be claimed as the 'belle indifférence' of Janet, but could just as easily be his habitual stoicism.

Examination of this patient revealed clear evidence of widespread vascular disease. His blood pressure is raised, a bruit is present over one carotid and a peripheral pulse in a foot is missing. The findings on examination of the eyes indicate that there is no damage to the peripheral visual mechanism, or to the visual connections with the brain stem, for the pupillary responses are all intact. The loss of the menace response supports his claim to be blind. His emotional response also suggests that his blindness is organic in nature. The likely diagnosis, therefore, is blindness due to ischaemia of the occipital poles of the cerebral hemispheres due to vascular disease. Such a syndrome can occur temporarily as a result of the vascular spasm of migraine, but this is not a relevant diagnosis here. Blindness due to vascular spasm associated with cerebral oedema may occur in hypertensive encephalopathy, and this syndrome can develop at relatively low levels of blood pressure if there is renal failure. The absence of significant retinopathy excludes this diagnosis, although it would be reasonable to check the blood urea.

Although not common, sudden blindness is a well-recognized complication of vertebrobasilar disease. Although it may be complete as in this case, commonly as recovery occurs the visual loss takes the form of an homonymous hemianopia, and at this stage macular vision may be better preserved than peripheral. The final recovery of vision is often surprisingly good, although the overall prognosis is poor as there is usually generalized vascular disease. If there is doubt as to whether sudden bilateral blindness is hysterical or due to occipital cortical damage, an EEG may help by showing abnormalities posteriorly and failure to respond to photic stimulation. A CT scan may confirm bilateral occipital lobe infarcts. Using the radiopharmaceutical HMPAO (Ceretec), SPECT scanning of the brain will show areas of reduced or absent blood flow in the occipital lobes.

> This patient's cortical blindness slowly improved over 3 weeks. A presumptive diagnosis of basilar artery thrombosis was made.

28

Dizziness

The complaint of 'dizziness' is common and it is essential to establish exactly what the patient means. This is sometimes a frustrating process for the doctor and the patient. Dizziness is a symptom that means different things to different people. Patients may use different terms such as giddiness, unsteadiness or light-headedness. One key feature to try and establish is whether the patient experiences a feeling of rotation or movement inside the head. The term **vertigo** should be reserved for this group of patients. The movement usually has a rotatory feeling to it or it may be a side-to-side movement. The patient may describe that their head is spinning or that the world is spinning; alternatively they may indicate that the feeling inside their head is like being on a ship, rocking from side to side. Vertigo is often accompanied by other symptoms such as nausea, vomiting and unsteadiness. These related symptoms may be very severe and disabling. The presence of such symptoms in a patient does not therefore require an additional explanation other than the vertigo.

If the physician is able to establish that vertigo is indeed present this is most useful since it narrows the differential diagnosis to a disorder of the vestibular system. This may be peripheral, i.e. labyrinthine, or central, in other words affecting the central connections particularly to the brain stem (see Box 28.1). If the patient feels dizziness but there is no sense of movement in the head, one of the commonest causes is **presyncope**: this is a reduction in cerebral blood flow that is not enough to cause syncope. This may occur in the setting of postural hypotension (which may be related to drug therapy) or in patients with cardiac arrhythmias.

It is important to note that no clear cause is found in a significant proportion of patients who complain of dizziness (usually without vertigo). In some of this group the complaint may be a symptom of a psychological disturbance.

HISTORY

If vertigo is present then it is more likely that there will be a peripheral vestibular disorder than a central cause. Peripheral disorders tend to be associated with features in addition to the complaint of vertigo. Patients frequently experience severe nausea, vomiting, sweating and significant prostration. An acute single attack of severe vertigo is typically caused by viral infection (vestibular neuronitis) or acute vascular lesions usually in elderly patients, for example occlusion of the internal auditory artery. The patient experiences sudden onset severe vertigo, nausea and vomiting. The patient finds it impossible to turn the head without precipitating severe vertigo. Typically the patient will lie motionless usually with the affected ear uppermost. Symptoms are usually severe for two to three days and then settle over the next few weeks to months. Vestibular neuronitis may sometimes be very slow to resolve with chronic unsteadiness lasting several months. With careful advice and rehabilitative balancing exercises the illness slowly resolves.

Some patients continue to experience recurrent attacks of vertigo which are particularly position dependent. This is called **benign positional vertigo**. In positional vertigo patients complain of recurrent acute episodes of vertigo in response to changes in head position. The episode of vertigo tends to be very short-lived and worse in the morning. The illness may be episodic with long periods in between runs of attacks. It is caused by damage to the otolith apparatus in the semicircular canals. At the bedside the diagnosis can be confirmed by rapidly laying the patient flat, from a sitting position, and turning the head to one side as described below. Occasionally positional vertigo may be caused by central (brain-stem) lesions.

Ménière's disease is a common disorder resulting in episodes of vertigo and is associated with deafness and tinnitus. Unilateral deafness is usually the first symptom often accompanied by low pitched tinnitus. Patients often describe a feeling of fullness in the ear. Episodes of severe vertigo usually develop some time after the onset of deafness and are often very disabling. Over the years progressive unilateral sensorineural deafness develops. Bilateral disease may sometimes develop. The combination of recurrent attacks of vertigo with progressive deafness should lead one to suspect the diagnosis. Hearing tests confirm sensorineural deafness and vestibular function studies demonstrate so-called canal paresis on the affected side. It is suspected that Ménière's disease is due to accumulation of fluid in the endolymphatic system. Structural pathology in the cerebellopontine angle, such as an acoustic neuroma, should also be considered; the deafness is usually progressive rather than fluctuating, as in Ménière's.

MRI brain imaging is used to exclude an acoustic neuroma. Patients with *cerebellopontine tumours* such as acoustic neuromas initially present with progressive deafness and intermittent vertigo. Tinnitus may also be present. As the tumour enlarges there may be compression of the brain-stem resulting in cerebellar ataxia. Raised intracranial-type headache may follow as a result of aqueduct stenosis and resulting obstructive hydrocephalus.

Central causes of vertigo result in dysfunction of vestibular connections within the brain-stem and their central connections. Such centrally mediated vertigo is much less common than the peripheral causes described. Often, there are other clinical and examination features of the central disorder which lead to suspicion of a central process. The commonest such disorder is *multiple sclerosis* in which plaques of demyelination interrupt the central vestibular connections. Occasionally isolated vertigo may be caused by temporal lobe epileptic discharges. Usually, however, the patient has other types of seizure which allow clarification of the diagnosis.

Vertebrobasilar ischaemia is often cited as a cause of vertigo, particularly in the elderly. While it is

true that impaired vertebrobasilar circulation may cause vertigo it is likely that this process is overdiagnosed as a cause of 'dizziness'. In order to be certain that such ischaemia is the cause of vertigo there should be additional clinical symptoms and signs which would point more strongly to impaired vertebrobasilar circulation. They include limb weakness or clumsiness, loss of vision, diplopia, ataxia, perioral numbness and dysarthria. These latter symptoms may be all caused by ischaemia of the structures supplied by the posterior circulation, that is the brain-stem, the cerebellum and the visual cortex.

In a large proportion of patients with non-specific dizziness a precise reason is not established. However, it is important to consider drugs, anaemia, postural hypotension and cardiac arrhythmias as possible causes. Patients with systemic infection may complain of non-specific dizziness but there are usually other clues to the infective process. Patients with anxiety states and depression frequently complain of dizziness or light-headedness. It is therefore important to consider psychological factors.

EXAMINATION

Physical examination

A full general examination is required, but attention must particularly be paid to the central nervous and cardiovascular systems, and also to the function of the auditory and vestibular mechanisms. Anaemia and polycythaemia must be looked for, and the blood pressure must be checked both lying and standing and, if indicated, after exercise. If the vertigo is related to exercise of the arms, the pressure should also be measured in each arm, as there may be a subclavian steal syndrome. All the pulses must be felt. A reduction of the carotid pulse or bruits heard over either the carotid or vertebral arteries will indicate extracranial cerebrovascular disease. One may also find an arrhythmia, which if intermittent can give rise to syncope or dizziness (see Ch. 24). Rarely, increased carotid sinus sensitivity may also give rise to such symptoms. In the heart there may be evidence of anaemia in the form of a tachycardia and apical systolic murmur. Movements of the cervical spine should be examined and the patient asked whether any position of the neck produces these symptoms.

In the general examination it is important to look for evidence of thiamine deficiency, as this will aid a diagnosis of Wernicke's encephalopathy. Most attention, however, must be to the central nervous system. In the majority of patients complaining of dizziness no abnormal signs are found that would suggest disease of temporal lobe, cerebellum, or brain-stem. If present, however, the list of probable diagnoses changes considerably. Thus infarction in the territory of the posterior inferior cerebellar artery, tumours of the cerebellar vermis, multiple sclerosis involving the medulla, brainstem encephalitis and basilar artery aneurysm can all give rise to recurrent vertigo, usually associated with other distinctive symptoms.

An important, although rare, cause of vertigo is a tumour of the cerebellopontine angle, the commonest being the acoustic neuroma. Although later on these will give signs of central damage from compression of the brain stem and hydrocephalus, every effort should be made to establish the diagnosis at an earlier stage while the tumour is still small. An important physical sign, absent in most of the other commoner causes of vertigo, is diminished corneal sensation and this must be always looked for with considerable care in all cases of dizziness.

Other important central nervous system signs in the diagnosis of dizziness are nystagmus and 8th cranial nerve involvement.

Nystagmus

This remains a physical sign that is often poorly elicited and analysed and its interpretation is perhaps the source of even more confusion. When testing for its presence the patient must not be asked to look to the extreme limits of his gaze, for then anyone may show spurious nystagmus. Furthermore at least 5 seconds should be allowed in each direction for it to develop. The presence of a few nystagmoid jerks, such as occur commonly in normal people when tired, should be ignored. If present, the position of the eyes when the nystagmus occurs, the deviation which produces the greatest amplitude, and the direction of the fast movement, should all be noted. Nystagmus is usually described by the direction of the fast component if present.

A number of types of nystagmus can be distinguished clinically. One is pendular nystagmus, where there is a rapid symmetrical horizontal oscillation on either side of the midline. This form of nystagmus is due to local ocular disease and is not important in the differential diagnosis of dizziness. The more common and significant form of nystagmus is jerk nystagmus, where there is a fast movement in one direction followed by a slow movement in the other. Jerk nystagmus can be present at rest or on deviation of the eyes, and can be horizontal, vertical, or rotary. Nystagmus of this kind always indicates disease of the labyrinth or its higher connections.

Dissociated or ataxic nystagmus is present when the abducting eye shows coarse and irregular nystagmus, while the adducting eye shows only a fine nystagmus associated with some degree of paresis of the medial rectus of that eye. It most commonly occurs in multiple sclerosis.

The eighth nerve

It is important to test both divisions of this nerve, whether or not the patient actually complains of deafness. Simple clinical tests can be surprisingly effective. Care must be taken to mask the other ear and also to exclude the presence of wax by inspection with an auroscope. At the same time obvious disease of the drum and middle ear can be excluded. If any impairment of hearing is found, Rinne's and Weber's tests should be done to differentiate between conductive middle-ear deafness and perceptive nerve deafness. Normally in the Rinne test the tuning fork can be heard twice as long by air conduction as by bone conduction from the mastoid. In Weber's test the tuning fork at the vertex of the skull will normally not be lateralized.

Investigation of labyrinthine function is rather more complex, and the caloric and rotational tests used are not normally performed as part of routine examination. The delineation in recent years of the condition of benign positional vertigo does, however, justify testing for positional vertigo and nystagmus as it can be done quickly and simply. Starting with the patient sitting on a couch, the head is turned to one side and then the patient is laid back with his head hyperextended over the end of the couch. Each side is tested in turn several times. The positive result obtained in benign positional vertigo develops after a latent interval of some seconds and disappears if the test is repeated several times (adaptation). The nystagmus is chiefly rotatory and is directed to the underlying ear. If, as in some less common cases, the positional vertigo is due to a central lesion of the posterior fossa the nystagmus appears immediately and does not show adaptation.

Simplified tests of caloric function can be used. One is to irrigate each auditory meatus in turn with 5 ml of 5°C water, the patient sitting upright with his head tilted 60° backwards. The time is noted to the onset of the typical symptoms of nausea and dizziness. There is horizontal nystagmus away from the side irrigated. Vestibular damage is indicated by a delay and reduction in the response.

SPECIAL INVESTIGATIONS

In the majority of patients these will not be needed. If any impairment of hearing is detected or suspected, this should be delineated accurately using the audiometer to measure the threshold at different frequencies. A valuable test is for loudness recruitment. Here the relative loudness of two sounds, one presented to the normal ear and one to the deaf ear, is assessed at differing overall levels of intensity. In some patients as the overall loudness is increased the difference between the two sounds decreases – the phenomenon of loudness recruitment. It appears to be due to a lesion producing selective destruction of the low intensity elements of the cochlea itself. Lesions of the cochlear nerve and central nervous system usually affect fibres from the low and high elements equally and then loudness recruitment is less likely to occur. The test is positive in all cases of Ménière's disease where the low intensity elements are especially affected. Loudness recruitment does not occur in cases of vestibular neuronitis, where the cochlea is unaffected and the hearing usually normal. It is positive only to a minor extent in a few cases of acoustic neuroma.

Caloric testing (Fig. 28.1) is based on the warming and cooling of the lateral semicircular canals by water, usually at 44° and 30°C. Convection currents are set up resulting in movement of the cupolas: the normal finding with cold water will be nausea, horizontal nystagmus to the opposite side, and falling to the stimulated side. With warm water, the opposite results are obtained. The exact onset and duration of the nystagmus can be assessed clinically or more exactly by recording electrodes around the eye – electronystagmography. The simplest and commonest abnormality which is detected is canal paresis, where the duration of the nystagmus is reduced when the affected side is irrigated by both hot and cold water. Canal paresis results from damage to the vestibular system, particularly to the cupolar sense organs or their connections. A second type of abnormality that may be seen is directional preponderance, Here nystagmus in a particular direction is reduced, while in the other direction it is increased. Such a pattern occurs particularly with lesions of the central connections of the labyrinth, the nystagmus being towards the side of the lesion. This pattern (rather more than the canal paresis pattern) may also occur with lesions of the cerebellum or the posterior temporal lobe if these involve vestibular connections.

Examination of the CSF will be of value in encephalitis and can help in the diagnosis of multiple sclerosis. In acoustic neuroma the protein content is usually markedly increased and the extent of the rise correlates roughly with the size of the tumour. In one series, however, 25% showed a normal protein.

Neuroradiology will be of little value in the majority of cases. X-ray of the cervical spine may show

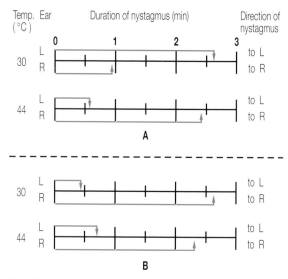

Fig. 28.1 Patterns of caloric response.

Normally nystagmus continues for 2–3 minutes and is equal on each side. Cold water induces nystagmus to the opposite side, hot water the reverse. In canal paresis the duration of nystagmus is reduced in the affected ear for both hot and cold water. In directional preponderance the duration of nystagmus is reduced when the nystagmus is provoked towards the side of the lesion.

A) Nystagmus is reduced in duration to the left, when either ear is irrigated. There is therefore directional preponderance to the right. This was due to a L temporal glioma.

B) Nystagmus is reduced when the left ear is irrigated by hot or cold water. This is left canal paresis, due to Ménière's disease.

the changes of cervical spondylosis, or the calcified arteries of extracranial cerebrovascular disease. Skull views are important in the diagnosis of acoustic neuroma, particular attention being paid to the internal auditory meatus. The slightest difference in diameter of the two canals is suspicious, as is any erosion or alteration in shape. Congenital or acquired lesions of the base of the skull may also be seen. If a space-occupying lesion of the posterior fossa is suspected then a CT or MRI scan should be obtained.

In those cases where episodes of cardiac arrhythmia are a possible cause of dizziness, ambulatory monitoring of the ECG will often allow a precise diagnosis to be made.

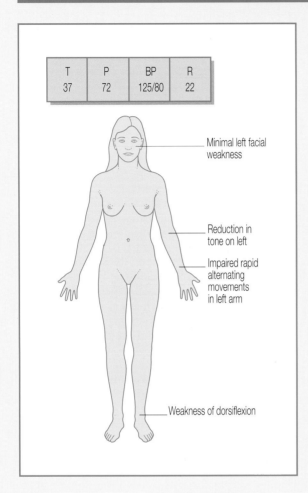

T	P	BP	R
37	72	125/80	22

Minimal left facial weakness

Reduction in tone on left

Impaired rapid alternating movements in left arm

Weakness of dorsiflexion

A 26-year-old housewife developed recurrent attacks of dizziness, which initially lasted for about one minute. During these attacks her surroundings appeared to move, but there was no actual rotation. She felt unsteady and had to sit down. The attacks began and stopped suddenly and occurred for no obvious reason. She had not noticed that any particular activity appeared to precipitate her attacks, which had occurred at all hours of the day. Over about 3 weeks they increased in frequency, until finally they were occurring hourly. With some of the attacks she had felt a little nauseated, but at no time had she vomited. There had never been any tinnitus or impairment of hearing. Over the same few weeks she also had the feeling that her walking was disturbed, and she had the sensation that she was being pulled to the left. She felt that her left leg was tiring more easily than normal, and she had noticed occasional cramps in the calf of that leg at night.

She was given symptomatic treatment with prochlorperazine and over the next week her symptoms improved considerably. The attacks of dizziness settled completely, although she continued to feel that her walking was not quite normal. However, a month later the attacks recurred and in addition she also noticed double vision. The images were only slightly separated and the symptom was more marked towards the end of the day when she was tired.

In the past she had always been well and had had no previous illnesses except appendicitis 4 years earlier. Her mother had suffered from 'sick headaches' for many years, thought to be due to migraine.

Because of the further development of her illness she was admitted to hospital for investigation. No abnormality was present on general examination, abnormal signs being confined to the nervous system. The fundi were normal, and examination of the cranial nerves revealed nothing except some degree of facial asymmetry which suggested the presence of minimal weakness of the lower half of the face on the left. Rapid alternate movements were a little impaired in the left hand, but she was a right-handed person. Tone appeared reduced in both the left arm and leg. There was some weakness of dorsiflexion of the foot on the left, and the left plantar response was equivocal.

Questions

1. What are the most likely causes of this woman's illness?
2. What further investigations may be of value in arriving at the diagnosis?

Dizziness

This woman's major complaint is of dizziness which is non-vertiginous in nature. Her attacks have no obvious precipitating cause and in particular there are no associated symptoms that might suggest disease of the middle or inner ear. If dizziness or vertigo occur for any reason there is commonly some nausea or vomiting and her feeling of nausea has therefore no extra significance. The disturbance of her gait is an important symptom. The feeling that her left leg tires more easily and the occurrence of occasional cramps raise the possibility of an upper motor neurone lesion involving that limb, although the sensation of being pulled to the one side while walking could also occur with a lesion of the cerebellum or its connections. The fact that her symptoms improved with prochlorperazine is of no value in establishing the diagnosis as this is a non-specific effect. Her walking would be unlikely to improve on such treatment and the fact that this also improved suggests that the natural course of her illness is fluctuant, and that a spontaneous improvement may be occurring. Her final complaint of diplopia also suggests, in this context, that there may be disease involving the cerebellum or its connections.

This overall pattern of symptoms is strongly suggestive of organic disease. Dizziness, ataxia and diplopia may occur in drug intoxication, for example with barbiturates, but would usually give rise to more symmetrical symptoms and not involve particularly one side of the body. It is likely therefore that some more localized pathology is present involving particularly the brain stem.

The findings on examination support this interpretation. The signs are minimal and their exact significance must initially be in doubt, but the asymmetry disclosed in the face, the arms and the legs all suggest organic pathology. The weakness and equivocal plantar response support the possibility of a left-sided pyramidal disturbance, while the impairment of rapid alternate movements and the reduction in tone may indicate an additional cerebellar lesion. The fact that both sets of signs involve the same side of the body suggests that they may be due to separate lesions, for unlike pyramidal signs resulting from a brain-stem lesion, cerebellar signs are ipsilateral.

A number of possible diagnoses must be considered. Brain-stem encephalitis is uncommon, most viruses showing more widespread neurotropism. There is usually some disturbance of consciousness and also symptoms such as headache due to raised CSF pressure. Ménière's disease is uncommon at this age and is usually associated with deafness and tinnitus and also would not explain the symptoms in the left arm suggestive of a cerebellar lesion.

The story is fully compatible with a diagnosis of multiple sclerosis and the time course of the first episode is quite typical. Vertigo is a well-recognized early symptom occurring in between 5% and 15% of cases. Less clearly defined dizziness is as common as true vertigo. A feeling of being pulled to one side is also described in association with vertigo. During an attack there will usually be nystagmus, and some cases may show a continuous dissociated (or ataxic) nystagmus. Such a finding is always highly suggestive of the disease but is not completely pathognomonic.

The diagnosis of acute vestibular neuronitis is rendered untenable by the presence of symptoms and signs elsewhere in the central nervous system. Acoustic neuroma must be considered in a case such as this, although the age of the patient and the time course of the symptoms would not support the diagnosis of a progressive space-occupying lesion. Furthermore the presence of cerebellar and possible pyramidal signs would be very unlikely in the absence of any evidence of damage to the trigeminal nerve.

In the investigation of this case, audiometry and caloric testing would be reasonable although not essential. They showed in fact no impairment of hearing, but bilateral reduction in caloric responses compatible with a bilateral brain stem lesion. EEG and isotope scan would be very unlikely to give information of value, both techniques giving little information about lesions in the posterior fossa. Vertebral angiogram is rarely required in this type of case. Occasionally these symptoms may arise from a basilar aneurysm, or vertebrobasilar angioma, but delay in establishing such a diagnosis is not usually of importance. These investigations were not therefore performed. Skull X-rays were done and were normal, and views of the internal auditory meati showed no evidence of expansion. An X-ray CT scan was also completely normal. A lumbar puncture revealed clear fluid at a normal pressure, with a free rise and fall on jugular compression. The number of white cells was slightly raised at $10/mm^3$. The protein was also a little increased at 50 mg/dl and immune electrophoresis showed a rise in IgG with discrete oligoclonal bands. There was impairment of visually evoked responses on the EEG compatible with retrobulbar neuritis.

> It was thought that the most likely diagnosis was multiple sclerosis, and this was confirmed by the later history of the patient and an MRI brain scan.

29

Headache and facial pain

HEADACHE

Headache is the commonest neurological symptom in the general population and in most people does not indicate serious neurological disease. In assessing the patient with headache the physician aims to classify the type of headache since this will direct treatment. In addition, those patients who have symptoms or signs which indicate they are more likely to have neurological disease need to be identified. One useful guide in determining the cause of headache is the time course. Headaches may be usefully separated into acute, subacute and chronic. Generally, patients with acute and subacute headaches are more likely to have significant pathology.

Acute headache

Subarachnoid haemorrhage. This is one of the most important causes of sudden onset headache. The patient may describe it like 'a blow to the head'. Nausea, photophobia and neck stiffness quickly follow the onset of the headache, these symptoms being caused by the presence of blood in the subarachnoid space. The headache usually becomes generalized. Some patients may lose consciousness at the onset of the headache and others may develop focal neurological signs such as dysphasia or hemiparesis. Neck stiffness is a common finding. Patients who have sustained large subarachnoid haemorrhages may develop subhyaloid retinal haemorrhages. Any patient giving such a history of acute onset headache must be investigated urgently to rule out subarachnoid haemorrhage. The main point of such urgent investigation is first, to establish if the patient has had a subarachnoid haemorrhage and second, to identify a potential source from which a further bleed may occur. The commonest source is a berry aneurysm in the circle of Willis. Rebleeds from such aneurysms are commonly fatal, hence the need for urgent investiga-

tion of such patients which may afford the opportunity to treat an aneurysm, if identified, before rebleeding occurs.

All such patients should have a CT brain scan. Since 10% of patients who have had subarachnoid haemorrhages are 'CT-negative' a normal CT does not rule out the diagnosis. Such patients should have a lumbar puncture at least 8 hours after the onset of the headache. This time period will allow xanthochromia to have developed if there has been a subarachnoid haemorrhage. The CSF should be examined spectrophotometrically for xanthochromia. A red blood cell count in sequential CSF samples taken at a lumbar puncture is *not* a reliable way of ruling out a subarachnoid haemorrhage in a CT-negative case. If a subarachnoid haemorrhage is confirmed the patient should have intra-arterial cerebral angiography to establish if an aneurysm is present. If an aneurysm is identified this should be treated either by neurosurgical intervention or by interventional radiological techniques. The choice of modality depends mainly upon the anatomy of the aneurysm.

Some patients seem to be prone to sudden onset headaches identical to a subarachnoid haemorrhage, although they do not develop neurological signs. On the first occasion a subarachnoid needs to be ruled out. This group have been termed '**thunderclap**' headaches. The precise aetiology of such thunderclap headaches is uncertain but it is possible that they represent a form of migraine.

Subacute headache

Any patient with a recent onset headache over the previous few weeks (i.e. subacute) must be evaluated with great care. Although it remains true that most patients with subacute onset headaches will not have major pathology, this is more likely than in cases of chronic headache. This is particularly the case if the patient has not previously been prone to headaches. Raised intracranial pressure headache and temporal arteritis are the most serious causes to consider.

Specific symptoms and signs that might indicate **raised intracranial pressure** should be sought. Typically, raised pressure headaches are worse on waking in the morning and often subside by the middle of the day. The patient may be woken from sleep by the headache. Patients may experience nausea particularly in the morning when they may also experience effortless vomiting. Raised pressure headaches may be helped significantly by simple analgesics such as paracetamol. Such a therapeutic response should therefore not mislead the physician. Indeed, benign headaches such as chronic muscle contraction tension headache usually do not respond to such simple analgesia.

Box 29.1 Headaches classified on the basis of time course

Acute headache
- Migraine
- Subarachnoid haemorrhage
- Intracerebral haemorrhage
- Meningitis
- Encephalitis
- Rapid increase in intracranial pressure
- Drugs – e.g. vasodilators
- Alcohol – 'hangover'

Subacute headache
- Raised intracranial pressure:
    tumour
    abscess
    subdural haematoma
    hydrocephalus
    benign intracranial hypertension
- Temporal arteritis
- Referred from other cranial structures e.g. sinuses, teeth

Chronic headache
- Continuous:
    muscle contraction – tension headache
    psychological – anxiety, depression, hypochondriasis
    post-traumatic
    referred – cervicogenic headache
- Intermittent:
    migraine

The raised pressure headache may be a generalized ache or may have a predominantly frontal distribution. It may be made significantly worse by manoeuvres which raise intracranial pressure, such as coughing, sneezing or bending over. The patient may or may not have neurological signs such as a hemiparesis or cerebellar ataxia. It is important that raised pressure can be present in the absence of papilloedema. Some patients who do have papilloedema complain of visual obscurations. These are transient disturbances in vision, usually a momentary darkening of vision, precipitated by performing manoeuvres which raise intracranial pressure. If a cerebral abscess is the cause of headache the patient may have pyrexia. All patients with symptoms suspicious of raised pressure, even in the absence of signs, need urgent investigation with brain imaging.

Temporal arteritis. This is an important cause of subacute onset headache in the elderly. Indeed, in any patient presenting over the age of 55 years with new headaches this condition should be considered. The risks of not making the diagnosis are of blindness from an ischaemic optic neuropathy and also of stroke. Patients may be generally unwell with systemic symptoms such as malaise, generalized aches and pains and weight loss. They complain of a persistent generalized headache sometimes with tenderness over the scalp. They may volunteer that pressure on the head when lying on a pillow or brushing the hair is unpleasant and tender. The temporal arteries may be tender and in severe cases there may be reddening of the skin overlying the artery. Some patients describe jaw claudication. An urgent ESR should be requested and, if elevated, a temporal artery biopsy should be done as soon as possible to confirm the diagnosis. Steroids should be commenced without delay if the ESR is elevated while waiting for the biopsy. If the diagnosis is correct the patient will notice a dramatic improvement in symptoms, usually within 12 hours of the first dose.

Chronic headache

Tension headache and migraine headache are the two commonest causes of chronic headache. Patients with these headaches never have abnormal neurological signs on examination. It is a useful working rule that patients who have experienced headache for more than three years without developing neurological signs will virtually always have one of these two types of headache. The diagnosis is based entirely upon a careful history. Distinguishing these two common causes of chronic headache is important because different treatments are appropriate.

Tension-type headache (also known as muscle-contraction headache). Patients with tension headache report daily headache with few pain-free days. It does not usually disturb sleep but builds up as the day progresses. It is commonly described as a pressure feeling on top of the head or as a band around the head like a vice. It is not accompanied by prominent nausea or vomiting, or visual disturbance. It is commonly the case that the patient manages to keep going in their normal activities despite the headache. Nothing appears to help the headache and many patients take large amounts of analgesics. There is evidence that chronic analgesic intake can itself produce headache (termed analgesic abuse headache) and therefore every effort should be made to reduce analgesic intake in this setting.

Underlying depression can be a factor in producing tension headache and a history suggestive of this diagnosis should be sought. In addition it can be a symptom of a chronic anxiety state and made worse with peaks of stress. There is evidence that the headache may, at least in part, be generated by continuous increased contraction of the scalp musculature.

The medication shown to be effective in a trial setting is amitriptyline. The mechanism is complex but this drug does have muscle relaxing activity as well as sedative and anti-depressant actions. Alternative, safe strategies, which some patients find helpful, include relaxation techniques, acupuncture and cranial massage. If they help, these modalities avoid the need for regular medication. Some patients who have experienced head injury, often minor, are troubled by continuous headaches with features very similar to tension headache. There may be associated symptoms such as light-headedness, dizziness and lack of concentration which amount to what is termed a post-concussion syndrome. These patients do not have abnormal neurological signs. Litigation is sometimes pending, but not always. The majority resolve, usually within 18 months, but they can become long term.

Migraine. Migraine is very common, affecting as much as 2% of the population at some time. It is an episodic headache disorder, unlike the continuous headache experienced by patients with tension headache. In taking the history it is useful to establish that the patient does have headache-free periods. Two common types of migraine are migraine with aura (previously known as classical migraine) and migraine without aura (previously termed common migraine). In both types the headache is similar. It builds up gradually and may be unilateral or generalized. At its height it is a severe throbbing headache often associated with nausea, vomiting, photophobia and phonophobia. Typically the patient cannot continue with their activities, may feel drowsy and simply wants to lie still and alone in a darkened room. Attacks usually last hours and may be as long as 3 days. In migraine with aura there is a characteristic set of symptoms prior to the onset of the headache – the aura. This is commonly visual. The patient might become aware of flashing, often coloured, lights in their field of vision. Various descriptions are given such as fortification spectra (zig-zag bright lights) and scintillating scotomata. Other auras include dysphasia, hemisensory, dysarthria, diplopia or ataxia. When present, the aura typically lasts no longer than 30 minutes. At the end of an attack the patient returns to normal and is then headache-free until the next attack. Some patients identify precipitants to attacks but this is not always the case. When present, known precipitants can be avoided. Precipitants relevant to some patients include certain foods (chocolate, cheese, red wine), stress, lack of sleep and menstruation (so-called catamenial migraine).

FACIAL PAIN

Facial pain, like headache, is a not uncommon symptom in the general population. Patients do not usually have any neurological signs and the diagnosis is often based on the clinical history. Pain in the face may result from disease in local structures (eyes, sinuses or teeth). The major sensory nerve supply to the face and oropharynx is from the trigeminal and glossopharyngeal nerves. Facial pain may result from direct damage to one of these nerves, in which case there will be neurological signs. Alternatively the patient may experience facial pain because the nerves seem to be hyperexcitable, but there are no abnormal signs. This latter group includes the neuralgias.

Local causes of facial pain

There are a large number of possible local causes. A careful history and examination will usually reveal the cause. In the causes outlined here there are no abnormal neurological signs.

- **Sinus infection** is a common cause of facial pain. The distribution of pain will depend on the sinus involved but most commonly the frontal or maxillary sinuses are implicated. Acute sinusitis can have an explosive onset with severe throbbing facial pain, increased by coughing or sneezing. It is sometimes exacerbated by lying flat. There may be tenderness over the sinus and the patient may be pyrexial.
- **Eye diseases** such as acute glaucoma may produce intense local eye pain with clouding of vision and represents an ophthalmological urgency. Iritis can also produce eye pain. Pain in the face on chewing (jaw claudication) is a particular symptom of **temporal arteritis** in the elderly. Pain on eating can also be seen in patients with salivary duct calculi in which case it is often unilateral.
- Pain due to **dental caries** can be severe and may be precipitated by extremes of temperature. This pain is usually felt in the teeth or gums.

Facial pain associated with neurological signs

Facial pain in the presence of abnormal neurological signs is always a cause for concern and one must suspect sinister pathology until proved otherwise.

Involvement of the **trigeminal nerve** by an infiltrative or compressive process produces ipsilateral facial pain. This is usually a continuous aching pain in the face, sometimes with superimposed jabs of neuralgic pain. Pathologies to consider include posterior fossa tumours (e.g. cerebellopontine angle tumours) or tumours involving the skull base (malignant meningeal infiltration). Post-nasal space tumours, such as squamous cell carcinomas, can also infiltrate the skull base. An ENT referral is therefore usually required to facilitate careful examination of this region. There may be additional cranial nerve signs in association with skull-base tumours (most commonly VI–X). When such processes impinge on the trigeminal nerve sensory functions tend to be lost initially and motor dysfunction follows. Loss of the **corneal reflex** is often the earliest sign of trigeminal nerve damage. If an infiltrative skull-base process is suspected, imaging of the brain and skull base, usually with contrast techniques, is required. CSF examination is often helpful and may reveal changes of a malignant meningitis (low glucose, high protein, raised white cell count with malignant cells on cytology).

Disorders of the intracranial and extracranial arterial vasculature may present with facial pain. Acute pain in the eye associated with a **third nerve palsy** is a recognized presentation of an expanding aneurysm of the posterior communicating artery.

A painful **Horner's syndrome** may be the presentation of a dissection of the internal carotid artery either in the neck or in its proximal intracranial portion.

Facial pain without neurological signs

There are a number of facial neuralgias, which present with facial pain, often of severe intensity. Generally, these neuralgic disorders are believed to represent increased excitability of structurally normal nerves.

Trigeminal neuralgia (tic douloureux). This is a cause of episodic unilateral facial pain usually presenting over the age of 40 years. The pain is usually confined to the second and third divisions of the trigeminal nerve. The pain occurs in spasms. The patient describes a shooting or lancing momentary pain of extreme intensity. Characteristically the pain is triggered by at least two of the following: eating, talking, washing the face, brushing the teeth, touching the face or exposure to cold wind. The patient may experience multiple episodes in a day. The illness is intermittent with bouts lasting days or weeks separated by prolonged periods of freedom. Neurological examination is normal. Medication such as carbamazepine or gabapentin is often helpful. Some patients require surgical ablation of the trigeminal nerve ganglion, but this may lead to trigeminal sensory loss.

Glossopharyngeal neuralgia. This has similar characteristics to trigeminal neuralgia but involves the glossopharyngeal nerve. Patients experience paroxysms of severe pain felt at the back of the throat, back of the tongue and deep in the ear. It is typically triggered by swallowing.

Post-herpetic neuralgia. The ophthalmic division of the trigeminal nerve is commonly involved in herpes zoster. Some patients go on to develop post-herpetic neuralgia after the initial zoster rash has recovered. There is a continuous burning pain with sharp jolts in the distribution of the ophthalmic division. Touching the face may trigger the pain.

Migrainous neuralgia. This disorder is considered to be a variant of migraine but has very characteristic distinguishing features. It is more common in males. Patients experience attacks of extreme agonizing pain centred around one eye, most commonly during the night. The patient is typically woken from sleep. At the height of the pain it might be described as 'the eye being torn out of the socket' or a 'hot poker in the eye'. Unlike migraine the patient will pace around in an agonized state. Some individuals will resort to banging their head against a wall to try and distract themselves from the pain. Examination during an attack will show reddening of the affected eye and the patient commonly complains of ipsilateral nasal congestion. The pain usually lasts for about an hour and then subsides. Typically patients experience nightly episodes of pain for a few weeks and are then pain-free for prolonged periods. Remarkably the pain seems to occur at the same time each night (hence the term 'alarm clock headache'). In a given individual it is usually the same eye which is affected in attacks. Anti-migraine drugs may help. In some patients it has been shown that high-flow oxygen can relieve an attack.

Chronic paroxysmal hemicrania. This disorder has some similarities to migrainous neuralgia. It affects women more than men. It causes sharp jolts of severe pain which are usually short lived. The pain is normally felt in one side of the head. Multiple separate attacks may occur in a single day; they may be episodic. Its recognition is important since complete resolution is usually achieved with indomethacin. Other medications seem to be ineffective.

Atypical facial pain

There remains a group of patients with facial pain that does not conform to any of the descriptions given above. They have no abnormal neurological signs. The term atypical facial pain is used to refer to this group. It is commoner in women and most complain of unilateral continuous facial pain on a daily basis unrelieved by any medication. These latter features are similar to tension headache. It is considered that in some of these patients depression and anxiety may be relevant factors. However, positive symptoms of these latter disorders should be present before concluding this is the case.

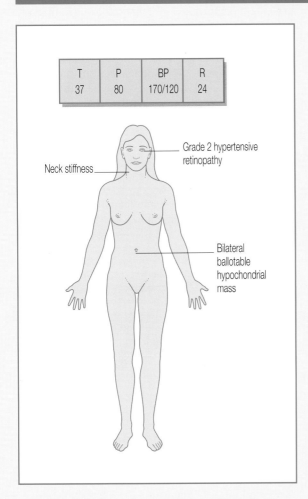

T	P	BP	R
37	80	170/120	24

Neck stiffness

Grade 2 hypertensive retinopathy

Bilateral ballotable hypochondrial mass

A 56-year-old woman developed a sudden onset headache while shopping. She described it 'like a sudden bang' on the back of her head. The pain stopped her in her tracks but she did not black out. She felt acutely nauseated and sat down. After a few minutes the pain subsided to a generalized dull ache. She was able to catch the bus home. On arriving home she was very nauseated and vomited several times. She became aware of an ache and restriction of movement in her neck in addition to a generalized headache. She presented to the casualty department of her local hospital five hours after the onset of the headache still feeling unwell.

She explained she had a previous history of hypertension, detected at a routine examination 2 years previously but not investigated, for which she took bendrofluazide. Otherwise she has been well in the past with no history of headaches. She had three brothers, one of whom received renal dialysis for polycystic disease, as did her father before he died from a heart attack. The patient had three adult daughters who were healthy; she did not smoke or drink alcohol.

On examination she was alert and orientated. She complained of a generalized headache which she described as tolerable. She had a mild ache in her neck which was exacerbated by neck movements. She was mildly photophobic. There were Grade 2 hypertensive changes in her retinae but no other cranial nerve signs. Neurological examination of her limbs was normal. Her blood pressure was 170/120. She had a palpable ballotable mass in her right hypochondrium and possibly in the left hypochondrium. The rest of the general examination was normal

Questions

1. What is the likely diagnosis?
2. What investigations are needed?

Discussion

Any patient who gives a history of a sudden onset headache must be considered to have had a subarachnoid haemorrhage until proven otherwise. It is particularly important to take the history very carefully. In this context 'sudden' means instantaneous. Some patients say sudden when they mean over the course of a few minutes or longer: the headache of a subarachnoid is truly instantaneous. The patient often describes it like a blow to the head 'like being hit with a hammer'. It is important to remember that patients with small (also known as Grade 1) subarachnoid haemorrhages can have no symptoms other than headache and may not necessarily have any focal neurological signs. Another possible cause to consider is an intracerebral haemorrhage in view of the history of hypertension. Although migraine can occasionally cause a sudden onset headache, there is no history of migraine headache, making this unlikely. It is essential to rule out more serious intracranial pathology before entertaining a diagnosis of migraine.

In the present case the patient felt nauseated and unwell but was able to make her way home. By the time she reached hospital she had developed some stiffness in her neck as well as headache. Examination confirmed neck stiffness but no other neurological signs. The absence of neurological signs does not rule out a subarachnoid haemorrhage and the presence of neck stiffness indicates that there may be subarachnoid blood present causing meningeal irritation. The absence of neurological signs would be unusual in a haemorrhage stroke, even if small. The abdominal signs suggest she may have enlarged kidneys and one should suspect polycystic kidney disease in view of the family history. This disorder is associated with intracranial berry aneurysms.

The priority in this patient is to perform a CT brain scan to look for evidence of a subarachnoid haemorrhage. If the CT brain scan is normal this does not rule out a subarachnoid haemorrhage and she should have a lumbar puncture at least 8 hours after the initial headache with analysis for xanthochromia. If a subarachnoid is confirmed intra-arterial angiography is indicated.

This patient's CT was normal but the CSF confirmed xanthochromia. An ultrasound of her abdomen showed bilateral polycystic kidneys. Angiography showed two aneurysms in the circle of Willis. She proceeded to neurosurgery and had both aneurysms clipped successfully with no recurrence of bleeding after many years' follow-up.

Weakness in the arms and legs

Weakness of the limbs may be part of any debilitating illness such as systemic infection or cancer, in which case there are usually pointers to this in the history. If limb weakness is the principal complaint, it is more likely that there is an underlying neurological disease. Some patients complain of 'weakness' when they actually mean unsteadiness or even numbness; detailed analysis of exactly what the patient means is therefore essential.

Neurological diseases that result in limb weakness are best understood on the basis of the normal neuroanatomy of the voluntary motor pathways. Normal muscle strength depends principally on normal function of a relay of four systems:

- the upper motor neurone system
- the lower motor neurone system
- the neuromuscular junction transmission system and
- the skeletal muscle.

Neurological diseases presenting with muscular weakness may do so by causing dysfunction at one or more of these four levels. Important causes of weakness affecting all four limbs include cervical cord diseases such as myelitis or cord compression, anterior horn cell diseases such as motor neurone disease, multiple radiculopathy, neuropathy, neuromuscular junction diseases such as myasthenia gravis or muscle diseases such as polymyositis or muscular dystrophies. In each case there will be important clues in the history and findings on examination which will allow a diagnosis to be made on clinical grounds alone in the majority of cases.

A CLINICAL APPROACH TO THE PATIENT WITH WEAK LIMBS

A careful history and subsequent examination will help to pinpoint which of the four sites in the voluntary motor pathway is involved. The time course of the onset of weakness is usually helpful in determining the possible aetiology. Generally, the rate of onset of limb weakness may be divided into acute, subacute and chronic categories.

Acute onset limb weakness

Acute onset of weakness affecting one side of the body is typical of a vascular event affecting the contralateral upper motor neurone pathways. For example a left middle cerebral artery occlusion will cause sudden onset weakness in the right arm and leg. There will often be an associated dysphasia, right homonymous hemianopia, right hemisensory loss and right lower facial weakness which aid the diagnosis. There will usually be upper motor neurone signs in the affected limbs. These are: a pyramidal pattern of muscle weakness, a spastic increase in muscle tone, tendon hyperreflexia and an extensor plantar response. However, in some acute stroke cases the affected limbs may initially be rather flaccid without hyperreflexia, although typical upper motor neurone signs usually subsequently develop.

Sudden onset weakness in all four limbs (tetraparesis) or in both legs (paraparesis) is seen in patients with spinal cord infarction, usually caused by occlusion of the anterior spinal artery. Such occlusion is more common in those with general atheromatous arterial vascular disease.

Patients with sudden onset paraparesis commonly have atheromatous disease of the abdominal aorta sometimes associated with an abdominal aortic aneurysm. Patients complain of the sudden onset of painless motor and sensory loss in the affected limbs. Bladder function is also commonly affected and urinary retention is usual. Examination typically shows a flaccid paralysis with reduced or normal tendon reflexes at first. Initially, the plantar responses may be flexor or absent. This phase of flaccidity, without clear upper motor neurone signs, is sometimes known as the phase of spinal shock. Subsequently upper motor neurone signs develop. Patients with anterior spinal artery occlusion typically have preservation of dorsal column function (i.e. vibration and proprioception) in the presence of marked loss of other sensory modalities such as pin-prick. Such patients often have a sensory level to pin-prick which may give an approximate guide to the level in the spinal cord at which the vascular lesion has occurred. The reason for preservation of dorsal column function relates to the normal arterial supply of the spinal cord. The anterior spinal artery is situated in a groove on the anterior aspect of the spinal cord and sends branches into the cord which supply the anterior two-thirds of the cord. Hence, virtually all spinal cord pathways except the dorsal columns are rendered ischaemic.

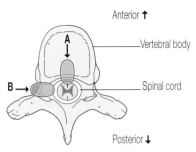

Anterior ↑

Vertebral body

Spinal cord

Posterior ↓

Fig. 30.1 The spinal cord may be compressed at any level along its course from C1 to where it ends at the L1/L2 level. Spinal metastases are a common cause of spinal cord compression. Such metasases may be deposited in the vertebral body and may compress the anterior surface of the spinal cord (**A** in figure). Alternatively metastases may compress the cord laterally via the intervertebral foramina (**B** in figure).

Subacute onset weakness in the limbs

Weakness which evolves over a few days or weeks has a much larger differential diagnosis. Important causes to consider include cancer (e.g. spinal cord compression from metastatic deposit), inflammatory disorders (e.g. viral myelitis, polymyositis) or immunologically mediated disorders (e.g. multiple sclerosis or myasthenia gravis). Cord compression requires urgent treatment and must be excluded quickly in all such cases. The two main patterns of subacute limb weakness are an upper motor neurone pattern or a lower motor neurone pattern.

Spinal cord disease. If the patient has upper motor neurone signs in the limbs a pathological process in the spinal cord should be suspected. The important causes to consider include spinal cord compression, viral myelitis or demyelination. It is important to remember that the spinal cord ends at the L2 vertebral level. It therefore follows that a lesion causing upper motor neurone signs in the legs (a spastic paraparesis) must be located above this vertebral level. Imaging of the thoracic cord and not the lumbar spine is therefore required in this clinical setting. Patients with thoracic spinal cord lesions develop weakness in their legs, usually with accompanying sensory symptoms of numbness and tingling. Bladder dysfunction is common and there may be frequency and urgency of urination or difficulty micturating culminating in urinary retention.

Tumours of the cerebral hemispheres and the meninges will not usually present solely as difficulty in walking. A well-recognized exception is a falx meningioma, which by pressing on the underlying leg areas of each precentral motor cortex may initially give rise to the symptoms and signs of a spastic paraplegia, mimicking a spinal cord lesion. Usually, cerebral tumours cause fits, symptoms resulting from a general rise in intracranial pressure, personality change, and focal symptoms and signs arising from damage and irritation at the site of the tumour. Hemiplegia is a common occurrence and its association with some of the other features mentioned will usually point to the underlying diagnosis.

Patients with viral myelitis or demyelinating myelitis affecting the spinal cord have a similar combination of motor, sensory and bladder symptoms as in patients with compressive lesions. However, back pain is not usually a prominent feature. Patients with viral transverse myelitis may give a history of preceding systemic symptoms to suggest a viral process. For example, glandular fever may be complicated by transverse myelitis. Previous episodes to suggest demyelination elsewhere in the nervous system, e.g. optic neuritis, point to a diagnosis of multiple sclerosis.

Examination of patients with a pathological process in the thoracic spinal cord will normally reveal upper motor neurone signs in the legs, namely increased tone in a spastic fashion, a pyramidal pattern of leg weakness (i.e. the lower limb flexor muscles are more affected than the extensors), brisk tendon reflexes, absent abdominal reflexes and extensor plantar responses. There may also be a sensory level: that is, a loss of sensation below the spinal cord level of the lesion. Such a sensory level may be dense, in which case all sensory modalities are lost below the level. More commonly the sensory level is subtle and may only be detected with vibration or pin-prick (pain) testing. It is often the case that a patient with a spinal cord lesion does not have all the upper motor neurone signs and sensory signs listed. It is common for spinal cord lesions to be partial in which only some of the spinal cord fibre pathways are interrupted. For example, some patients have predominantly upper motor neurone signs but no sensory signs. The reverse may also occur. There may be localized tenderness in the back over the site of cord compression caused by a metastatic tumour or an infective process such as an epidural abcess.

Imaging (ideally MRI) of the spinal cord is mandatory to rule out a compressive lesion in any patient with a spastic paraparesis. This should be arranged as a matter of urgency once the diagnosis is suspected. It is particularly important to rule out a compressive lesion before bladder function is lost (that is, before the patient is in urinary retention) since in the context of a compressive lesion, once bladder function is lost, it is unlikely to return even if the compression is relieved surgically. A common error is that the physician directs imaging to be undertaken of the wrong part of the spine. Patients with a spastic paraparesis are often transferred to neurology centres having only had

Box 30.1 Important causes of a bilateral pyramidal lesion affecting the lower limbs

- Cord compression
- Trauma
- Multiple sclerosis
- Transverse myelitis
- Cervical spondylosis
- Motor neurone disease
- Vitamin B_{12} deficiency
- Cerebrovascular disease
- Spinal vascular disease
- Falx meningioma

lumbar spinal imaging which is illogical, since the cord ends at the L2 vertebral level.

If MRI imaging excludes cord compression it may show abnormalities in the substance of the cord which suggests viral myelitis or demyelinating myelitis. The typical changes seen are high signal changes in the substance of the cord on T2 weighted images. If there have been previous clinical episodes suggestive of multiple sclerosis an MRI brain scan should be performed. This may show typical white-matter lesions consistent with a diagnosis of multiple sclerosis.

CSF examination should be undertaken once a compressive lesion is excluded. In viral myelitis there will usually be normal glucose, a raised protein and an elevated white cell count (often over 200 predominantly or exclusively lymphocytes). In addition, PCR amplification of viral gene sequences can be performed on the CSF. If the presence of viral DNA/RNA is confirmed this is helpful in diagnosis. In demyelination due to multiple sclerosis the white cell count, although raised, is usually lower than in viral myelitis (usually less than 100 lymphocytes). Electrophoresis of CSF will normally detect oligoclonal bands in multiple sclerosis.

Peripheral neuropathy. The main neuropathy which evolves in a subacute fashion is **Guillain–Barré syndrome** (GBS). In GBS patients may give a history of a preceding infectious illness 2–3 weeks before they develop neurological symptoms. The first symptoms are often sensory and may comprise tingling or numbness in the feet. Motor symptoms soon develop initially in the legs and later in the arms. Back pain is a prominent early feature, which may precede the neurological symptoms. This is often severe and radicular in nature and may be misdiagnosed as sciatica.

Neurological examination shows signs of a mixed peripheral neuropathy which is mainly motor and which often affects the lower limbs to a greater extent

than the upper limbs. Typically there is flaccid lower motor neurone weakness with loss of reflexes. Particular care should be taken to assess bulbar function and respiration in patients with GBS. In severe cases, usually with significant upper limb weakness, there can be marked bulbar and respiratory muscle weakness. Ten per cent of GBS patients still die in the acute phase of the illness, often because the severity of respiratory muscle weakness has not been appreciated until the patient has a respiratory arrest. A bedside assessment of respiratory muscle strength is therefore mandatory in all cases. This is best achieved by measuring the vital capacity which in an average adult male is usually greater than 5 litres and in an average adult female is above 3 litres. If there is a falling trend in vital capacity or it is less than 1.5 litres the patient should be transferred to intensive care with a view to elective ventilatory support. Bulbar function can be assessed simply at the bedside by listening to the speech, observing the palatal movements and by observing the patient swallow a sip of water.

The diagnosis of GBS is confirmed by electrophysiology which normally shows changes of a demyelinating neuropathy. CSF examination is also helpful and normally shows an elevated protein, often above 1 g/dl, but with a normal cell count and glucose.

Myasthenia gravis. Patients with **autoimmune myasthenia gravis** often give a subacute history of painless limb weakness without sensory symptoms. The clinical hallmark is fatiguability, a symptom the patient will usually volunteer. For example, they may describe being able to start a repetitive activity but being unable to complete it because their muscles seem to get 'weaker and weaker'. Ocular involvement at the onset is common and is a distinguishing feature from most other causes of subacute weakness. Occasionally patients with Guillain–Barré syndrome may have ocular muscle weakness; this is known as the Miller–Fisher variant. However, unlike myasthenic patients the tendon reflexes are absent. Diplopia and ptosis are much more common in myasthenia. Bulbar weakness may be present and the patient may have fatiguability of chewing, swallowing or talking. They may find it difficult to hold a long conversation or to complete a meal. Because of fatiguability, and also because the symptoms may fluctuate considerably over time, there is commonly a long delay before the diagnosis is made.

Examination in a case of generalized myasthenia might reveal ptosis and diplopia. Neck flexion weakness is common and there might be variable degrees of weakness in the limbs, which might be global or mainly proximal. Muscle wasting is not usually a feature. Reflexes are preserved. Fatiguability can be demonstrated at the bedside by repetitive activity. For example asking the patient to abduct the shoulder 20 times and then comparing the strength with the opposite shoulder which has not been exercised. The diagnosis can be confirmed by electrophysiological testing (specifically repetitive stimulation EMG studies and also single-fibre EMG studies). In the majority of cases a pathogenic antibody can be detected in blood; this is most commonly the acetylcholine receptor antibody.

Inflammatory myopathies. **Inflammatory diseases of skeletal muscle** often evolve in a subacute fashion. The commonest forms are dermatomyositis and polymyositis. The patients typically have a proximal distribution of muscle weakness. They therefore notice symptoms such as difficulty getting out of chairs or climbing up stairs. They may complain of difficulty with tasks that involve lifting their arms above their head such as grooming. In severe cases the bulbar and respiratory muscles may be involved. Muscle pain is a feature in only a minority of patients and its absence certainly does not exclude the diagnosis. Examination typically shows proximal limb weakness with preserved reflexes and normal sensory testing. There may be the typical rash around the eyes (heliotrope) or over the dorsal aspect of the knuckles in dermatomyositis. Dermatomyositis in adults can be a paraneoplastic phenomenon (bowel and lung cancer in particular). This is more likely in older patients and a general physical examination should be undertaken with this in mind. In a minority of patients inflammatory muscle disease is part of a generalized autoimmune disorder and there may therefore be evidence of other autoimmune diseases such as rheumatoid arthritis or SLE. In all forms of polymyositis muscle wasting develops if active disease is present for more than a few months. Investigation should include blood creatine kinase measurement, EMG studies and a muscle biopsy. The CK is usually elevated in the region of a few thousand units (normal less than 150 units), the EMG is myopathic and the biopsy will confirm inflammatory infiltrates in the muscle. A tissue diagnosis is essential before commencing potentially hazardous immunosuppressive drugs such as steroids and azathioprine.

CHRONIC LIMB WEAKNESS

Although the disorders described above typically evolve over days and weeks there is some overlap with the disorders described in this section which normally evolve over weeks and months. For example some cases of polymyositis and myasthenia gravis may evolve with a more chronic time course. The commonest neurologi-

cal disorders causing limb weakness which evolve over a chronic time course include motor neurone disease, most neuropathies and many genetic muscle diseases (such as the muscular dystrophies).

Motor neurone disease. This disease is characterized pathologically by premature degeneration of populations of motor neurones. The precise mode of clinical presentation depends on which populations of motor neurones are involved. Broadly, there are three main populations: upper motor neurones located in the motor cortices, lower motor neurones in the brain stem (the bulbar motor neurones) and lower motor neurones located in the anterior horn of the spinal cord. Although patients tend to present with symptoms and signs chiefly due to loss of neurones in predominantly one of these three regions there is overlap. Indeed, careful examination will show that most patients have a combination of upper and lower motor neurone signs and indeed this combination of signs is an important clue to the diagnosis.

Patients with a bulbar presentation may present with dysphagia, dysarthria or a change in the quality of their voice (dysphonia). Examination will often show fasciculation in the tongue. Fasciculation is a lower motor neurone sign which is often particularly prominent when the site of the lower motor neurone lesion is at the level of the motor neurone cell body. There may be a slurring dysarthria and nasal speech. The cough may be weak.

In the spinal muscular atrophy variant the main signs are lower motor neurone signs in the limbs reflecting predominant degeneration in the anterior horn cells. Patients complain of weakness, and muscle cramps are a common feature in this form of the disease. Fasciculation is prominent and the weakness is often global but asymmetric. The reflexes are typically lost and sensory testing is normal.

In the predominantly upper motor neurone variant (**amyotrophic lateral sclerosis**) the patient may present with asymmetrical upper motor neurone signs in the limbs.

Some patients present with a weakness and wasting and lower motor neurone signs in a single limb (so-called monomelic motor neurone disease). Careful investigation is required in this group of patients to rule out another cause such as multiple radiculopathy. Poliomyelitis can also result in a weak and wasted limb but the distinction is usually clear since polio is typically a childhood event and the limb changes are therefore usually of long standing.

As the disease progresses all patients develop a combination of upper and lower motor neurone signs. In some patients upper motor neurone dysfunction may affect the bulbar motor system. Such patients may have a characteristic strained dysarthria and prominent emotional lability (this combination is known as a pseudobulbar palsy).

At presentation other diagnoses may need to be considered. For example, a patient may present with a predominant spastic paraparesis in which case spinal cord imaging may be needed to rule out a compressive lesion. Bladder involvement is not a feature of motor neurone disease but is common in compressive spinal cord disease and this may therefore be a helpful pointer. Imaging of the spinal cord is still required. Electrophysiological studies are helpful since they can confirm denervation in the presence of normal nerve conduction, a combination of changes characteristic of anterior horn cell disease. Such changes are often detectable by EMG even before lower motor neurone signs are evident clinically and this may be particularly helpful in achieving a diagnosis in a predominant upper motor neurone presentation. Sometimes it is only by following the patient up that the diagnosis of motor neurone disease becomes clear. This is usually because with time the patient who was initially monomelic lower motor neurone develops upper motor neurone signs. It is important to remember that the sensory system is not involved and therefore sensory signs are not compatible with the diagnosis.

There are a large number of causes of **peripheral neuropathies**. Important causes include diabetes, excess alcohol, vitamin B_{12} deficiency, drug exposure (e.g. cytotoxics used in cancer), paraneoplastic and genetic.

Most of these common causes result in mixed peripheral neuropathies in which the patient has a combination of motor and sensory symptoms and signs. When the motor component of the nerves is significantly involved the patient complains of weakness. This typically begins in the distal lower limbs. The patient may describe weakness around the ankle which is a reflection of distal muscle weakness. Later the upper limbs are affected, again starting distally.

Examination of gait is essential. There may be a bilateral foot drop gait due to anterior tibialis weakness. The patient may have difficulty standing on tiptoe reflecting weakness of plantar flexion. There will be other lower motor neurone signs including loss of ankle reflexes and, later, other lower and upper limb weakness. Depending on the degree of sensory nerve involvement there may be sensory signs such as reduced pin-prick and light touch. Initially this is in a stocking distribution but later may spread to the hands. The combination of distal weakness and sensory symptoms should always make the clinician suspicious that a neuropathy is the cause of weakness in a patient.

The muscular dystrophies

The commonest genetic muscle diseases are the muscular dystrophies. There are many types but the commonest are Duchenne, Becker and myotonic dystrophy. Duchenne and Becker are disorders affecting males caused by different mutations in the gene on the X chromosome which codes for a vital muscle membrane protein called dystrophin. Boys with **Duchenne dystrophy** develop proximal lower limb weakness soon after walking. They have prominent calf muscles and contracted Achilles tendons causing them to 'toe walk'. The calf enlargement is termed pseudohypertrophy since it is caused by replacement of the damaged muscle by fat and fibrous tissue which is functionally useless. The disease progresses rapidly and the proximal upper limb muscles are soon involved. Most boys are wheelchair-bound in their early teens and usually die from cardiac and respiratory muscle involvement in their late teens or early twenties.

Becker's dystrophy may be considered as a 'slow motion' version of Duchenne. The age at onset is later, often in the teens, and the progress is much slower. The pattern of muscle involvement is similar. Patients often have very prominent bulky calf muscles which is a clue to the diagnosis as is a family history. The diagnosis is confirmed by a combination of finding a very elevated creatine kinase (often many thousands), muscle biopsy and genetic testing.

Myotonic dystrophy is the other common genetic muscle disease. Unlike most other muscle diseases, which present with proximal weakness, patients with myotonic dystrophy have distal muscle weakness and wasting. This is often mild or moderate but rarely severe. The patients may notice weakness of hand-grip and a foot-drop gait. The latter would normally lead to suspicions of a neuropathic process, as described above. In addition to this distal weakness there is often facial weakness and bilateral sternomastoid muscle weakness and wasting.

One of the important clinical features is myotonia. Myotonia is the inability of a contracted muscle to relax at the normal rate. Patients notice they have difficulty releasing their grip when opening jars or doors. It can usually be demonstrated clinically by asking the

Box 30.2 Important causes of peripheral neuropathy

- Diabetes mellitus
- Acute post-infective polyneuritis (GBS)
- Vitamin B_{12} deficiency
- Chronic alcoholism
- Polyarteritis nodosa
- Carcinomatous neuropathy
- Drugs, e.g. vincristine, vinblastine

patient to clench the fist very tight and then to open it rapidly. The patient is unable to rapidly extend the fingers and does this only very slowly. In addition to these muscle features patients with myotonic dystrophy have a number of other symptoms which indicate that this is a multi-system genetic disease. Indeed it is not uncommon for patients to present to medical specialties other than neurology. Common systemic features include premature cataracts, premature frontal pattern balding, mild mental retardation, diabetes mellitus, subfertility, cardiomyopathy and gastrointestinal dysmotility. The diagnosis is often straightforward on clinical grounds alone. This is an autosomal dominant disorder and there is often a family history which can aid the diagnosis. The genetic defect (a trinucleotide repeat expansion near a protein kinase gene on chromosome 19) leading to the disease is known and genetic testing is available.

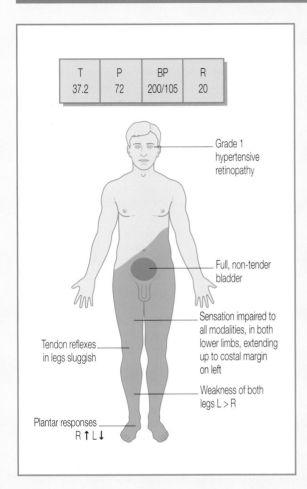

T	P	BP	R
37.2	72	200/105	20

Grade 1 hypertensive retinopathy

Full, non-tender bladder

Sensation impaired to all modalities, in both lower limbs, extending up to costal margin on left

Tendon reflexes in legs sluggish

Weakness of both legs L > R

Plantar responses
R ↑ L ↓

A 49-year-old businessman consulted his general practitioner because of low lumbar pain which had come on gradually over the previous 10 days. The pain was dull and aching and had developed after a long car journey. It troubled him especially at night and also if he coughed or strained. He had continued working during this time, taking large amounts of aspirin. Initially this controlled the pain but had subsequently proved ineffective. Furthermore, over the preceding few days the pain had begun to spread into his right buttock and down the back of the right thigh.

In the past he had been generally well except for a previous episode of back pain 8 years ago which had responded to bed rest. He was known to be mildly hypertensive and had been taking a thiazide diuretic for several years. He smoked 20 cigarettes daily and drank fairly heavily, mainly in the context of his job. His father and one brother had both died from myocardial infarction.

Examination revealed an obese man, pulse 72 regular. Blood pressure 200/105. The fundi showed Grade I changes. There was loss of the normal lumbar lordosis and the lumbar spine was a little tender on percussion. Straight leg raising on the right was limited to 60° and on the left to 80°.

He was admitted to a private nursing home for bed rest and over the next 2 weeks his symptoms and signs improved rapidly.

Routine investigation showed: Hb 16.5 g/dl. WBC and differential normal. ESR 28 mm in 1 hour. Urea 4.8 mmol/l. MSU: normal. CXR showed slight cardiomegaly but was otherwise clear. X-ray of the spine showed early spondylitic changes, with narrowing of the disc spaces of L4/L5 and L5/S1.

He was being considered for discharge when he complained that for the previous 24 hours he felt his legs had become weak and that he had difficulty in walking to the toilet. He had also noticed some hesitancy in his micturition. He had not passed urine for 12 hours.

Examination (see diagram) revealed a full bladder which was not tender. The prostate appeared normal. There was weakness of both legs, more marked on the left, tone was not obviously abnormal, and the tendon reflexes in the legs were sluggish. The plantar response was thought to be extensor on the right and equivocal on the left. Sensory testing revealed some impairment of all modalities in both lower limbs, and this extended up to the costal margin on the left. No abnormality was found in the upper limbs.

Questions

1. What are the likely reasons for this patient's sudden deterioration?
2. What would be your immediate management?

Early in his illness the patient was thought to have a mechanical derangement of the lumbosacral region; probably a prolapsed disc with root pressure. The story he gave was completely compatible with such a diagnosis, both in the nature and site of his pain, its relationship to coughing and sneezing (manoeuvres which raise the CSF pressure) and its pattern of radiation. Prolapsed intervertebral disc (PID) is undoubtedly the commonest cause of such a syndrome, but it is important to remember that many other disease processes can produce nerve root compression and present in a similar manner.

His obesity and the fact that he had suffered an episode of back pain in the past support the diagnosis of PID, while the findings of local tenderness, loss of the lumbar lordosis, and limitation of straight leg raising are indicative of local pathology with root irritation. His investigations are also compatible with this diagnosis, except that the ESR is a little high. His initial management, therefore, with bed rest was reasonable. Usually this would be combined with a low-calorie reducing diet, sedation and analgesia.

His obesity, heavy cigarette smoking, hypertension, and bad family history also suggest that he is a candidate for vascular disease and that the rare condition of spinal artery occlusion must be considered.

The deterioration which occurred shortly before his discharge is obviously a very sinister event. The difficulty with micturition, the extensor plantar response, and the sensory level suggest a lesion involving the spinal cord rather than the nerve roots. This could obviously not occur with a disc lesion at the level of L5/S1. Higher disc lesions may occur but are very rare.

The common causes of a clinical picture of this type are very varied. Trauma is a frequent reason, but is self-evident and not relevant here. Demyelinating disease, either the common multiple sclerosis or the rare variant neuromyelitis optica may present in this way. However, there have been no previous episodes of neurological disease, there are no signs of lesions elsewhere in the nervous system, and he is a little old for this disease.

Furthermore, it would not explain his initial presentation with back pain and root irritation.

A transverse myelitis can result from infection. This may occur as a result of local infections, either tuberculous or pyogenic, spreading to involve the cord and its blood supply, or it may be as a complication of one of the common exanthemata such as herpes zoster. There is no history of recent infection in this patient and such an interpretation is unlikely.

Neoplastic disease may involve the meninges either directly or by spread from the vertebral bodies. This can result from disseminated carcinoma, and may also be a complication of the lymphomas and leukaemias. Initial presentation of the disease with a neurological syndrome such as cord compression is well recognized, and must certainly be considered here. He is a heavy smoker and carcinoma of the bronchus is not excluded by a single normal chest X-ray. Primary tumours of the meninges and nerve roots such as meningioma and neurofibroma can cause spinal cord compression, but usually there is a longer story of progressive disability.

The most important investigation in this patient is further radiology. Myelography should be performed. In addition to showing any block, it may, by indicating the exact site of any pathological lesion, also suggest its nature.

Radioisotope scanning of the skeleton may show evidence of any disseminated malignancy and is more sensitive in showing metastases than conventional radiology early on. If leukaemia or lymphoma is suspected a marrow aspiration is indicated.

In this patient lumbar puncture showed the typical changes of spinal block and myelography showed that this was due to an extramedullary, extradural lesion at the level of D6. Emergency laminectomy at this level revealed extensive tumour tissue spreading from the vertebral bodies, and histology showed this to be probably anaplastic carcinoma of the bronchus. This was confirmed by the later progression of the disease.

31

Movement disorders

The term 'movement disorder' relates to those neurological diseases in which the patient experiences a disturbance of movement. This disturbance cannot be attributed to weakness or sensory loss. In general, movement disorders are caused by diseases which result in dysfunction of the basal ganglia. The basal ganglia are grey-matter structures located deep within the brain; they are also sometimes termed the deep nuclei. The basal ganglia have complex connections to many parts of the CNS including the cerebral cortex, the cerebellum and the spinal cord. The main function of the basal ganglia is to control voluntary movements.

In general, patients with movement disorders present with one of two broad categories of symptoms, either hypokinetic or hyperkinetic. Hypokinetic movement disorders are characterized by a poverty and slowness of voluntary movements which may amount to an akinetic rigid syndrome. In contrast, patients with hyperkinetic movement disorders experience excessive abnormal and uncontrolled involuntary movements also termed dyskinesias. There are five main types of dyskinesia: tremor, chorea, myoclonus, tics and dystonia.

HYPOKINETIC MOVEMENT DISORDERS

Parkinson's disease

Idiopathic Parkinson's disease is the commonest hypokinetic movement disorder. It usually begins over the age of 40. It is a slowly progressive degenerative disease of the basal ganglia. Degeneration begins in dopamine-producing cells located in the substantia nigra which send axonal projections to the basal ganglia. The symptoms are therefore due to a deficiency of brain dopamine. The precise cause of the dopaminergic cell degeneration is unknown and there is no laboratory test for Parkinson's disease. The diagnosis is achieved by careful consideration of the patient's symptoms and signs and also by the response to dopaminergic drugs.

The characteristic clinical features are resting tremor, general slowness in all voluntary movements (bradykinesia), postural and gait abnormalities and muscle rigidity. The typical tremor is mainly present at rest, often asymmetrical and described as 'pill-rolling' in nature. Many patients also have a tremor of the outstretched hands (known as a postural tremor), but the resting tremor is generally the most prominent. The tremor is intensified by mental or emotional stress but disappears during sleep.

One of the most disabling symptoms for patients with Parkinson's disease is the general slowness in all voluntary movements (bradykinesia). They experience a slowness to initiate and execute all movements. The more complex the movement the greater the effect of bradykinesia. Repetitive movements tend to become progressively slower often also reducing in amplitude. A common consequence of this is that the patient may notice the tendency of their writing to become smaller (micrographia), at first most noticeable towards the end of a sentence.

Movements required to produce facial expression are reduced and the patient typically has a blank, expressionless facial appearance, often leading to a mistaken diagnosis of depression. The gait in Parkinson's disease is typically slow. The patient walks without swinging the arms and tends to lean forwards with a stooped posture taking small shuffling steps. As the patient walks there is a tendency to try and catch up with their displaced centre of gravity resulting in the gait becoming faster and faster – this is termed festination. Some patients experience episodes of freezing during walking in which they become rooted to the spot.

Muscle rigidity is usually present from an early stage and affects axial muscles (in other words, the muscles around the vertebral column) and limb muscles. Axial muscle rigidity typically causes difficulty turning, either when walking or turning over in bed for example. Limb muscle rigidity may be appreciated if the examiner passively moves a joint. For example, if the examiner passively flexes and extends the wrist he or she will become aware of a uniform resistance to this movement because of an increase in muscle tone rigidity. This is quite different to the non-uniform resistance to such movement in the patient with a pyramidal increase in muscle tone (e.g. a stroke patient) where there is 'clasp-knife' rigidity. This increase in muscle tone in patients with Parkinson's disease is sometimes termed lead-pipe rigidity or an extrapyramidal increase in tone (to distinguish it from a pyramidal increase in tone). The combination of resting tremor and lead-pipe rigidity is sometimes termed cogwheel rigidity.

The diagnosis of Parkinson's disease is usually straightforward when the patient has the combination of features described. In the early stages of the disease the diagnosis may be more difficult. A positive response to the administration of a dopaminergic drug can be helpful.

In addition to idiopathic Parkinson's disease there are a number of other disorders which may result in a very similar clinical picture and therefore need to be considered in the differential diagnosis. It is helpful to divide the differential diagnosis into two groups – those patients with Parkinsonism and those with Parkinsonism 'plus'. The term Parkinsonism is used to refer to patients who have the characteristic features of idiopathic Parkinson's disease. In addition to idiopathic Parkinson's disease the most important cause of Parkinsonism is neuroleptic drugs (so-called drug-induced Parkinsonism). The term Parkinsonism 'plus' is used to refer to patients who have not only the typical features of idiopathic Parkinson's disease but also have additional clinical features not present in idiopathic Parkinson's disease.

Drug-induced Parkinsonism. A number of drugs block dopamine receptors in the basal ganglia and may result in Parkinsonism. The most important group of such drugs are the neuroleptics. These drugs are most commonly used in psychiatric practice to treat patients with psychotic illnesses such as schizophrenia. Commonly used drugs include phenothiazines such as chlorpromazine, butyrophenones such as haloperidol, thioxanthines such as flupentixol and benzamides such as sulpiride. These drugs may be used in other settings: for example chlorpromazine may be used to calm the acutely agitated or aggressive patient and metoclopramide (a benzamide) is an anti-nausea drug in common use. It is therefore important to take a careful drug and psychiatric history in any patient presenting with Parkinsonism.

Box 31.1 Causes of Parkinsonism and Parkinsonism 'plus'

Parkinsonism	Parkinsonism 'plus'
• Idiopathic Parkinson's disease	• Progressive supranuclear palsy (Steele–Richardson–Olszewski disease)
• Drug-induced Parkinsonism	• Multiple systems atrophy
• Wilson's disease	• Corticobasal degeneration

Wilson's disease

Wilson's disease is an autosomal recessive disorder of copper metabolism. The primary abnormality is an inability to excrete copper because of defective transport. Copper is consequently deposited in large amounts in various body tissues. In the brain, copper is particularly deposited in the basal ganglia causing neuronal damage. This often results in movement disorders. Parkinsonism is one of the commonest consequences, although other movement disorders such as dystonia or tremor may occur. Parkinsonism due to Wilson's disease develops early – often before 20 years. Since idiopathic Parkinsonism is generally a late onset disease (after 40 years) any patient presenting with young-onset Parkinsonism should be screened for Wilson's disease by performing copper studies. The serum caeruloplasmin is elevated and the free serum copper is usually reduced. Copper is also deposited in Descement's membrane in the cornea. This results in a characteristic greenish-brown pigmentation around the margin of the cornea – the Kayser–Fleischer. This is a clinical indication of the diagnosis.

Steele–Richardson–Olszewski syndrome

This is an uncommon neurodegenerative disorder characterized by bradykinesia and muscle rigidity (particularly axial), usually without tremor. The main distinguishing clinical feature from other forms of Parkinsonism is that the patients develop a very specific disorder of voluntary eye movements known as a **supranuclear gaze palsy**. This results in the patient being unable to voluntarily direct gaze. Initially this is impaired in a vertical direction and later in a horizontal direction. Ultimately the patients can only direct gaze by turning their head. The symptoms do not respond to dopamine.

Multiple systems atrophy

Patients with multiple systems atrophy usually exhibit an akinetic rigid syndrome similar to idiopathic Parkinson's disease, but they also have additional clinical features. These may include prominent autonomic failure or prominent cerebellar ataxia. These patients are not responsive to dopamine and the disease usually progresses much more quickly than idiopathic Parkinson's disease.

Corticobasal degeneration

In this rare neurodegenerative disorder there is neuronal cell loss in parts of the cerebral cortex as well as in the basal ganglia. Patients therefore present with focal cortical defects in addition to an akinetic rigid syndrome. The commonest presentation is a combination of apraxia (caused by neuronal cell loss in the parietal cortex) and Parkinsonism.

HYPERKINETIC MOVEMENT DISORDERS – THE DYSKINESIAS

The initial step in assessing a patient with a hyperkinetic movement disorder is to observe the abnormal involuntary movement the patient exhibits and decide into which of the five main categories it falls. Having categorized the dyskinesia the differential diagnosis of that dyskinesia should be considered. The common causes are outlined below.

Tremor

Tremor is usually a rhythmic sinusoidal movement. It is helpful to determine when the tremor is maximal. Three main types of tremor are distinguished on this basis: rest tremor, postural tremor and action tremor. The commonest cause of a **rest tremor** is idiopathic Parkinson's disease and is typically pill-rolling in nature (i.e. a pronation-supination movement at the wrist). The commonest **postural tremor** is known as essential tremor (also known as familial tremor). Essential tremor is maximal on adopting a posture, such as holding the hands straight out in front. It usually begins in the hands but may spread to involve the legs and head. Patients complain of difficulty holding drinks and spillage and untidy writing. Some patients find alcohol improves the tremor. Essential tremor often runs in families as an autosomal dominant trait. Physiological tremor is also a postural tremor. Under normal circumstances it does not cause any functional disability. However, in states of anxiety or in thyrotoxicosis it may become more prominent. **Action tremor** (also called intention tremor) is caused by disease of the cerebellum and its connections to the brain stem. Typically patients experience tremor as they approach a target object. This is usually demonstrated by asking the patient to touch their own nose and then to touch the examiner's finger held in front of the patient. Such patients develop tremor as their finger approaches the target and often miss the target. Common causes of action tremor include multiple sclerosis and alcoholic cerebellar damage.

Chorea

Chorea is a series of jerk-like semi-purposeful movements that flit from one part of the body to another.

They are continuous and random. Any part of the body may be affected including the face. The actual movements are usually small: for example, small flicking movements of the fingers or twitching movements of the face. Causes include Sydenham's chorea, which follows streptococcal rheumatic fever, and Huntington's chorea. Systemic disorders may also cause chorea: these include thyrotoxicosis, polycythaemia rubra vera, hypoparathyroidism, systemic lupus erythematosus and the anti-phospholipid syndrome.

Huntington's chorea is an autosomal dominant neurodegenerative disorder. Typically it develops in the mid-30s and comprises a triad of chorea, psychiatric disturbance and dementia. It is relentlessly progressive and death usually occurs 10–15 years after the onset.

Myoclonus

Myoclonic movements are brief shock-like movements. The muscle jerks are intermittent, unlike the continuous movements in chorea and may result in large movements as well as small movements. Myoclonic jerks may affect one part of the body (focal) or be generalized. Myoclonus may occur in diseases in which there is degeneration of the cerebral cortex such as Alzheimer's disease and Creutzfeldt–Jakob disease. It may also be caused by systemic metabolic disorders including uraemia, hepatic failure (asterixis is a form of myoclonus), respiratory failure, hypocalcaemia and drugs (e.g. phenytoin).

Tic

Tics are small jerk-like movements which usually affect the face and to a lesser extent the upper limbs; tics do not usually affect the lower limbs. The main distinguishing feature from chorea and myoclonus is that they are repetitive and stereotyped. Typical tics in the face include repetitive blinking, sniffing or lip smacking. Tics are common and may be a transient disorder in childhood or may be part of a more generalized behavioural disorder which is probably genetic (Gilles de la Tourette syndrome).

Dystonia

Dystonia is characterized by sustained, often irregular, muscle spasms which are frequently prolonged and of longer duration than the movements in chorea, tics or myoclonus. Typically agonist and antagonist muscles co-contract, resulting in distorted and awkward body postures. Dystonia may be confined to one part of the body (focal dystonia) or may be generalized affecting the entire body. Hemidystonia, in which one side of the body is affected, is also recognized. The commonest focal dystonia affects the neck and is known as torticollis (also commonly termed 'wry neck'). In most cases the cause of focal dystonia is unknown but genetic factors are thought to be important. Most generalized dystonias begin in childhood and are often disabling. Several genetic variants are recognized. If hemidystonia is present there is a high probability that there will be structural pathology in the brain, e.g. a stroke or a tumour on the contralateral side.

SUMMARY OF THE CLINICAL APPROACH TO THE PATIENT WITH A MOVEMENT DISORDER

In the patient presenting with an involuntary movement disorder the first step is to decide if there is a relative lack of movement (a hypokinetic disorder) or an excess of involuntary movements (a hyperkinetic disorder). The commonest hypokinetic presentation is Parkinsonism. There may be a history from the patient and relatives of a general slowness in motor tasks such as walking, dressing and eating. The voice often becomes quiet (hypophonia) and relatives often note the blank face. The patient may complain of a resting tremor which may particularly interfere with writing resulting in micrographia. If Parkinsonism is suspected from the history, clues to the possible aetiology should be sought. A drug history should be obtained with particular attention to neuroleptic drugs. In patients under the age of 40 years Wilson's disease should be excluded. Idiopathic Parkinson's disease typically develops over the age of 55 years and slowly progresses over 10–15 years. More rapid progression over just a few years is more suggestive of Multiple Systems Atrophy (MSA) or Progressive Supranuclear Palsy (PSP). Falls within the first two to three years are unusual in idiopathic Parkinson's disease but common in MSA and PSP.

When examining a patient with a history suggestive of Parkinsonism the cardinal signs of tremor, rigidity, akinesia and postural instability should be sought. The presence of at least three of these four features strongly suggests that the patient has Parkinsonism. The presence of additional clinical features may help to determine the cause of the Parkinsonism, for example the typical supranuclear gaze palsy in PSP or postural hypotension suggesting autonomic dysfunction in MSA. Kayser–Fleischer rings may be visible at the bedside using a direct ophthalmoscope, although slit-lamp examination is often needed. Limb apraxia in combination with Parkinsonism suggests corticobasal degeneration.

In patients presenting with hyperkinetic movement disorders clinical observation is usually the first step. This will usually allow the precise type of hyperkinetic disorder to be determined. Tics predominate in the face and upper limbs. They are momentary twitching movements. In the face they may result in transient eye closure or movements of the mouth. If tics are observed, additional behavioural features of Gilles de la Tourette syndrome should be sought. Patients with chorea have jerk-like semi-purposeful movements that flit from one part of the body to another. Unlike tics they are not restricted to the face and upper limbs but may affect lower limbs as well. The sustained spasms of dystonia, resulting in awkward contorted body postures, is usually easy to distinguish from other hyperkinetic movement disorders. In the patient with tremor it is helpful to observe the upper limbs in three different postures; at rest, with sustained posture and with repetitive finger–nose testing. The extrapyramidal tremors, such as in Parkinsonism, are typically maximum at rest and diminish with movement and posture. In patients with essential tremor, adopting sustained postures, such as the arms outstretched, maximizes the tremor. Cerebellar (intention) tremors are most evident on finger–nose testing.

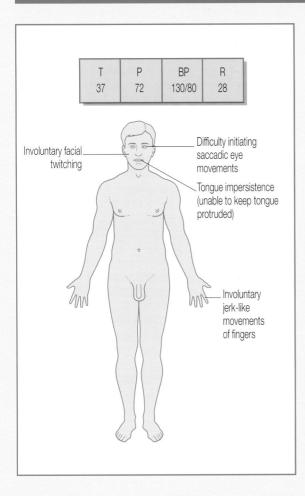

Involuntary facial twitching

Difficulty initiating saccadic eye movements

Tongue impersistence (unable to keep tongue protruded)

Involuntary jerk-like movements of fingers

T	P	BP	R
37	72	130/80	28

A 43-year-old tax accountant presented at the request of his wife. The patient himself did not see any need to come to the doctor and was rather irritated by his wife's insistence. His wife explained that her husband's personality had changed gradually over the preceding 18 months. He had become more irritable and moody. She described that he seemed to have lost interest in family life and also in his previously enjoyed hobby of fishing. He was more impatient and frequently chastized his three children for no good reason. They had become more cautious about upsetting their father. His wife had also become aware of a decline in her husband's work performance. Clients had been phoning their home complaining about errors in tax returns. His wife was also concerned that her husband's alcohol intake had increased substantially and he was drinking a bottle of wine on most days. She commented that he seemed to have become generally 'twitchy' and was always 'on the move', even when sat down. The patient denied these symptoms and explained that he felt his wife was rather neurotic.

Fifteen years earlier the patient had had a bout of severe depression with psychotic features and had been under the care of a psychiatrist for one year. He had received chlorpromazine for 10 months. The patient was one of three brothers aged 33, 43 and 50 years respectively. He had lost contact with his older brother many years ago but his wife had heard a rumour that he was in prison. The patient's mother was alive and well at the age of 72 years but his father had died in a road traffic accident at the age of 32 years. Nothing was known about the patient's father's biological parents as he had been adopted.

On examination the patient had a jocular, slightly disinhibited, affect. He appeared generally anxious and could not sit still. His gait was normal but as he walked there were involuntary jerk-like movements of his fingers. There were similar twitching movements of his face particularly when he closed his eyes. In his cranial nerves he had a full range of eye movements but did have difficulty initiating gaze to either side and had to blink in order to initiate gaze. When asked to protrude his tongue he was unable to maintain this for more than a few seconds after which his tongue would retract. The rest of the neurological examination was normal, and general physical examination was normal.

Questions

1. What is the most likely diagnosis?
2. What further investigations would you undertake?

Discussion

The history of change in personality and loss of interest in activities might suggest that the patient is developing a psychiatric illness such as depression. Alternatively, these symptoms, particularly with a suggestion of disinhibition, might suggest a frontal lobe disorder such as frontal lobe dementia or even a frontal lobe space-occupying lesion. The fact that his wife has brought him to the doctor but the patient does not feel there is anything wrong is significant. This indicates that the patient does not have insight into the changes which his wife has observed. Such a lack of insight should always make the physician suspicious that there is indeed an organic disease present. While the history given by the wife raises a number of possible diagnoses outlined above, the examination findings are very suggestive of one particular diagnosis.

The patient has a movement disorder characterized by involuntary jerk-like movements affecting his hands and face in particular. In addition, it is observed that he cannot sit still and his wife has noticed that he is generally 'twitchy'. These observations all indicate that the patient has chorea. There are a large number of causes of chorea and the following should be considered: hyperthyroidism, polycythaemia rubra vera, hypoparathyroidism, systemic lupus erythematosus, and anti-phospholipid syndrome. There may be additional clinical clues on examination to each of these. However, in this case the combination of psychiatric symptoms and chorea strongly point to a diagnosis of Huntington's chorea. The cranial nerve examination also points to this diagnosis. Difficulty with initiating gaze and difficulty keeping the tongue protruded (tongue impersistence) are highly suggestive of Huntington's chorea.

Huntington's chorea is an autosomal dominant disease with full penetrance. New mutations in the Huntington's gene without family history are exceptionally rare and one might therefore question the diagnosis in the apparent absence of the family history. However, on closer scrutiny there are features in the family history which are suspicious and which are not uncommonly seen in families with Huntington's chorea.

First, the patient's father died at a young age, 32 years, following a road traffic accident. Since the symptoms of Huntington's chorea typically develop over the age of 35 years it is possible that the father was a gene carrier but died before he manifested any symptoms. Since the patient's father was adopted it is not possible to establish whether there was any preceding family history in the patient's father's side of the family.

The patient's mother is well at the age of 72 years so it is unlikely that she is the gene carrier since she would almost certainly have developed symptoms by this age.

Second, there is the rumour that the patient's brother may be in prison. Some patients with Huntington's disease commit crimes because of their disturbed psychiatric state. It is a possibility that this may be the case with the patient's brother.

The patient should have a brain scan to exclude frontal lobe pathology such as a space-occupying lesion or focal atrophy that might be seen in certain dementias. The brain scan is generally normal in Huntington's disease except in the late stages when caudate atrophy may be seen. The definitive test to confirm the diagnosis is to sequence the Huntington's gene on chromosome 4. Patients affected with Huntington's chorea have an expanded triplet repeat nucleotide sequence (CAG) within this gene. It is important to obtain the patient's consent to having this test and that he is counselled fully about the implications of a positive gene test result for himself and for his children. Since this is an autosomal dominant condition any offspring of an affected individual are at a 50% risk of inheriting the disease gene and therefore of developing the disease.

> The patient had an MRI brain scan which was normal. He consented to the genetic test, which was positive confirming a diagnosis of Huntington's chorea. It transpired that his brother did indeed have the same disease. The patient subsequently developed worsening chorea and dementia and eventually became bed-bound. He died from the complications of immobility at the age of 54 years.

32

Haematuria

The passage of blood in the urine is an important symptom of disease of the kidneys and urinary tract. It is more often detected on urine examination than it is reported by patients. About 5 ml of blood in a litre of urine are visible to the naked eye. After some hours the blood appears as a brown discoloration rather than a red colour recognizable as bleeding. For this reason the symptom may not be reliably reported in a patient suspected of renal or urinary disease. Other substances may colour the urine red, including drugs such as phenindione and rifampicin, and foods such as beetroot. When there is intravascular haemolysis, free haemoglobin may be present in the urine and myoglobin may be passed in rhabdomyolysis.

The routine tests for blood in the urine used in the clinic depend on the reaction of haemoglobin with o-toluidine. If positive the test should therefore lead to the urine being examined for red cells which will be absent in haemoglobinuria. Microscopy should be performed on freshly voided urine since red cells lyse when the urine stands for some time. Microscopy may also show red-cell or white-cell casts, which are important indicators of renal disease. An experienced microscopist may be able to give a more precise indication of the cause of the bleeding. When red cells are extruded through the glomerulus they take on bizarre forms whereas frank bleeding from a tumour or inflammation leads to red cells with a normal morphology.

Tests for protein in the urine will not always be positive if there is a positive test for haemoglobin. This is because bleeding alone may not produce enough protein in the urine to give a positive test unless there is about ten times the amount of blood required to give a positive test for blood i.e. about 40–50 ml. If protein is present in a lightly bloodstained urine this is an indication that the cause is at the level of the glomerulus.

Some of the most important causes of haematuria are shown in Box 32.1. The confirmation that there is blood in the urine should be followed by taking a detailed history that is relevant to these causes. Pain in the loin may indicate a stone, infection or tumour in the kidney or ureter. Frequency and dysuria, a renal tract infection, difficulty in passing urine, urgency and poor stream may be caused by prostatic hypertrophy or cancer. The passage of frankly bloodstained urine in the absence of other urinary symptoms suggests a tumour or polyp in the bladder or a renal carcinoma. Chronic analgesic taking may point towards renal papillary necrosis which may present with haematuria or colic as the papilla is passed into the ureter.

Physical examination is likely to be unrewarding. An elevated blood pressure raises the possibility of a primary renal disorder such as glomerulonephritis or pyelonephritis. There may be signs of a generalized bleeding disorder, such as bruising or purpura (see Ch. 19). There may be enlargement of one or both kidneys suggesting a renal tumour or polycystic disease respectively. There may be tenderness over the bladder prostate or kidney suggesting the possibility of infection at one of these sites.

Further investigation will depend on the age of the patient and the associated physical signs, as well as the urinary findings. It is useful to consider the clinical approach according to the presentation. Fig. 32.1 summarizes an approach to investigation.

Symptomless haematuria

In young people it is very likely that recurrent isolated haematuria will not have an identifiable cause. If there are red-cell casts and abnormal shapes it is likely that the cause is glomerular. There are three common forms of glomerular disease that are responsible: **IgA nephropathy** typically occurs in men aged 20–30; they have episodes of pharyngitis and myalgia followed within 24 hours by frank haematuria lasting 2–6 days. The episodes are recurrent and may be accompanied by hypertension and impairment of renal function. The urine contains dysmorphic red cells and casts of red and white cells. The episodes remit spontaneously but recur. With time there may be a slow decline in renal function, although this may happen quickly in a minority of patients. The cause is unknown but the lesions are thought to be deposits of IgA immune complexes. Dense deposits of IgA are present in the mesangium. There is segmental glomerular damage, and proliferative changes including crescent formation are often present. Similar pathology occurs in **Henoch–Schönlein purpura** which is also accompanied by haematuria and urinary casts. In this disorder the cutaneous lesions and joint symptoms usually indicate the diagnosis. The renal disease is more severe in adults.

Another glomerular condition presenting as repeated episodes of haematuria with normal renal

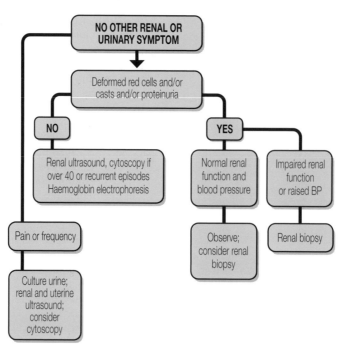

Fig. 32.1 A guide to the investigation of haematuria.

Box 32.1 Causes of haematuria

Tumours
Kidney
    hypernephroma, transitional cell carcinoma
Bladder and ureter
    transitional cell carcinoma, squamous carcinoma,
      polyps, in situ carcinoma
Prostate carcinoma

Glomerular pathology
    IgA nephropathy, glomerulonephritis, vasculitis,
      Henoch–Schönlein purpura

Renal medullary disorders
    Papillary necrosis (sickle cell disease, analgesics,
      diabetes)
    Medullary sponge kidney

Infection
    Pyelonephritis, cystitis, prostatitis, tuberculosis,
      schistosomiasis

Stones and trauma

Coagulation disorders

Factitious

---

function is the condition known as **benign familial haematuria**. In this condition there is microscopic haematuria which is persistent. Renal function is usually normal and there is usually a family history. Renal biopsy, not necessary if there is a clear family history, shows thin basement membranes without inflammation.

A less common familial form of glomerular disease which may present as haematuria, usually inherited as an X-linked dominant trait, is **Alport's syndrome** of glomerulonephritis and bilateral sensorineural deafness. This typically presents as gross haematuria in the first years of life and continues as microscopic haematuria and proteinuria. The renal disease usually presents before deafness is clinically apparent. In patients from Africa the possibility of **schistosomiasis** must be borne in mind, especially if the haematuria occurs at the end of micturition. The centrifuged urine may contain the eggs of *Schistosoma haematobium*. African patients may have **sickle-cell trait** which predisposes to renal papillary necrosis. In sickle-cell trait the sickle screening test is positive and haemoglobin electrophoresis shows 30–50% HbS.

If the urine contains red cell or white cell casts and abnormal red cell forms, it is likely that the cause is at the level of the glomerulus. The presence of proteinuria will support this and tests for renal function may be abnormal. A renal biopsy may be necessary for diagnosis if a glomerular cause is suspected and there is not a clear familial history. If there are no casts or abnormal red cell forms it is common to perform a cystoscopy preceded by an intravenous urogram (IVU) but it is very likely that no abnormality of the kidney or urinary tract will be found in European patients below the age of 40.

In patients over 40 the possibility of a tumour as the cause of haematuria is much greater. The commonest renal cancer is renal carcinoma or hypernephroma. The tumour usually presents with haematuria or pain in the loin. A mass may be palpable on examination. Systemic manifestations may be present such as fever, hypercalcaemia and erythrocytosis. The diagnosis is made by ultrasound examination of the kidney. Transitional cell carcinoma may arise in the renal medulla, along the ureter and in the bladder. The presentation may be with bleeding or with pain especially when ureteric obstruction occurs. Bladder polyps frequently bleed. Carcinoma of the prostate may invade the urethra and present with bleeding.

In each case the bleeding is of fresh blood without casts or deformed red cells and usually without significant proteinuria unless the bleeding is heavy. Investigation includes ultrasound examination of the kidney, cystoscopy and biopsy and occasionally intravenous urography.

Haematuria with associated symptoms

Pain and haematuria. Renal pain is usually a dull pain felt in the loin. It may occur with bleeding into a tumour, pelvicalyceal stones, blood clot in the renal pelvis, bleeding into a cyst in polycystic disease and acute pyelonephritis.

Ureteric pain is felt as renal colic – typically agonizing causing restlessness, nausea and sweating. It is usually caused by a renal stone and there may be associated bleeding. Blood clot can itself cause renal colic, for example from a renal tumour or papillary necrosis. A particularly difficult diagnostic problem is presented by patients who have recurrent attacks of renal loin pain associated with haematuria with no cause being obvious clinically. The patients are usually young women and there may be a history of previously diagnosed renal stones; investigation is unproductive of a diagnosis. The history may sometimes be complicated by heavy analgesic use. The question of factitious haematuria may be raised, especially if the patient has medical knowledge or employment. The symptoms may respond to analgesics and tend to remit over a period of years.

Frequency and haematuria. Infection of the lower urinary tract often causes frequency and may cause haematuria if the mucosa is sufficiently inflamed. Acute infection may be superimposed on other bladder pathology such as a tumour or chronic infection with tuberculosis or schistosomiasis. Urine culture will usually give a diagnosis, but if the bleeding is extensive, or if it occurs in a man cystoscopy will be indicated.

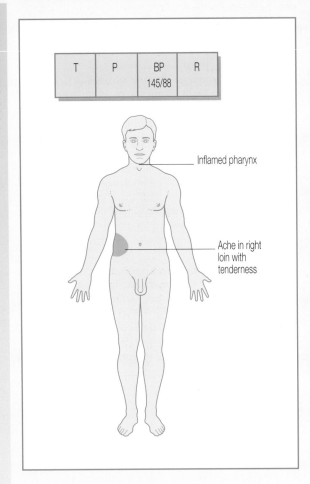

T	P	BP	R
		145/88	

Inflamed pharynx

Ache in right loin with tenderness

A 22-year-old male technician in a hospital biochemistry department consulted his family doctor with the complaint that he had passed bright red blood for 2 days some 10 days earlier. He had noticed the symptom after

he had developed a sore throat and muscle aches and pains. Subsequently his upper respiratory symptoms had settled and the urine had returned to a normal colour. There were no abnormalities on physical examination; his BP was 126/84. The urine contained no blood or protein. Urine culture was sterile and blood urea and electrolytes were all normal.

In the past he had suffered from episodes of severe headache for which he regularly took paracetamol or ibuprofen. These headaches had the features of tension headaches, tending to be felt in the vertex of the skull and made worse by stress. There were no migrainous features and no relevant family history.

He was advised to return to work and to report any further symptoms. He was well until 7 months later when he had another episode of upper respiratory infection again accompanied by fever and 24 hours of blood-stained urine. These symptoms passed quickly and he did not consult his doctor until 8 months later when he had a severe sore throat and bright red blood in the urine accompanied by aching in the right loin. On this occasion he was tender over the right kidney, BP was 145/88, there was blood in the urine on routine testing with a trace of protein. Blood urea and electrolytes were normal, as was the full blood count. ESR was 34 mm/1 h.

Questions

1. What is the differential diagnosis?
2. What further investigations are necessary?

Discussion

Recurrent haematuria occurring in a man of this age, accompanied by symptoms of acute upper respiratory infection, point to a diagnosis of IgA nephropathy. This would be the starting point in considering the case. There are, however, other features of the illness that raise the possibility of other diagnoses. He has had aching in the right loin which is not usual in IgA nephropathy and may indicate local renal pathology such as infection, tumour or stone. He works in a biochemical laboratory in a hospital and has a history suggestive of tension headaches for which he was taking an unspecified amount of analgesics. These features raise the possibilities of analgesic consumption associated with acute papillary necrosis and of factitious haematuria in a medical laboratory worker.

Physical examination on the second attendance revealed a mildly raised blood pressure. This may indicate underlying renal pathology such as glomerulonephritis, or may be due to anxiety. The slightly raised ESR is compatible with an inflammatory process in the kidney but otherwise uncontributory except that it makes a factitious cause less likely.

The trace of protein in the urine supports a glomerular cause of the haematuria. The next step should be microscopy of the centrifuged urine and its examination by a skilled interpreter. This may show red cell casts and deformed red cells if there is a glomerular cause of the haematuria. White cell casts would also strongly suggest a glomerular cause. An ultrasound of both kidneys should be performed to determine if there is dilatation of the renal pelvicalyceal system suggestive of obstruction due to stone or a necrosed papilla. This examination will also be valuable to exclude a tumour or polycystic disease. Urine culture should be performed to exclude acute infection.

If the ultrasound is normal and there are casts or abnormal red cells in the urine consideration would need to be given to a renal biopsy at some stage. It may be reasonable to postpone this for the time being if he is not too anxious about the diagnosis, but careful observation of renal function and blood pressure will be necessary in view of the slightly elevated values at the last consultation.

> Examination of the centrifuged urine showed deformed red cells and some red cell casts. An ultrasound of the kidneys showed no abnormality. Urine culture was sterile. His blood pressure returned to normal. He elected to forgo a renal biopsy. In the next 2 years he had two further attacks of haematuria and finally had a renal biopsy when his serum creatinine was found to be slightly elevated. The biopsy showed typical changes of IgA nephropathy.

Polyuria

Thirst and drinking habits are greatly influenced by social factors, and therefore the daily urine output varies greatly from one individual to another. Polyuria as a symptom means that the patient considers he is passing more urine than he should. There may or may not be associated frequency of micturition, or nocturia. Frequency – which is a common symptom of urinary tract infection – is not the same as polyuria, although the two symptoms may be confused by the patient. If the patient who has noticed polyuria has not also developed an increased thirst, then – with a few important exceptions – the complaint is unlikely to have an organic basis. The cause of polyuria can often be determined by the history and physical examination alone.

THE REGULATION OF PLASMA OSMOLALITY

A normal person's intake of water is greatly dependent on social and cultural habits. The sensation of thirst does not relate precisely therefore to any single physiological event. It is of course true that dehydration will give rise to thirst, but the strength of the response will vary greatly from one individual to another. There is no sensation which restrains a fully hydrated person from continuing to drink.

If there is excessive loss of water from any cause, the osmotic pressure of the plasma rises (this is measured in milliosmoles/kg and is termed osmolality). This rise in osmolality causes a sensation of thirst and the release of ADH. ADH binds to a receptor (designated the V_2 receptor) on the distal tubule and collecting ducts, and increases reabsorption of water through a cyclic AMP-mediated mechanism, the urine becoming concentrated with a high osmolality. Conversely, if more water is drunk than is needed to replace obligatory losses, plasma osmolality falls. ADH release is inhibited, and a dilute urine (with low osmolality) is passed (Fig. 33.1).

Diabetes insipidus

Diabetes insipidus can arise if there is either no effective ADH formation or release – such as occurs in pituitary tumours – or if the formation and release of ADH is normal but the kidneys are unresponsive to its action: 'nephrogenic' diabetes insipidus. Both these

---

Box 33.1 Causes of polyuria

1. Primary polydipsia
Psychogenic

2. Lack of ADH
Post-surgical
Pituitary tumours
- craniopharyngioma
- secondary carcinoma, e.g. breast, bronchus
- histiocytosis X

Pituitary granulomas
- sarcoid
- tuberculosis

Hypothalamic or pineal germ cell tumours

Familial
- autosomal dominant
- autosomal recessive

Vascular
- post-partum pituitary
- infarction

Infective
- viral meningitis and encephalitis

Unknown cause

3. Failure of renal response to ADH
Primary nephrogenic diabetes insipidus
Renal tubular diseases
- chronic renal failure
- Fanconi syndrome
- sickle-cell anaemia
- amyloidosis
- myeloma
- obstructive myopathy
- Sjögren's syndrome

Metabolic abnormalities affecting renal tubule
- hypokalaemia
- hypercalcaemia

Drugs affecting renal tubule
- lithium
- demethylchlortetracycline

4. Osmotic diuresis
Diabetes mellitus
Chronic renal failure
Mannitol

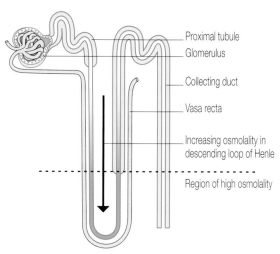

Fig. 33.1 Mechanism of concentration and dilution of the urine. In the region of high osmolality ADH increases the passage of water out of the collecting duct.

Labels in figure:
- Proximal tubule
- Glomerulus
- Collecting duct
- Vasa recta
- Increasing osmolality in descending loop of Henle
- Region of high osmolality

conditions result in the formation of large amounts of dilute urine and result in polydipsia. In the case of nephrogenic diabetes insipidus, there will be no, or diminished, response to injected ADH, while in pituitary diabetes insipidus the kidney should respond by producing a concentrated urine.

In pituitary diabetes insipidus the hypothalamic–pituitary system in which the anti-diuretic hormone is produced is damaged. This may be by tumours, both hypothalamic and pituitary such as pinealomas, gliomas, chromophobe adenomas and craniopharyngiomas. Granulomatous diseases such as sarcoidosis and Langerhans cell histiocytosis (eosinophilic granuloma) may involve the pituitary fossa and the hypothalamic region. Acute viral infections in childhood may be followed by diabetes insipidus. It is important to note that some hypothalamic tumours may destroy the 'thirst centre' in addition to the posterior pituitary. These patients are in serious difficulty because they pass large amounts of dilute urine (due to ADH lack) but feel no thirst. They are therefore liable to great increase in plasma osmolality, with marked hypernatraemia. This can lead to irreversible brain damage and death. In contrast, if the posterior pituitary is destroyed by a tumour, the diabetes insipidus tends to improve when there is subsequent destruction of the anterior part of the gland. This may be due to lack of adreno-cortical hormones which are necessary for the excretion of a water load. The commonest causes are post-surgical and 'idiopathic' cases which are usually on the basis of autoimmune destruction of the posterior pituitary.

Nephrogenic diabetes insipidus may similarly arise from many causes (see Box 31.1). It can be inherited as a familial sex-linked condition without evidence of other renal disease. The condition is due to a mutated V_2 receptor which is unresponsive to ADH. The female carrier may have impaired urine concentrating ability. Failure of renal concentrating ability may be due to renal failure, to renal tubular damage by deposition of amyloid or of immunoglobulin light chains in myeloma. Drugs (lithium, demethylchlor-tetracycline, amphotericin, glibenclamide) may also cause nephrogenic diabetes insipidus by interfering with the cyclic AMP mechanism. Failure of renal tubular concentrating ability occurs in the Fanconi syndromes, in sickle-cell anaemia and can follow the relief of chronic obstruction to the urinary tract.

Electrolyte disturbances are important causes of failure in concentration ability of the kidney. Hypo-kalaemia, caused for example by purgative addiction, or diuretic therapy are not uncommon causes. The latter may be accompanied by a total unresponsiveness to administered ADH. The polyuria caused by hypokalaemia, however, may in part be due to increased thirst, the reason for which is not known. Hypercalcaemia is another common cause of failure to concentrate the urine. With all these causes a failure to drink water leads to water depletion and pre-renal renal failure. This is especially likely to occur when patients are unwell because of the underlying disease that has provoked the abnormality or the drug use.

Compulsive water-drinking, or psychogenic polydipsia, is characterized by the passage of large amounts of dilute urine due to the high fluid intake. The patient says that she has great thirst, but this has no basis in organic disease. Although a history of attention-seeking symptoms is common, there may be no other psychiatric abnormality and the true nature of the polyuria may be difficult to uncover. Sometimes the patient gives herself away by having periods when the urine output is normal, or by not having thirst or polyuria at night.

HISTORY

The patient's age is important. In children, diabetes insipidus may follow exanthemata, a fracture of the base of skull, or be due to eosinophilic granuloma. Diabetes mellitus may occur at any age, and associated infection and weight loss will strongly suggest this disease. Chronic renal failure is notoriously difficult to diagnose clinically, and polyuria, often with nocturia, may be the presenting symptom of a patient whose kidney disease is already well advanced. Failure to concentrate the urine is particularly characteristic of the renal lesion found in sickle-cell anaemia, and other features suggesting this disorder may be present.

Compulsive water-drinking can prove a difficult diagnostic problem, and a careful enquiry must be made into the patient's past and present mental state. Of particular importance is a history of great fluctuation in the severity of symptoms, with periods of remission and relapse. Both these features are unlike diabetes insipidus, but are frequent in compulsive water-drinking.

Hypokalaemia causes impaired renal concentrating ability with resulting polyuria. Longstanding diuretic therapy, ACTH secreting small-cell carcinoma of the bronchus and prolonged diarrhoea may all be causes of potassium deficiency. A history of the drugs the patient is taking must therefore be obtained, together with details of any respiratory or alimentary disturbances. Hypercalcaemia may cause polyuria, and the associated abdominal pain, constipation and vomiting may suggest that the serum calcium is elevated, as may a history of renal stones. Hypothalamic tumours may present with headache and failing vision together with diabetes insipidus. Polyuria may also accompany the early stages of pregnancy, and occasionally occurs in thyrotoxicosis, but there will usually be other features suggesting these possibilities.

PHYSICAL EXAMINATION

Rapid weight loss in a young adult suggests diabetes mellitus. Chronic renal failure is often accompanied by anaemia, and acidotic respiration may be present. Much information may be obtained by looking at the eyes. Exophthalmos may occur in eosinophilic granuloma and may be unilateral or bilateral. The cornea may show calcification, which may accompany hypercalcaemia from any cause. It is best seen at the lateral aspects of the corneo-scleral junction. The visual fields may reveal bitemporal hemianopia if a pituitary tumour is present, although in hypothalamic tumours the field defect is often less characteristic. On ophthalmoscopic examination, there may be dot-shaped haemorrhages and exudates in patients with diabetes mellitus, or the changes due to hypertension which often accompanies chronic renal diseases.

Signs of peripheral vascular disease and of motor and sensory neuropathy can occur in diabetes mellitus. Tendon reflexes are often lost in hypokalaemia from any cause, and there is commonly profound muscular weakness and abdominal distension. In the abdomen, the presence of masses in the loins will suggest polycystic disease of the kidneys.

INVESTIGATION

Many of the causes discussed above are easily diagnosed clinically and by routine investigations. Examination of the urine is an essential preliminary. If the polyuria is due to diabetes mellitus, this will be obvious, while the presence of proteinuria suggests renal disease. The specific gravity of the urine gives some information since it is low in compulsive water-drinking and diabetes insipidus and often 'fixed' at about 1010 in chronic renal failure.

A chest X-ray may show a carcinoma of the bronchus, pulmonary sarcoidosis, as a cause of hypercalcaemia, or the deposits of eosinophilic granuloma in the bones. Measurement of the blood urea and electrolytes are obviously required as a test of renal function and to detect hypokalaemia. If hypokalaemia is present, estimation of the urinary electrolytes in a 24-hour collection will help to show whether or not it is due to a renal loss of potassium. If the hypokalaemia is the result of diarrhoea for example, then there will be renal conservation of potassium. If it is due to hyperaldosteronism or a renal tubular defect, then the urinary excretion will be inappropriately high. The serum calcium should be measured. If it is high, then this may be due to a variety of causes such as hyperparathyroidism, metastatic carcinoma, sarcoidosis or vitamin D intoxication.

If an abnormality is discovered by these investigations, then clearly further investigation will follow a variety of different paths.

There remains the more difficult problem, which is the diagnosis of pituitary diabetes insipidus, nephrogenic diabetes insipidus and the distinction between these conditions and compulsive water-drinking (primary polydipsia).

Further investigation

The basic techniques of investigation of these patients are accurate fluid balance measurements and careful estimations of plasma and urine osmolality. The following is a scheme of investigation (Fig. 33.2).

Measurement of fluid intake and output, and plasma and urine osmolality. This will give an estimation of the degree of polyuria and polydipsia and forms a useful baseline for assessing treatment.

Wide daily fluctuations of intake and output are suggestive of compulsive water-drinking. Often a patient's pattern of water-drinking allows them to sleep at night. The urine osmolality should be low constantly in pituitary and nephrogenic diabetes insipidus (usually below 170 mmol/kg). The plasma osmolality,

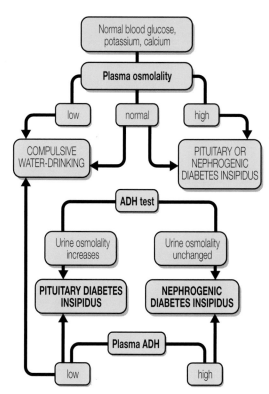

Fig. 33.2 A guide to the diagnosis of polyuria due to diabetes insipidus or primary polydipsia.

clearly differentiate compulsive water-drinking from the other two types of disorder. This is often the case, but unfortunately any patient who has been passing large amounts of dilute urine for long periods of time develops a partial unresponsiveness to the action of ADH and so fluid restriction in a patient with compulsive water-drinking may not always lead to the production of a normally concentrated urine. In addition patients with partial nephrogenic or cranial diabetes insipidus are sometimes able to concentrate their urine after a prolonged period of fluid restriction. The test can cause considerable distress and the information obtained from it can often be gained in other ways.

The response to ADH. If the diabetes insipidus is 'nephrogenic' then there will be little or no response to administered ADH (usually administered as its analogue DDAVP – desmopressin). If the patient has pituitary diabetes insipidus or psychogenic polydipsia, there should be a response to ADH with the production of a concentrated urine and a fall in plasma osmolality. The hormone is given and the urine and plasma osmolality are measured over a 6-hour period. Because there may be an acquired resistance to the action of ADH in patients with pituitary diabetes insipidus and compulsive water-drinking (due to a fall in osmolality in the renal medulla after a long period of polydipsia), this test may have to be carried out over several days, careful watch being kept on plasma osmolality to avoid over-hydration, which is particularly likely to occur in patients with psychogenic polydipsia. Patients with polyuria due to hypokalaemia or hypercalcaemia also fail to concentrate their urine when ADH is administered.

Assay of plasma ADH. Although the previous tests will usually differentiate between pituitary and renal diabetes insipidus and psychogenic polydipsia, they do not always do so. Reliable assays for ADH are now available. In renal diabetes insipidus the plasma levels of ADH are raised, while in pituitary diabetes insipidus or compulsive water-drinking the levels are low. In pituitary diabetes insipidus ADH levels do not rise normally after fluid restriction or infusion of hypertonic saline and a rise in plasma osmolality.

on the other hand, is normal (270–290 mmol/kg) or high (290–310 mmol/kg) in these two disorders, because a slight degree of dehydration is usually present. In compulsive water-drinking the urine osmolality is also low, but values are often variable while the plasma osmolality is normal or low (250–270 mmol/kg) because there is often some degree of overhydration.

Water-deprivation test. In this test, fluid is withheld until 3% of the body weight is lost. In a patient with pituitary diabetes insipidus or nephrogenic diabetes insipidus there is only a small rise in urine osmolality, and large volumes continue to be passed. The patient feels ill and thirsty and plasma osmolality rises above normal levels. It might be thought that this test will

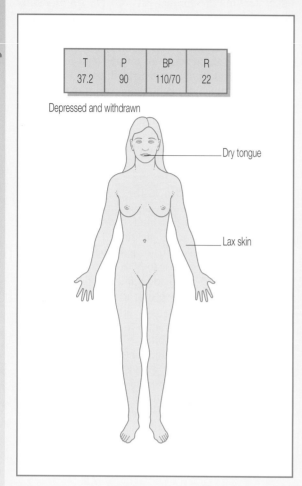

T	P	BP	R
37.2	90	110/70	22

Depressed and withdrawn

Dry tongue

Lax skin

A woman lawyer aged 35 presented with gradual alteration of mood, lethargy, depression and amenorrhoea of 6 months' duration. She had always been well apart from two attacks of frequency and dysuria 4 years earlier, which had been successfully treated with antibiotics. During the previous 6 months she had lost all interest in her family, and her work had suffered greatly. Friends and colleagues had noticed that she had become forgetful, and that she had become prone to bouts of crying for no clear reason. There were no other specific symptoms. She had two children aged 10 and 8 years.

On examination she seemed depressed and withdrawn. She had impairment of recent memory and had difficulty in doing simple arithmetic. There were no localized neurological signs. The tongue was dry and the skin was lax. While in hospital it was noticed that she was getting up at night to pass large quantities of urine. Her family then reported that she had complained of passing more urine than usual for several weeks previously. Urine analysis was normal; specific gravity 1.006.

Questions

1. How would you account for the change in her personality?
2. What investigations would you perform?
3. What is the probable cause of her illness?

Discussion

The history suggests organic brain disease, for it is unlikely that depression alone would account for the intellectual impairment. The combination of this with polyuria is in favour of a hypothalamic tumour, or an electrolyte disturbance. Hypercalcaemia may cause mental changes and polyuria. Hypernatraemia can be caused by excess water loss if the patient does not drink enough to maintain water balance, and may also cause dementia. This latter situation can occur in any process where there is destruction of the hypothalamus such as in granulomas, craniopharyngiomas or gliomas. A pituitary–hypothalamic disturbance is also suggested by the amenorrhoea. There is nothing to suggest nephrogenic diabetes insipidus, diabetes mellitus, or chronic renal failure. Compulsive water-drinking would not account for the memory loss and amenorrhoea. Furthermore the patient did not herself complain of thirst and polyuria, as do patients with compulsive water-drinking. The most valuable initial investigation would be chest and skull X-ray, which might show evidence of a granulomatous disease or tumour in the pituitary region. Serum calcium must be estimated, and blood urea and electrolytes measured. Measurement of urine and plasma osmolality will be useful further investigations. Examination of the visual fields by perimetry may provide additional evidence of a field defect due to a tumour.

The most probable cause of her illness is a lesion in the hypothalamic and pituitary region causing failure of ADH release and dementia. The tumour may well have damaged the hypothalamic thirst centre, resulting in a failure to drink in response to the dehydration caused by progressive urinary water loss. The dementia may be due in part to hypernatraemia. There is no evidence from the history or examination to suggest hypercalcaemia, but this remains a possibility.

> This patient had histiocytosis X involving the pituitary–hypothalamic region with a diabetes insipidus-like picture but without any sensation of thirst. The resultant hypernatraemia had led to dementia which reversed when she was rehydrated (the serum sodium was 170 mmol/l).

Index

Note: The text makes comprehensive reference to the figure numbers and to the relevant material in those figures. Therefore, figures appearing on a different page to the related text have usually not been given an additional page reference. Only important items mentioned exclusively in figure legends have been given page references. 'vs' indicates the differentiation of two conditions.